P9-DWI-791

Praise for *Younger Next Year*

"One long, exuberant New Year's resolution."
— *New York Times*

"Brain-rattling, irresistible, hilarious. If you're up for it, it could change your life." — *Washington Post*

"A twenty-first-century fountain of youth."
— *Kiplinger's Retirement Report*

"From the trenches, a real practicing doctor teaches us that normal aging is NOT normal. Harry's Rules light the path to renewed vitality, and his action steps **will change your life.**" — MEHMET OZ, MD,
coauthor of *YOU: The Owner's Manual* and
YOU: On a Diet; director, Cardiovascular Institute,
Columbia University Medical Center

"I am fifty-four years old and have been on your program for ten months. I purchased a heart monitor, hired a trainer, and exercise for at least forty-five minutes, six days per week. I have lost over thirty pounds and still enjoy my wine. **I want to thank you for writing the book that reached me. It was not too late.**" — STEVE M.

"An extraordinary book. . . . It is easy to read, the science is right, and if one follows Henry Lodge's and Chris Crowley's recommendations, both **mental and physical aging can be delayed.** I wish my patients would follow their advice!"
— K. CRAIG KENT, MD,
chief of vascular surgery,
New York–Presbyterian Hospital

"A **high-octane** approach to keeping lean, fit, and active as we age." —PETER SCARDINO, MD, Department of Urology, Memorial Sloan-Kettering Cancer Center

"I can't thank you enough for turning my life around. I read *Younger Next Year* about eight months ago, it struck a chord, and I started a serious workout program. **I've lost sixty-one pounds** to date and need to shed another eighteen to reach my goal. Great work, and thanks for adding a number of years to my life." —KEITH V.

"I'm glad I read your book in my late thirties. I have that much more time to prepare for the aging process and establish good habits—and **I have built more aerobic endurance than I had as a teenage athlete!**" —ANGELO N.

"**You've put the spring back in my husband's step** and his posture improves daily. It didn't hurt me to read your book, either." —BETSY A.

"A must-read for any woman with a special man in her life. Lively and entertaining, it is packed with important information to help men **live longer, healthier, sexier**, and more vibrant lives." —HILDA HUTCHERSON, MD, codirector, New York Center for Women's Sexual Health; author of *What Your Mother Never Told You About S-e-x*

"**A breakthrough book** . . . written in a lighthearted, humorous style, [its] serious intentions underscore excellent advice." —*Frequent Flyer*

"With optimism, insight, and humor, Crowley and Lodge provide sound information and practical suggestions for **living a healthy and active later third of life.**"
— ALLEN ROSENFIELD, MD,
dean, School of Public Health, Columbia University

"Your book changed my life, and I gave many copies to friends. One gave it to her seventy-five-year-old father, who is on oxygen. **He was so inspired that he started walking laps around his dining table**, carrying his tank with him."
— ELAINE R.

"Men apparently are reluctant to ask for directions, but can they resist advice regarding their well-being? I think not. Here is a book full of sound information, thoughtfully **provocative, fresh, and witty.** And better yet, you don't have to be a man to find this book useful."
— JAMAICA KINCAID,
author of *Annie John* and
The Autobiography of My Mother

"**A powerful message** . . . for all concerned with living long and well, a book in plain English that weaves knowledge of medicine and evolving science together with concrete advice and a thoughtful perspective."
— HERBERT PARDES, MD,
president and CEO, New York–Presbyterian Hospital

"Written with a sense of humor in a chatty style that's easy to read . . . **full of important advice** to heed now in order to stay healthy and fit well past one's retirement years."
— *The Detroit News*

"*Younger Next Year* has changed my life and outlook in countless positive ways. My dad, who died a couple years ago at age ninety, was a star basketball player and a golfer who believed he could continue to improve until his very last days. He worked out every day of his life and was way ahead of his time.

Shortly after his death, I happened to pick up your book. **It was like my dad speaking to me, telling me it was time to get moving.** I realized that though my job and four kids kept me busy, the wee hours of the morning could rejuvenate my physical and mental well-being. I am now up six days a week before work to swim, run, spin, or do weights." —BONNIE B.

"We owe it to ourselves to know that **we have the choice to age in good health.** This book tells you about it. Read it."
—JOHN S. REED,
former chairman, New York Stock Exchange; former chairman and CEO, Citicorp

"*Younger Next Year* will fill you up with facts. But these facts are fun to learn because they are important and because they are **described with great joy and passion.** I was astonished by how well [the authors] wove sophisticated concepts such as the emotional brain, inflammation, nutrition, and metabolism, into the fabric of everyday life."
—GERALD D. FISCHBACH, MD,
director, National Institute of Neurological Disorders and Stroke, National Institutes of Health;
dean, Faculty of Health Sciences and the Faculty of Medicine, Columbia University

"As a nurse practitioner, I would highly recommend your books to any and all adults. Your wonderful books actually have a very real potential to make a huge difference. **Our obese nation needs this NOW!**"

— DEBBIE B., RN, MS, NP

"One of our highest recommendations so far on growing old gracefully. . . . Dr. Lodge, a prominent MD, focuses on developments in cellular and evolutionary biology. Crowley, his guinea pig, is a firm believer in Dr. Lodge's science and very good at convincing the reader that, if you're a fifty-year-old man, you'd be an idiot not to start following the rules as soon as possible. . . . **Should be read avidly by anyone growing older as well as forward-thinking youngsters.**"

— *Kirkus Reports*

"This may sound a bit odd, but I get great—I mean really great—motivation from reading and rereading this book. **I just completed my seventh time reading through it cover to cover.** I do not find it boring even after all those times. In fact, every time I pick up on something that I sort of glossed over on a previous visit. It's incredible, but with each reading I get more committed (maybe even more compulsive) about keeping this new lifestyle going. And working to get better at it little by little. So if you find yourself slipping a little on the exercise, or the nutrition, or maybe a little discouraged about making connections and commitments, sit down and read through the book again. It's amazing the effect it has on your motivation."

— TOM C.

"Not a week goes by that I do not utter a silent prayer of thanks that *Younger Next Year* came into my life. **You guys are saving the world, one body at a time.** I was on the StairMaster today with my heartbeat at 140. One minute after quitting my heartbeat was 92. I'm three weeks from my sixty-second birthday. You guys belong in the pantheon of the Olympic gods for giving all of us 1) hope and 2) a plan of action."
— T. GUERRANT

"Chris Crowley [and] Dr. Henry Lodge are on a mission to change your life. **What sets the book apart is its ebullient personality** . . . [blending] very practical how-to advice with hilarious personal anecdotes."
— LISA MILLER, *Newsweek*

"I turned my life around when my physician told me I was headed down a destructive path. I then read the wisdom put forth by Chris and Harry. My next physical blew my doctor away. **I am seventy-four and in better shape than when I was fifty."**
— JACK S.

"I've been sticking to the program since last July. **I've lost twenty-three pounds and can now run three miles without dying.** Lifting the weights, too. It's truly changed my life. THANK YOU!"
— ANONYMOUS

"I'm almost fifty-seven and have been following the program for about eighteen months. Over the years I've read a ton of self-help books, but *Younger Next Year* is **the only one that has definitely and positively changed my life."**
— MIKE T.

"A friend recommended this book last August. I read it, paid attention, started the hourly exercise program, and took the advice to start something new. In late September I took my first ballroom dance lesson, something I had been telling friends and family that I always wanted to do. **It has literally been life-changing.** My body is different, slimmer, more muscular, better toned; my posture is upright. The challenge to learn how to dance is huge—it incorporates my brain, my mind, my body. After four months, I entered the ballroom competition in Nashville; two months later the competition in St. Louis—and did fine. I dance four times a week and practice moves every day.

None of my clothes fit anymore. I have more energy, I look better, feel better, am competing with people ten and fifteen years younger than I am. I'm sixty-eight.

I am realizing that *Younger Next Year* is not just the title of a book, and am hugely grateful to the friend who told me about the book, and to Chris and Harry for writing it."

—ANNE

"A must-read" for everyone who is interested in being active and living well when they are seventy, eighty, and ninety-plus."

—FAITH PULIS,
CEO/president, The Thoreau Club

"*Younger Next Year* **delivers the goods**. Confronting the myths and realities of aging, it is a treasure trove of life-enhancing recommendations that prove the so-called inevitabilities of middle age are not inevitable at all."

—DAVID J. DEMKO, MD,
editor in chief, *AgeVenture News*

"Three years ago, I was a chronic asthmatic—overweight, out of shape, highly stressed, and not having much fun. Today, **life is fun again**. I compete in masters and corporate track and field (sprints, shot, and discus). The fountain of youth is not a myth."
— AL U.

"I have lost fifty pounds over the last nine months by eating less, moving more, and changing the way I think. I am sixty-two and look better and feel better and have more energy than I have in the last fifteen years."
— RON T.

Younger
Next Year®
for Women

Live Strong, Fit, Sexy, and Smart—Until You're 80 and Beyond

Chris Crowley & Henry S. Lodge, MD
with Allan J. Hamilton, MD
foreword by Gail Sheehy

Workman Publishing ▪ New York

Copyright © 2004, 2005, 2019 by Christopher Crowley and Henry S. Lodge

Preface © 2007 by Christopher Crowley and Henry S. Lodge

Younger Next Year® is a registered trademark of Christopher Crowley and Henry S. Lodge

All rights reserved. No portion of this book may be reproduced—mechanically, electronically, or by any other means, including photocopying—without written permission of the publisher.

Published simultaneously in Canada by Thomas Allen & Son, Limited.

Library of Congress Cataloging-in-Publication Data is available.

ISBN 978-1-5235-0793-1

Cover photo credits:
Clock: © Can Stock Photo Inc./Andrey Kuzmin
Runner: ArtFamily/Shutterstock

Workman books are available at special discounts when purchased in bulk for premiums and sales promotions as well as for fund-raising or educational use. Special editions or book excerpts can also be created to specification. For details, contact the Special Sales Director at the address below, or send an email to specialmarkets@workman.com.

Workman Publishing Co., Inc.
225 Varick Street
New York, NY 10014-4381

workman.com
youngernextyear.com

WORKMAN is a registered trademark of Workman Publishing Co., Inc.

Printed in the United States of America
First printing November 2019

10 9 8 7 6 5 4 3 2

To our beloved Harry Lodge,
Whose brilliance, compassion, and charm
embraced and enhanced every life he touched.
We will always be grateful.
—C.C.   L.Y.

Introduction
to the Second Edition

've had a ton of good luck in this life—an embarrassing amount of it, really. But none of it better than when I found Dr. Harry Lodge to be my internist and persuaded him to write *Younger Next Year* with me. It changed my life.

I'd had the basic idea (the very basic idea) when my wife, Hilary, and I moved out to Aspen, after twenty-five years of practicing trial law on Wall Street. (I'd always wanted to be a ski bum for a bit, and now I could afford it— *such* a good idea.) But it was always clear that I needed a heavy scientist or doctor as coauthor. So, once I got serious, we moved back to New York and started looking. I found Harry. Then things got real.

It took forever to find him (the story's in the book) and even longer to persuade him to write the book. He was, after all, a rock star in his field, the founder (in his late thirties!) and head of a twenty-two-doctor practice with ties to Columbia Medical School and in tremendous demand. (He later became a full professor at Columbia, a rare honor for a practicing doctor.) So he was already stretched. But he loved the idea of the book—the idea that profound behavioral change, especially the development of a serious exercise habit, could have an astonishing impact on health, wellness, quality of life, and aging. (Avoid 70 percent of normal aging until close to the end; avoid 50 percent of the worst diseases and accidents forever.) He loved it because he had understood it so well for years and because it was at the heart of his theories about how to practice internal medicine. He was just about the only internist in New York who paid as much attention to behavioral issues (exercise, your work life, stress, your sex life, general *engagement)* as to conventional medicine. Because he believed that those things had more of an impact than conventional medical issues. The notion of telling that story to a broader public was a powerful temptation. Also, I had been in the business of persuading people to do stuff for a long, long time, and I leaned on him awfully hard. So I pushed; his natural inclinations pulled. And he finally agreed, poor bugger.

I say poor bugger because doing this book would be like taking on a second full-time job for a guy who was already frantically busy. It could have been a draining horror, but it wasn't. Quite the contrary, it was a joy for both of us. First, we became friends almost at once—close friends before long. That made all the difference. Intellectually, our minds worked similarly (a high level of skepticism and analytical rigor), and we saw the book in almost exactly the same light. Finally, our senses of humor jibed perfectly. In the book, I'm the funny one. In life, it may have been Harry. Beyond that, we discovered we had grown up just two miles (and twenty-five years) apart, on the ocean, north of Boston. In the end, that year turned out to be about the most fun either of us had ever had.

At one point the thought was that I could do the lion's share of the work, especially the writing. That turned out to be nonsense. Harry wasn't the kind of guy to delegate that way, especially when it came to something he cared so much about. In the end, we both wrote it. That is, we wound up writing alternate chapters, telling the same story but in very different voices and in very different ways. That doesn't sound very promising, but apparently it had a certain charm. Finally, the message—that you had an unimagined degree of control over your own aging, health, and quality of life—was plenty seductive. *Everyone* wants that, especially the type-A execs and professionals to whom we seemed to appeal. As of this writing we have sold well over two million copies in some twenty languages. And—if our mail is a reliable indicator—we have changed an awful lot of lives. The book became—and has remained—a cult book for a lot of people, especially those over forty.

The book came out in January 2005. We were on all kinds of national TV shows and so on, and it quickly became a *New York Times* bestseller. Everyone seemed to like it, and, I confess, we liked it, too. Harry is the least vain man I've known, but once—when I was trying to persuade him to do a follow-up book—he said, "No, we've written one perfect book. That's enough."

Wow! "One perfect book," huh? Even I—the vain one—might not have said that, but it wasn't totally ridiculous. We did about what we had set out to do. We took what we both believed to be a truly important and deeply under-appreciated concept—the notion that behavioral change can have a more profound impact on wellness, quality of life, and aging than anything else—and told it in such a way that a lot of people took it in. It is still the only book on the subject. Interestingly—considering that it went against the grain of traditional medicine, which mostly ignores behavior—no one disagreed. No one in the medical field, no one in other sciences, no one at all. And the popular response could not have been warmer.

Here's another nice thing: Despite the fact that the original book was novel and cutting-edge, it has stood up remarkably well. Nothing we wrote—nothing Harry predicted or we both recommended—has turned out to be wrong or needed to be amended. In fact, as more research has gone on, the book's conclusions just get stronger. And more important, new studies come out all the time, and the reports on them breathlessly point out that it makes a ton of sense to do this or that. And it's the same exact stuff we wrote fifteen years ago. That is a treat, believe me. And all that credit—let us be clear—goes straight to Harry. Harry had written at one point that some of the minor stuff we wrote might turn out to be wrong but that the major themes would stand up. Well, he was wrong about that: None of it turned out to be wrong. That's downright eerie.

At this point, you may reasonably ask (perhaps with a touch of irritation), If the book is so amazing and you two are such great guys, how come you're writing this new version or revision or whatever it is?

Fair question. And the answer is that this is not a revision or re-edit. No changes have been made to the science and advice in the old text, including our ages at the time we wrote it; there are only additions. Instead of a "revision," this is a "completion" of the original story. Looking back, it's clear there were a couple of glaring omissions in the original book. They're glaring now, but they weren't then. Because back then, there was no science on the subject of cognition and how exercise and emotional connections affect it . . . not even a level of speculation ripe enough to include. So some stuff had to be omitted. But today, the "omissions" are driving us crazy. That's why we did this edition, to put in a little new (and incredibly important) material.

But before we turn to that, it's time to strike a dark note. A terribly dark note. As many of you will have heard, Harry Lodge died three years ago at the age of fifty-eight of a fast-moving prostate cancer. Most prostate cancer is not lethal; this version was very lethal indeed. He had taken good care of himself; he was a passionate follower of the *Younger Next Year* regimen, and he followed all the regular medical steps for a man his age. When the cancer was discovered, he had superb medical care, obviously, and everything possible was done. He lived longer than he might have, but the end came shockingly fast. His doctors and closest friends knew it was probably coming, but it was still all but impossible to accept. Still is. He was *so* alive, and he had so very much more to do, both in his amazing career and in his private life. It was hard to conceive of his being taken away at that absurdly early stage. But it happened, and a lot of people were absolutely heartbroken.

This edition of the book is dedicated to Harry, obviously. And it is beyond fitting. First, because the new chapters (there are only two of them, but they are a big deal) are so well aligned with his interests and character. Harry's friend, the matchless Allan Hamilton—another polymath, like Harry, but this time in the field of neuroscience and brain surgery—graciously stepped in and wrote the chapter that finishes the book. But in a way, it is also Harry's work. Harry's work in the sense that he had a great interest in the impact of behavioral change on energy, mood, resistance to stress, and cognitive effectiveness. Those are Allan's great topics. As you'll see in my new chapter, Chapter 20, Harry had written quite a bit on the subject. He would have been delighted to have Allan take up the baton. (Among other things, Allan was a passionate admirer of *Younger Next Year,* and had bought cartons of copies for colleagues, friends, and every single one of his patients!) And it may be worth noting that Harry would almost certainly *not* have presumed to write the chapter himself, because—as he once said of nutrition—he was only a "student" of the subject, not a master. Allan is most assuredly a master. He has taught it and lived it all his life, as a University of Arizona professor (in an astonishing *four* areas) and a brain surgeon. He has also thought endlessly about its consequences for individuals and the society. He is the perfect guy to "complete" the original book, as you'll soon see in his chapter, Chapter 21.

It is important to say that the idea of creating this new edition *and* of recruiting Allan Hamilton was Laura Yorke's. Laura was our agent for the first book, but her contributions went way beyond that. She also had a lot to do with its organization. On the extremely rare occasions when Harry and I disagreed about something, she arbitrated—with amazing fairness, when you realize that she and Harry were falling in love with each other at the time. It was a hell of a year, as I said before, and the great highlight for Laura and Harry had to be the fact that they fell in love and consecrated their union as soul mates. She is Harry's literary executor. She connected with Allan Hamilton, and she is the one who persuaded him to do his chapter. She also persuaded our publisher to go forward with the project. As ever, she was a key player in the whole business.

Allan's chapter contains some remarkable and powerful stuff. For example, he says that behavioral change will have a more profound effect than anything else on what

I think of as the executive functions—energy, optimism, decisiveness, interest, and, most of all, sheer cognitive intelligence. He says that sheer intelligence can be increased by as much as 10 percent; that's amazing. There will be similar gains in the other executive functions. And he says of Alzheimer's—which we were always told we could do nothing about—that the risk of getting it can be reduced by *half*. And these amazing changes will come—not through conventional medicine, for which we are so grateful—but from serious behavioral change. It is *Younger Next Year* taken to a new level.

Years ago, a reader wrote to us about *Younger Next Year*. He told us about the changes he'd made, and the consequences. And he finished by saying, "Life is fun again." We get a ton of wonderful letters, but that one may be my favorite. I hope this new edition will give a significant number of people a reason to read it. Or read it again. And I hope that a few of you will be moved to say, "Life is fun again."

Foreword

When I first met Harry and Chris, the authors of this extraordinary book, I thought I might impress them by casually dropping the fact that I was going off on a five-day bike trip in Maine. Chris gave me a high five—"Fabulous!" He is a ferocious biker himself, who warms up in the winters by biking daily up and down the Berkshires so he and his wife will be ready to go howling around the mountains of Europe in summer, following the Tour de France route.

"What do I need to do to train?" I asked.

"How long do you have?"

"I just finished my book. I leave in three days."

His rugged face collapsed. "You'll just have to suck it up this time. But next time, you might enjoy it."

The cycling outfit I toured with in Maine, Summer Feet, is small. I mean, really small. Only three cyclists showed up for the week: Chris Hedges, a fellow author and toughened war correspondent, his young and very tall wife, Kim, and myself. Our two guides, Norman and Rae, were both muscle-bound Mainers. First thought: *These are all demon uphillers; I'll either have to find the coastal evacuation route—it must be flat—or get off in the middle of the hill, throw my hand in the air, and shout, "Taxi!"*

But it turned out that Christopher and Kim, like me, love books even more than biking. So we turned the trip into something like pedaling with Proust, thoroughly enjoying our twenty miles a day of cycling on the sylvan roads of Acadia National Park and circling the jagged fjords of Schoodick Island. Each day was pleasantly punctuated by breaks for reading and discussing our favorite authors. I came home without a single pain or strain.

But once home, foolishly thinking myself now fit as a biker chick, I plunged into a boot camp aerobics program at the YWCA. After the first day, a knee locked up, one hip listed, and every rib felt like a chicken bone poking in my sides. I went back to look at Harry and Chris's book again.

"We urge you not to start gradually," they had written. "You might think about a 'Jump-Start Vacation'—a trip where exercise is the central activity." They had even suggested going on a bike tour in New England. Okay, did that, then what? "It is far better to make a sharp break with the past and a serious commitment to the future," they had written. "Jump in for the rest of your life." Ah, that was the meat of their message . . . "the rest of your life." Never mind the first few days of muscle protest; it will get better and easier.

I read the manuscript of this book while I was finishing a book of my own, and *Younger Next Year for Women* sounded as if it might be a companion volume. My book, *Sex and the Seasoned Woman*, is about sex, love, dating, and new dreams among women over forty-five. It is based on interviews with over two hundred women who belong to a new universe of lusty, liberated boomer babes—some married and some not —who are unwilling to settle for the stereotypical roles of middle age. Today's women in their mid-forties, fifties, and sixties are at the peak of their lives. They consistently tell me that they are happier and more productive than they have ever been before. Among my subjects in their seventies to nineties, I have found many who are younger in mind and body than their average peers, and some who remain seductresses, dazzling to both men and women.

It is the seasoned woman who knows best how to resonate with her sexuality. Happily, Harry and Chris point out that committing to regular exercise is the foundation of positive brain chemistry, which leads directly to burning fat, heightening your immune system, improving your sleep, and toning up your sexual desire and response. Sounds like a pretty good prescription for chasing away the menopausal blues!

Okay, you might ask, What do two guys know about menopause? As the author of *The Silent Passage*, I wondered myself.

Chris Crowley is a guy's guy with a Dionysian flush to his face. He's a recovery case, years younger at seventy than when he retired from a Wall Street law firm and began wondering who the hell he would be, once stripped of his professional status. He started the usual slide into fat and foolishness but caught himself and reversed direction. Seriously: he now looks like a fifty-year-old hunk.

Dr. Harry Lodge is only forty-seven, a rod-straight prepschool prototype, just as good-looking and intense as Chris, but a medical practitioner, teacher, and man of science. He tells readers that after fifty we start to decay.

Yes, *decay*. Unless we signal our bodies to keep growing by exercising six days a week—yes, *six days*—our bodies head downhill after fifty. Exercise provides the signal that jolts our cells into repairing and renewing themselves and releases the chemicals that bathe our brains in positive feelings. You may not want to hear this advice, but you know it's true. Some need it more than others.

Kids, you know who you are.

Harry the doctor provides solid data and vivid descriptions to back up the two major points in this book—points I make in my own book and illustrate with dozens of women's life stories: Seventy percent of aging after fifty is governed by our lifestyle. Half of all of the sickness and serious accidents we are told to anticipate after we turn fifty can be virtually eliminated, if we learn how to live younger.

The authors of this book and I are on the same page when we project a vision of women's years after menopause. I call it a Second Adulthood. Harry and Chris call it "the Next Third of your life." They project that there are "thirty years to live after menopause and [that] they can be some of the best of your life." We differ only on the numerical projection.

Why only thirty years?

The fastest-growing segment of the American population is people over one hundred. This population will only swell, driven by boomers who have the good fortune of unprecedented levels of education, income, a keen awareness of good health habits, and access to cutting-edge medical resources. The MacArthur Foundation's studies on aging predict that, of the seventy million boomers born between 1946 and 1964, approximately three million will live to the age of one hundred, or beyond.

Will you be one of them?

You could be if you honor the house that you live in—your body. As an eighty-five-year-old marathon runner once told me, "We are all like snails, we carry our houses with us." Our body holds the remarkable ability to repair and renovate itself, provided we help it rather than letting it go to seed. If, as we age, we concentrate on the three "F's"—Family, Friends, and Fun—and keep our minds alive with new challenges and new vistas, there's no telling how long the current generations of women might live.

My own profession is one of the most prone to physical deterioration. A writer sits, tensely hunched over the keyboard, for hours at a time, butt spreading, gut wound like a garden hose, and lungs hanging limp as yesterday's balloons. All of us sit too long in front of our computers, at work and at home. Sure, we promise our physical therapists and ourselves that we'll get up and do cat stretches every hour. But honestly, how often do we unwind?

I developed a good habit in my fifties: When I finished writing a book, which was every two or three years, I would go to my favorite health ranch for a week. But after finishing a harrowing book about the families of 9/11 victims, *Middletown, America*, I didn't go. It was a big mistake. More than ever, I needed rejuvenation, spiritually as well as physically, as we all do after a period of great emotional exertion. Instead, I kept getting worse. I had a cranial sacral treatment, where a practitioner listened with her hands and felt the energy and rhythmic patterns in my body's fluids. She looked grim.

"Have you had a trauma lately?"

"No." (It didn't occur to me that I had experienced a vicarious trauma.)

She told me that the important fluids that are supposed to circulate between my head and tail were moving very sluggishly, indicating that my immune system was very weak. My husband asked, "Why don't you go to the ranch?"

Off I went. It was winter, but Rancho la Puerta is in Mexico and always mild. This is the *ur* fitness camp, started in the 1940s and spread over several miles beneath a spiritually charged mountain rendered sacred by Native Americans. I've always enjoyed hiking the mountain before dawn and walking to classes along the paths of the ranch, swooning from the potpourri of herbal shrubs. But on the first day of that stay, as I reprised my old routine, I was in for a rude surprise. Dinner ended at seven-thirty that evening, as usual, and I had about a quarter of a mile to walk back to my villa. Halfway there, I completely ran out of gas. I seriously considered lying down on the ground and going to sleep. That was a shock. But a good shock.

I made a vow then to come to the ranch once a year to get that physical jump start and spiritual refreshment I missed after finishing the 9/11 book. My new annual retreat would act as a reminder of all the good habits of mind and body I have learned at the ranch over the years. I experienced, firsthand, that the aftereffects of giving my body daily aerobic exercise, making my muscles dance, rising early and retiring early are the best medicine for depression. They are also natural and powerful stimuli to pursuing a more passionate life.

So this time, after finishing my latest book, and after my cycling trip and the painful introduction to aerobic boot camp, I decided to act on the powerful message in *Younger Next Year for Women*. I went to Rancho la Puerta for a week and "jumpstarted" the exercise program I'm committed to continuing through my Second Adulthood. (Well, maybe modified a little.)

My bag didn't arrive. I had to sit in the San Diego airport for five hours waiting for it. By the time I finally arrived at the ranch, my legs were tingling from the lack of movement beginning at four that morning. So I went for a brisk two-mile walk around the ranch, picked some of the purple grapes ripening on the vines, sat and read on my terrace, had a banana and a glass of water, and lay down at 8 p.m., thinking that I'd just catch a catnap. I didn't stir until four in the morning. It was wonderful.

Starting off with that mini fast and the restful eight hours of sleep, I attacked the day with a tremendous appetite for every kind of movement the ranch could offer. After a three-and-a-half-mile hike around the mountain, I went to circuit training for a combination of strength-training with little aerobic bursts; from there to Pilates for tightening in the core; then off to yoga for seventy-five minutes of breathing and stretching. By lunchtime, I felt strong and happy but—surprise!—not hungry. So I skipped the soup and had a little jicama and edamame salad and a rice-stuffed pepper. Then on to Tai Chi and a nap by the pool.

That night, I gave an hour lecture and still had enough gas left over to read myself to sleep at eleven o'clock. The wonderful paradox I'd discovered is that the more calories I burned, the less I seemed to need. As long as the body's metabolism has a new spark plug, all batteries are recharged and you're in an enthusiastic, supportive, and aesthetically pleasing environment, it's easy to exercise and eat well. You know you're going to get enough sleep and you're not going to be asked to speed up finishing that report, so you can do without the third cup of coffee, the glass of wine, or the chocolate-chip cookie.

The next afternoon I was somberly doing Tai Chi, rocking silently from foot to foot, when I heard something far more primitive going on in the gym next door. The women who emerged after that class were all laughing uproariously and practicing a noise that sounded like Roxie Hart in *Chicago*: "AAGGHgggghhhhmmmmmmmm ..."

"What were you doing in there?" I asked.

"Strip dancing."

The next day I decided to let the Tai Chi people levitate into higher consciousness; I wanted to get down with the girls who strip-danced. The teacher, Demetrius, a young African American man with an impish smile, told us right off the bat: "Strip off your usual identity. Throw it away. Decide who you're going to be today. Is it going to be Beyoncé? Gypsy Rose Lee? Whoever ..." He pulled on a wig: "I'm Ginger."

Demetrius gave us a chair to make love to. We had to choose a gauzy wrap and strike a sexy pose behind a folding metal chair. Then he put on music from the movie *Moulin Rouge* and taught us to do those moves you've seen a thousand times.

At five foot four, with enough years on me to rate senior movie fare, I'm never going to move like Nicole Kidman. Neither, presumably, are you. But it didn't matter one bit. There were women in the class who were in their seventies and eighties, along with a lot of beauties who were celebrating their fiftieth year. And nobody was looking at any of us—we only had eyes for Demetrius and ourselves.

With one hand on the back of our chairs, we listened as Demetrius counted down, "Five-six-seven-eight," and we were off strutting a Janet Jackson walk around the chair, then hanging off the back of it, grinding our hips to one side and the other and then down in a hammocky swivel.

Well, every woman in the room began to shake her booty, dangle her ornaments, and toss her head in that slave-to-love swing, all while stroking her chair like Brad Pitt was sitting right there. Before you knew it, we were on our backs, kicking our legs and pulling up with a long, erotic moan, "AAGGHggghhhhmmmmmmmmm . . ." You have never seen so many middle-aged women vamping. With the sarongs wrapped around our fannies or swirling around our necks, we shamelessly stroked our hands up and down our inner thighs, over our tummies and breasts, flinging our arms high in the air with squeals worthy of Marilyn Monroe.

Ladies, under the skin, we are all natural strippers. So why not show it?

Demetrius told us stripping is good for releasing your inner goddess. I say, it's more of a release for your inner harlot. And it's a heck of a lot more fun than doing squat thrusts in a sweaty gym.

Invite your partner to watch you chair-dance. I guarantee you will feel younger. And so will he.

So, make up your mind to follow the gung-ho practices this book recommends and then find your own ways to jump-start growth. (I know I've found mine!) But whatever you do, don't let this become just another exercise book, gathering the dust of unread guilt. Use it as a kind of bible; reread a few pages now and then, to remind you of the central commandment:

Jump in for the rest of your life.

GAIL SHEEHY
East Hampton, New York

Acknowledgments

First, special thanks, as ever, to Harry, who has been a joy to work with, a flawlessly sane collaborator, and about as good a friend as you could hope to have. Not so common, I'm told, in the literary collaboration business.

We have had a world of wonderful help on this book, but a handful of people deserve special mention. Again, my list starts with Alexandra Penney, who said from the beginning that Harry and I had to write this book and who gave me the resolve to go forward with it. Laura Yorke and Carol Mann of the Carol Mann Agency have had everything to do with getting this book started, shaped, and published. Beyond that, Laura has been informal editor, confidante, and close friend, and has pitched in and given major help on the editorial side. But the heavy editorial lifting has, of course, been done by our editor, Susan Bolotin, who had unusually broad and important responsibilities on this book, and she carried them off flawlessly, quickly and kindly. Special thanks, too, to Lynn Strong, our copy editor, and to Megan Nicolay, person-of-all-work at Workman, who, among other things, drew the indispensable "Healthy ... Dead!" charts.

My thanks again to all the people who were helpful on the first version of this book, and to the following who were particularly helpful on this one: Lois Smith Brady, Bobo Devens, Tina McDermott, Polly Guth, Tukey Kofend, Elena and Michael Patterson, Ranie Pearce, Marni Pillsbury, Mary Ross, Ton Ton Russell, Helen Ward, and Woody and Priscilla Woods.

Finally, profound thanks to my wife, Hilary Cooper, who is the virtual coauthor of all my chapters. She has been unflagging in her support, intense in her interest and sound in her judgment. As with my life, she has made all the difference. — C.C.

Chris has my eternal gratitude for having the idea for these books, for talking me into writing them with him, and for becoming one of my closest and dearest friends in the process. His wife, Hilary, has also been a constant source of support and strength in both literary and life matters. Carol Mann has done a superb job as one of our agents, and had the vision and talent to see the potential in this book. Suzie Bolotin is an extraordinary editor, and has been unstinting with both her advice and her time.

Many people have helped along the way, but I owe special thanks to my parents and siblings, who have always been there for me and have my love and respect in every way. To Laura Yorke for being not just my agent but my partner in love and in life, and to my children, Madeleine and Samantha. To my colleagues at the Columbia University Medical Center and New York Physicians, who are the best one could ask for. Ellen Randall and my sister Felicity gave invaluable advice and feedback, and I owe a special debt of gratitude to Ashley Mui and Maria Camacho for coping with all the challenges I gave them with consummate skill, endless patience and good humor.

Finally, as with the first book, I owe the biggest debt of all to my patients, who have enriched my life and taught me the true meaning of courage, compassion, optimism, strength, and, most of all, grace. — H.S.L.

A special note is due from both of us to Workman Publishing. It is a special place, where teamwork is truly celebrated and where the whole is always greater than the parts. Everyone we have come in contact with has been talented, hardworking, dedicated, and enthusiastic. We were going to thank them all by name, but then we realized that the success of the book is equally due to the efforts and enthusiasm of the people we don't see, who pore over the layout until it is just right, tirelessly promote the book in market after market, or do all the hundreds of other things that make a book succeed. The bottom line is that we are sharing our remarkable adventure with the entire company, and we appreciate the efforts of every single person there. Thank you all. — Chris and Harry

Contents

Introduction

This is a book that can change your life. It will tell you how you can turn back your biological clock and be functionally younger next year and for years to come. A heady claim, but a deadly serious one.

There's a curious thing, however. This is a book for women, and yet it's written by two men: Harry, a forty-seven-year-old doctor who is not an expert in women's health, and Chris, his seventy-one-year-old friend, patient, and "demo model." Let us explain. First, we published *Younger Next Year*, a deeply optimistic book about the new science that is transforming aging in America. While most of the information in it applies equally to women and men, we cast it as a man's book, largely because we presented our program through the lens of Chris's life—and Chris, no matter how you look at it, is not a woman.

The book became a best seller and has changed the way a lot of people lead their lives. But as the book's success grew, so did our conviction that we needed to get our message across to women as well. We knew that women, who continue to buy the book for their husbands or lovers, their brothers, fathers, or friends, loved it. They told us they had no trouble reading a "man's book" . . . and no trouble enjoying Chris's rough-and-tumble approach. It turns out they'd had enough Jergen's Lotion poured on their heads by the women's magazines to last a lifetime, so blunt felt good. Still, they kept asking us when we were going to write a woman's version. Why should they have to read over some guy's shoulder?

We decided to give it a shot. As a first step, we checked the bookstore. There were aisles and aisles of books for women about disease: books, many of them excellent, about breast cancer, ovarian cancer, depression, osteoporosis, heart disease, stroke, Alzheimer's, and menopause (which is not a disease but is often treated as one). But nothing about *health* . . . nothing about just how terrific the thirty-plus years after menopause can and should be. And that's when we went to work.

We took the original *Younger Next Year* and Harry added the information women need about menopause, osteoporosis, and a few other gender-specific issues. Chris rewrote his chapters to reflect the very different angle from which women approach aging. But we did not rewrite the biology or the fundamental advice. We didn't have to. Chris is still the floor model for the simple reason that *the biology of health is virtually identical between men and women.*

Think about that for a moment. Disease is often gender-specific, but health is gender-neutral. Biological responses to disease and to medications are different. Things like breast cancer and osteoporosis are obvious, but heart disease—the number one killer of women—is essentially a different disease for women. Different symptoms, different tests, different treatments. But great health—and the optimism, energy, strength, and focus that go with it—is gender-neutral. And great health is what this book is all about.

A final point. The two of us are absolutely messianic about the importance of changing the way we live and age in this country. The way we do it now—our idleness, isolation, obesity, illness, and apathy—is a disastrous waste. An outrage, frankly. Women, we sense, are quicker to pick up on that than men. They seem to *know* something is wrong and to be more interested in change. They are quicker to go to the gym or the yoga studio . . . quicker to find new ways of connecting and committing to others. Quicker to weed out the absolutely rotten food in their diets. Women are, in a word, "naturals" for the kind of change we're talking about. We hope that you will read our book, enjoy it, and then join the revolution.

CHRIS CROWLEY AND HARRY LODGE
New York City

PART ONE

Take Charge of Your Body

CHAPTER ONE

The Next Forty Years

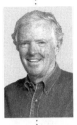

Okay, you're a terrific woman, maybe in your late for-ties, maybe your early sixties, and your life has gone pretty well. You have good energy, decent gifts, and right now you seem to be heading into a particularly nice stretch. The kids are getting big or are gone. Old Fred, if he's around, is taking care of himself, and the relationship is taking some nice turns, getting a little calmer. For some reason—menopause or whatever—you feel as if it's time, at rather long last, to look after yourself and your own serious business. Time to take your own affairs, your own life, your own needs in hand and *do something*. Maybe something pretty big.

There's a lovely quote from Isak Dinesen that goes, "Women, when they are old enough to have done with the business of being women, and can let loose their strength, may be the most powerful creatures in the world." You may feel that you're never going to be "done with the business of being a woman"—maybe you don't want to be—but you know what she means and you know that it's true. And nice. Very nice.

Harry (that's Henry S. Lodge, MD, my doctor, coauthor, and close pal) and I have been picking away at this project for several years now, and we have talked to an awful lot of women your age and older. We have come to realize just how right Isak Dinesen may be. Unlike men, who are often getting a little shaky as they approach their sixties or retirement age, many women are feeling more independent, more optimistic, more *powerful*. Freed from lots of the caregiving, and perhaps some other stuff that Dinesen may have had in mind, they are liberated to look at other, possibly larger, issues. Such as themselves. Not out of selfishness or narcissism, but out of *interest*. They're not going to shove Old Fred out of the boat, you know, but they're not going to lose track of themselves anymore, either. I spend a lot of my time with women—especially able and ambitious ones—and I see it and hear about it *all* the time. It is exhilarating, it is striking, and it is very different from what we hear from men.

Men may be at the actual height of their careers and powers, but they're uneasy, too . . . starting to worry about what's going to become of them next, when they hit sixty, or retirement. When they no longer have the lifelong robes of Office, Job, and Position in which to wrap and comfort and define themselves. They're starting to wonder, ever so slightly, just who the hell they are under that blanket. Or who they're going to be in the Next Third of their lives when they have to take it off and hand it to someone else.

All generalizations are flawed, but women seem to see the situation differently. For one thing, few women have the luxury of wearing one lifelong robe. They slip into one role after another, juggling and doing the best they can. Few have the time to fall in love with themselves as the Great This or the Important That. And so, after whatever detours life has thrown their way, women are nowhere near as likely as men to stew about what's going to happen next. To lift Faulkner out of context, women don't just "survive," they "prevail." Which makes them a lot readier than many of their spouses or lovers to tackle the next phase, whatever it is. So, you ask, what's next? What about this Next Third you mention? And how about this business of getting younger next year? Is it true? Is it for me? And what do I do?

That, of course, is what the whole book is about (and yes, you bet it's true ... and absolutely, it's for you). But before we get to that, let's talk for a minute about what you think you know about the aging process ... the pictures you carry around in your head. They are probably not that great. You've been reading and talking a lot, and everywhere you look, there are these scary problems, fluttering down like feral birds at the edges of an uneasy garden party. You know you're supposed to live a long time, but it may not be that much fun. Runaway osteoporosis after menopause. Breast cancer. Epidemic levels of heart attacks and strokes. Failed retirement plans and a good chance of dying broke. Failed marriage, loneliness, and the utter impossibility of finding sex after sixty. Hell, after forty. And other, formerly nameless horrors like *incontinence*, for God's sake. There's June Allyson (who was so young and whom I loved so *achingly* when I was ten) talking on TV about incontinence. Yikes! You may be led to have visions of yourself as an old woman, bent double over her cane in some lonely place ... looking for all the world like the old girl in the gingerbread house with the wart on her nose. Or maybe a bag lady in New York, shuffling along with mountains of crap, muttering strange incantations under her breath. Great.

So look, could you use some good news? Fine, try this: That's not going to happen to you. Not even close. Bad things do happen to some older women in America. Bone loss is a terrible problem. Heart attacks and strokes are the great killers of women. Lots more women than men *do* die broke. (More women than men die rich, too; however, that's another matter.) But the terrible things are probably not going to happen to you. Because the worst things turn out to be voluntary. You do not have to go there. So don't.

Two amazing numbers, right up front: 70 percent of aging, for women as for men, is voluntary . . . you do not have to do it. And you can also skip 50 percent of all the sickness and serious accidents you'd expect to have from the time you turn fifty to the day you die. Skip 'em. Altogether. Harry will explain the details later on, but for now just remember those numbers. They're numbers to live by, and they're real.

In fact, the Next Third of your life — and that's what we're talking about here — can be absolutely terrific. Instead of getting old and fat and ridiculous in the thirty- or even forty-some years after menopause, you can remain essentially the same person you are today. It's better than that. Learn some of the new science that Harry is going to talk about in the rest of the book, then do some of the hard stuff that will seem obvious after that . . . and most of you can be functionally younger next year and for a good many years to come.

That sounds like baloney or hype, but it is literally true. Limited aspects of biological aging are immutable. Like the fact that your maximum heart rate goes down a bit every year, and your skin and hair get weird. So you're going to *look* older. Tough . . . what did you expect? But 70 percent of what you *feel* as aging is optional. No joke. No exaggeration even. There's a new, tough game out there. And congratulations: You are eligible to play. You just have to learn how.

Again, here's what you *think* you know: You turn fifty-five or sixty and your feet are on the slippery slope...the remorseless slide into old age, foolishness, and death. Every year a little fatter, slower, weaker, more pain-racked, more apathetic. You can't hear and you can't see. Your hips go... your knees. You develop that becoming "widow's hump" because your bones are turning to chalk. You get petulant, except when you're absolutely furious, which is half the time. Your conversation goes stupid and you start calling strangers "dear." You don't have any money, and your muscles look like the drapery in *Great Expectations*. You break your hip...go to the Nursing Home. Here's the graph:

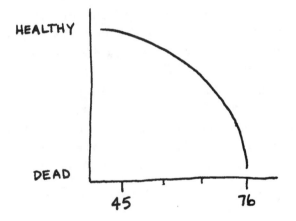

That can certainly happen. In this country, it often does. But it's a choice, *your* choice, not a sentence from on high. It's a choice that *you* control by how you are living right now. And it is not the only choice. You can, just as easily, make up your mind—and tell your body—to live as if you were forty-five or fifty for most of the rest of your life. If you're willing to send your body some different signals, you can get off the slippery slope. You can stay on a gently tipped plateau until you're eighty and beyond. Way beyond. There are women out there skiing slalom races in their late eighties; I've seen it with my own eyes. Harry has a patient who is playing tennis in her late nineties. And other older women are biking in the steep hills outside Barcelona, where the real pros train. Not just crawling along, either, like little old dollies, but doing it. *Going for it. Having a major good time.* Amazing sight, believe me. I travel in these circles and I see it *all the time.* Honest.

And there are other older women who are not interested in athletics but who are *still* in great shape and having a vigorous, amusing, deeply sensual (and often sexual) old age. So here's the lesson of the book: You do not have to get old the way you think. You can do all the same things, almost the same way. Bike, ski, make love. Make sense! Roughly the same energy . . . roughly the same pleasure. Roughly the same woman. In fact, if you're a bit of a mess right now, you can become a radically *better* woman over the next few years and *then* level off. No kidding. I might kid you a little, to keep your spirits up, but not Harry. If Harry says you can do all this, it is simply true. A lot of the book is in my words, but Harry sets down the heavy timbers. I tell the stories. Harry tells the truth. You'll see.

At the worst, Harry says, it can look like this:

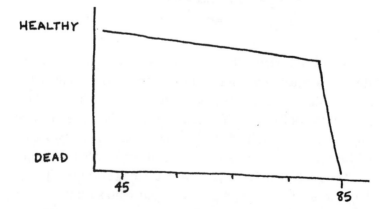

And for 95 percent of you it can look like this:

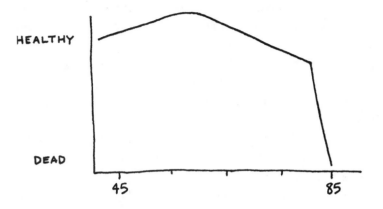

If you haven't been there, you cannot imagine how important the difference is between either of these last two curves and the one on page 7, because you probably can't imagine how bad "normal aging" is in this country. Take it on faith for a minute: normal aging is pretty grim, and the difference between the curves is profound. We are *begging* you, Harry and I, we are *begging* you to get off the slippery slope. It will make a fundamental change in how you look at aging and how you feel and who you are in the Next Third of your life.

You Do Have to Age, but You Don't Have to *Rot*

Harry and I want this book to be fun for you . . . want you to sail right through it before you realize just how serious we are. But let us have a candid moment. We are deadly serious. The stakes here — the potential changes in the rest of your life — are enormous. Think again about those numbers I mentioned: 50 percent of all illness and injuries in the last third of your life can be *eliminated* by changing your lifestyle the way we suggest. Not delayed until you are a little older . . . eliminated! By the way, 70 percent of premature death is lifestyle-related (like dying after you break a hip). "Premature" means before you are deep in your eighties or—if you're in your forties now— your nineties.

And, again, 70 percent of the "normal" decay (that's the *rot*) associated with aging . . . the weakness, the sore joints, the lousy balance, the feeling crappy . . . 70 percent of that horror can be forestalled almost until the end. *That is a huge difference in how you lead your life and who you are.* Believe me, it's true. I have had some interludes of normal aging in my life, when my joints hurt so much that regular walking was painful and I looked for the cutout in the curb so I wouldn't have to "step up" three inches to get on the sidewalk. Think about that. Think about being so weak that you have to rock just a little to get out of a normal armchair. *That stuff happens. It happened to me. It will happen to you. It really, really will. And it doesn't have to.*

All this sounds extreme, but it is not. Harry—whose credentials are bulletproof—knows and will tell you about the emerging science to prove it. It is head-turning. I will tell you about the life. I may not be as good a model for women as I am for men, but men and women are mostly in this Aging Boat together. My stories—about skiing like a maniac at seventy and taking long, scary bike trips and all that—could just as well be coming from a woman. There are plenty of women my age doing the same thing. Most of the women in my bike group are in their sixties and they go *howling* along, in the mountains of Austria, out west, all over the place. It could just as well be a woman talking when

I say I am functionally *younger* today than I was ten years ago. So extrapolate a little . . . this is not chest-thumping nonsense from some delusional old guy, this is a preview of your own story.

What I Bring to the Party: A Report from the Front

Okay, let's talk about structure. My part here is simple: I have lived through my sixties and I have been retired for a while. At seventy-one, I have absorbed and followed the message of this book for a number of years, and I am prepared to tell you the exact truth about the process. Mine is the report from the front. Optimistic, sure, but honest and unadorned. Not a woman's report, but still relevant because, as I say, we're in this Aging Boat together. Same joints, same gut, same apathy, same drifting mind. Unless we do some stuff I happen to know about.

Here's the good news. I have done pretty well. Not stunningly well: I am not thirty-eight. But way better than I expected: I am functionally a surprisingly healthy fifty . . . more healthy aerobically, I recently learned, than most fifty-year-olds. And this despite the following truths: I am an indifferent athlete at best. I am hugely self-indulgent (at one point I was forty pounds overweight). I drink almost every day, and I am hardwired for pleasure. Absolutely hardwired. But once I got it into my head what the stakes were and how modest the commitment was—compared to the results—I was there. I made a job of it. You've made a job of a lot of different things in your life. Make a job of this one, too . . . arguably the most important job you've ever had. You're a lifelong juggler: okay, get one more ball in the air. Learn to handle it, and you won't have to turn into a helpless old lady.

And here's another nice thing. The *process* is pretty good fun. (By the way, the appetite for and appreciation of this stuff is gender-free.) Some of the process—the exercise part, maybe—sounds appalling and you'll think we're kidding. But it isn't and we're not. I wouldn't have done some of the stuff we're going to urge on you for a month, let alone years, if it weren't fun, but mercifully it is. Slightly addictive, as a matter of fact. We'll explain. It's tough, but it's fun, and it works. How do you like that?

What Harry Brings to the Party: The Truth

Harry is the real McCoy. A board-certified internist and a gerontologist, he has long been ranked as one of the best doctors in America in national surveys. He is the head of a cutting-edge, twenty-three-doctor practice in Manhattan and on the clinical faculty of Columbia University's College of Physicians and Surgeons. Importantly for us, he is also a serious student of recent developments in cellular and evolutionary biology. His is the report on that science—which has not yet made its way into the medical journals and won't for a while—and on what he has learned from his own profound experience treating patients in their fifties, sixties, and beyond for the last fifteen years. The science is heavy, but Harry makes it accessible and persuasive. Okay, sort of accessible. But when you read his chapters, the logic—indeed, the near-necessity—of embracing his suggestions becomes clear and doesn't sound crazy at all.

By the way, the science is sufficiently new that Harry—a profoundly conservative man in this area—warns that some of what he says will turn out to be wrong as research goes forward. But not the basic themes. The revolution in aging that he talks about is here, and the science is real. Harry makes it clear that there are remarkable forces in your body—in your cells, all over the place—that are at work all the time, building you up or tearing you down. Darwinian forces—preservation-of-the-species stuff—that have everything to do with who you are and how you live. In his chapters (we more or less take turns), he tells you what they are and how they work. He also tells you how to manipulate and redirect them to your own ends. Like holding age at bay to a remarkable extent and for a very long time. Not completely and not forever, but a lot more than you can believe right now.

What you'll learn is partly what you have always known: There are tides in our lives that carry us forward or back. When you're a kid, the tide is behind you and you go forward regardless. Stronger, more coordinated, better focused . . . better able to understand and cope. But at some point the tide inside your body goes slack and the free ride is over. And then, in an instant, it turns against you. You get a little weaker, your balance is funny, your bones turn out to be frail . . . you can't remember things. And it begins to look as if before long the tide will be running pretty hard. And it's going to sweep you up on the rocks. Where the gulls are waiting. And the crabs. To eat your wattles and your gut. And your eyes. Take the guck out of your nose and your hair to make a nest. Go up there and eat you. Sorry.

But the interesting thing, Harry says, is that the tide is not that strong. It looks strong, because it's so steady . . . so remorseless. But it is not strong. It is manageable, in the sense that you can turn its relentless power to your own purposes. Like using the terrifying force of a wind that is rushing you toward the rocks to sail *into* the wind and safety. Harry's chapters are not frilly. And Harry is not a breezy guy. But he's awful smart and his stuff is worth a close study. All he wants you to do is change the way you live. Fundamentally and forever. And he cares like crazy. We both do, as a matter of fact. We want desperately to have the Next Third of your life be absolutely terrific. Read this book closely and maybe that's what you'll want as well.

Meeting Harry and Getting a New Start

went to Harry because a pretty redheaded skin surgeon named Desiree told me to. She had just taken off half my nose with a local anesthetic and I was still crazy about her, which requires a certain charm. I had just moved back to New York from Colorado, where I'd gone to be a ski bum for a couple of years when I first retired. (I couldn't afford it when I was a kid because I got married at nineteen and had three children before law school.) Anyway, I asked Desiree if she could be my doctor and she said no, but she had just the guy. Smart, decent . . . a terrific person. A WASP, she said, but not a dope, as if that had to be cleared up. He'd been her teacher of something in medical school and I'd like him.

So there I was in Harry's examining room, wary as a cat. Because (a confession) I don't like doctors. I don't like the haughty way they say, "Hi, Chris . . . I'm Doctor Smith." (I'm "Chris"? And he's "Doctor Smith"? What's that all about? And why do I always have to wait an hour to get this abuse?

Lawyers don't do that. Doctors, man! And then the stuff they do to you!)

Harry has lovely manners and is a conspicuously decent guy. I am still wary. We've just been through all this terrible stuff. He's drawn gallons of blood . . . taken long, dubious looks in my ears and down my throat . . . asked lots of vaguely scary questions. And, of course, stuck his finger up my butt. Finally, it's the old "Why don't you put on your things and come into my office and we can talk a minute."

You just know he's going to say, "Uh, listen, I found a little lump up your butt . . . the size of a pomegranate, actually. Probably nothing, but there is some gangrene, so let's get you booked into the hospital and . . ." I go into his office, and no, he has not found the pomegranate yet. In fact, he says, I am in fairly good shape. Overweight but not bad. The fact that I get regular exercise helps a lot.

Harry is tall and oddly shy for a guy running this big practice. He looks at his computer a lot while he's talking to you. You wouldn't say nerdy, because he's actually kind of handsome, if you think about it. But . . . well, "nerdy" might cross your mind. He was a serious oarsman in college and looks it. Women find him attractive, for some reason. But he dresses and carries himself so that I think "New England frump." Which, of course, is fine by me because I look about the same. I once had a male secretary who said, "Chris, you wear your clothes as if you hate them." Harry and I were cut from the same rumpled cloth in the same part of the world, the North Shore of Boston, five miles and twenty-five years apart. He drones on. Numbers, parameters. Blah, blah, blah.

Then, because I'm interviewing him for the important position of becoming my doctor, I say, "So, what is it about the practice of medicine that you like most?"

He stops, but only for a second, as if he's been waiting to talk about it. "What I really like is the notion of long-term relationships with patients and keeping them in good health. Not just curing disease but promoting health, which is a different thing. I would like to help them have a better life, not just cure them of this and that."

Bingo! "What do you mean?" I ask innocently.

"Well, I've always been interested in aging as well as internal medicine. I actually got board-certified in both, although I'm not sure how separate gerontology is from internal medicine." Then he turns and, very quietly, drops the bomb. "What I am sure of is that there is a fundamental revolution at hand in the way people age." He pauses and thinks how to get at it. "In the old days . . ." And he goes into the business about the slow, steady curve from fifty to death on the one hand and the new plateau on the other. Actually draws the lines in the air with his hand. "And you could be on the frontier of that change."

"Me?"

"Yeah. With your numbers . . ." He fools around with the computer. "Yup, this is pretty good. Uh, you don't smoke, and with these numbers and a more aggressive exercise habit, you could go on about the way you are today until you're, say, eighty. Maybe ninety. In fact, if you do a few things, you can actually be functionally younger. You're already in better shape than most of the men who come in here for the first time, but yes, you could be younger next year in all the ways that matter. Younger next year and for quite a few years to come."

I go over and sit in his lap. "True?"

"Yeah. You ski. Well, you can ski hard through your seventies. Slow down and eventually go to cross-country at some point in your eighties. Bike . . . you can do that forever.

There will be a certain decline eventually, but basically you can be as athletic, vigorous, and alert as you were at fifty until you're eighty or older. And for the first five or more years you can be functionally younger."

"What do I have to do?"

"It's hard to summarize, but there are three things." Did you ever notice how there are always three things? "Three things," he says. "Exercise. Nutrition. And commitment."

"The biggest one—and the biggest change for most people—is exercise. It is the golden key to great health. You should exercise hard almost every day of your life. And do strength training, lift weights, two or three of those six days. Exercise is the great key to aging. This long slide . . ." again, the arching curve with his hand in the air, "can simply go away. Or go up for quite a while. And you can be yourself for the rest of your life."

I have about four hundred questions but, uncharacteristically, I sit and wait.

Harry goes on. "Nutrition, too. You should eat the way you know you should eat but probably don't. If you possibly can, you should get down to your true weight. You're . . ." peek at the screen, "one ninety-four. You should be . . . what? What's your normal weight? One seventy-five?"

"One sixty-five, I guess. Maybe less. I rowed a little in college at one fifty-five and weighed about that until I was in my forties."

"Okay, if you could get back to one seventy someday, that would be great, but don't stew about it. It's much more important to exercise, regardless of what you weigh, and then learn to eat rationally from here on out. Quit eating the things that you know are rotten for you, like fast food and lots of fats and simple carbs. And eat less of everything." He says dieting is dumb and doesn't work, but my weight will drift down, over time, if I exercise the way I should and quit eating junk.

"Booze?"

He looks back at the screen. "Social drinker," he quotes me from the questionnaire. "Two drinks a night." Then those lovely manners cut in and he does not lean across the desk and shout "LIAR!" He just does the familiar thing about how a glass or two of wine is good but more than that is a negative. A lot more can be a real negative. Obviously.

"Commitment." He shrugs, as if to say this next part is harder to talk about. "What I mean is, you have to be involved with other people. And you have to care about something. Goals. Charities . . . people . . . family . . . job . . . hobbies. Especially after retirement, you have to dig in and take hold or things can take some bad turns." He stops, stuck for a minute, struggling a little. "It's specific to you, obviously. And it's awfully hard to generalize, but there have to be people and causes you care about. Doesn't seem to matter much just what they are. They don't have to be important to society or make money, as long as they're important and interesting to you. As long as you have some passion for them. There have to be people you care about and a reason to keep yourself alive. If not . . ." a little smile, "you'll die."

"That's it?" I ask.

"In a nutshell, yeah."

"Okay." I'm ready to go. "How much exercise? What do I eat?"

But that's the rest of the book. You are going to like it. It's going to save your life.

CHAPTER TWO

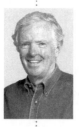

Lunch with Captain Midnight

efore we get serious and turn this over to Harry, let me ask you a couple of odd questions . . . and plant some notions that can just tick along beneath the surface while we talk about other things. We'll be going on for a good many chapters now about physical exercise and what it does to your body and your mind to keep you from aging. It is new, complicated, and terribly important stuff . . . the center of gravity of the book, really. But not the *only* stuff.

Later, Harry is going to tell you some wild things about how mammals are actually hardwired to function in pairs and groups. How we have this separate limbic brain for it. I didn't know I *had* a limbic brain until I met Harry, but it turns out I do. And it matters like crazy. You've got one, too. It's the brain that sends powerful messages that make you feel good when you touch someone . . . when you connect with and love other people. Or dogs. Dogs work fine. And it's the brain that can kill you dead if you get isolated. Because we are pack animals and are not meant to be alone. Anyhow, no details now . . . just a couple of impertinent questions.

Like: How's your husband? Or your lover or best friend . . . whoever you got? Whoever's got you? How's he or she doing with your aging? Or his or her own? Or retirement? Is he basically life-affirming or has he had about enough? Does he like you? Do you like him? What do you really think of each other, anyway, now that you're getting older? And the payoff question: Is your union strong enough so it can be made into a foundation for the two of you as you face the very different life that's coming at you both, at about a hundred miles an hour? Can you use the old stones? Use the old beams? Use the old love? Are you in this thing together?

Here's why I ask. It's too damn hard to be alone in the last third of our lives, that's why. And marriage helps. Unless it's just god-awful, in which case, the hell with it, though even a moderately good marriage can be a mighty help in the stretch that's coming up. Not the only way, for sure: close pals and family can be a complete and satisfying substitute. Which is a good thing, because 25 percent of women in America are not married in this Next Third. And most will be alone for a stretch at the end. But marriage has . . . oh, a special place, and should not be chucked out lightly.

One of the interesting things we learned in the course of doing this book is that there are a tremendous number of divorces after sixty and that women initiate two-thirds of them. It makes a certain amount of sense, when you think about it. A lot of women, as they come into their own in their fifties and sixties, are feeling that they've had enough of caregiving for a while. They're ready to focus some of their new confidence, their new *power,* on their own interests and goals. For many, that new focus means dumping Old Fred.

All of a sudden it occurs to them that Old Fred (who is leaking testosterone, big time) maybe wasn't such a giant in the first place. Now he's retiring . . . and he'll be home for lunch? How's that going to be? Will he adapt to his new life . . . get real . . . get a smaller job . . . get new interests? Or will he show up, like Captain Midnight, thinking he's doing you a hell of a favor just by showing up? For lunch!

You can just see it, can't you? He's bored stupid and scared to death, but he's still throwing his weight around and telling you what to do. Because maybe he was the main wage earner for a while and he still thinks he's The Great Guy. Or maybe because he was working in an *office,* you know, while you were at home, doing whatever you were doing. Eating Pop-Tarts and staring at the plumber's butt, he assumes. Or because he never took the time to figure out what you do in *your* office. So now he's going to do two things: he's going to try to depend on you for everything, and he's *still* going to try to give you some much needed advice on how to run your life. Can you hack that? Maybe not. Maybe it makes some sense to get the hell out.

But, gee, go slow. It's *so* much easier to do this aging number together as a couple. You can do it alone, of course, and eventually you may have to. But there's no rush. And there are compelling reasons not to.

I am an optimistic sort, and you should be, too. Much the best approach to life. But let us have a candid moment. Turning sixty can be awful damn bad sometimes. There are almost certain to be financial reversals . . . maybe a touch of sickness, an accident. And some people actually *die* in their sixties. Not hit by cars or knocked off their bikes. Just die, of seminatural causes. Like heart failure and cancer-of-the-this-and-that. It is highly unlikely that *you* will die, of course; I understand that. Especially if you do the things that Harry and I talk about. But death is out there. You keep hearing the waterfall in the distance, and you wonder all the time, What's that noise? And of course you know perfectly well. Scary. Very, very scary. And it's nice to have company. Preferably someone you know pretty well. Like Old Fred. You're going over the falls alone, you poor darling. Me, too. But it's nice to have company for as long as you can. Especially when you're lying there, listening to that cataract in the night. We are pack animals. Snuggle up.

Jessica Alone

Let's stop all this chat about marriage for a sec to remind ourselves that women can do awfully damn well alone, if that's the hand they're dealt. Here's an example. One of our pals—let's call her Jessica—was "alone" for the last forty years of her life, in the sense that her marriage ended and her kids grew up. She died last year, heart-breakingly young at eighty-something (it was the classic tangerine-in-the-brainpan; otherwise, she was in great shape). A small woman, she was a limbic giant all her life.

All right, the lessons. First, she *did* stuff, partly because she had to make a living. She was an editor for a while. Then she had a shop for years, where she sold goofy clothes and Mexican doo-dahs. She started a weekly show on the tiny TV station in her town. Lots of local news, lots of gossip, lots of dogs, for some reason. She had dinner parties all the time, even though she was a wretched cook. She was so serenely uninterested in her limitations that she wrote and published a cookbook just before she died. She did stuff, no matter what.

Second, she worked hard at nurturing and growing a circle of friends. She'd meet people on the *street,* and the next thing they knew, they were invited to dinner. One of the great risks in life is that you run out of friends. Jessica did not let that happen.

Third (these are *lessons,* remember), she worked hard at keeping herself in great shape. Thin and strong, she exercised steadily and skied hard most of her life. Lots of yoga, too. At a dinner in her late seventies, she would startle new friends by asking them to reach down and feel her thigh . . . see how strong she was. She was proud as punch and she should have been.

Next, she had great élan, great courage, great humor. She'd had some rotten luck as a younger woman, some truly rotten luck. And she just shook it off after some mourning. Got on with her life when a lesser person might have been eyeing the oven.

Finally, she *looked* and *sounded* as if she were a sexual or at least a sensual being until pretty late in the game. Not a necessary element for a great life, but a help if you have the good luck to be that kind of girl. Jessica got a late start. She used to say that during War War II, when she was in the Red Cross, she was the only virgin in the European Theater of Operations. As time went on, she said, that ceased to be true . . . whether because more virgins were brought in or for other reasons was never made clear. Later in life, she complained that appropriate men were thin on the ground, but there were a few. I remember, when she was in her seventies, a famous *Life* photographer came through town (they were pals from way back when). I don't know that anything happened, but she *did* disappear for a couple of days. The little rascal.

She was game all her life. Game for everything. And her

life was good. Good for her, great for us. So let's be clear when we talk about the joys of marriage. It ain't the only way.

Homesteading:
Marriage in the Next Third

B ut it's a pretty good way. And if your experience has been a bit harrowing so far, bear in mind that marriage in the Next Third is going to be quite different, maybe better, and certainly more important. If you happen to be blessed with a relationship that can bear some weight, or if you can retool and reinvent what you've got so that it can take the strain, then the great likelihood is that you two are going to be each other's primary resource for a long damn time . . . perhaps most of the rest of your lives. Primary company, primary joint-venturer, primary encourager or dissuader—the works. For an awful lot of you, it's going to be a huge part of the social structure for a while. Your husband may try to make it his *entire* social structure—an insupportable idea that he'll have to get over. The best relationship in the world cannot, and should not, be a substitute for everything you or he got out of your jobs. That's nuts. But it's going to be a primary resource, almost for sure. So we suggest that you start the emotional negotiations early. You are real partners now, whatever it's been like in the past. Talk as openly as you can and figure out who's interested in doing what, who can bear what loads. And do new stuff together. Think, for example, about the hellish exercise program that Harry and I will be touting in the rest of this book. It is so much more fun to do it together. Easier, too.

Give you an example, close to home. When Hilary and I met, the gag was that she never went outdoors, except to go to clubs, and only wore black. We moved to Colorado and she shrugged off that persona like Superman changing in a phone booth. In a heartbeat she was skiing, hiking, biking, and Lord knows what. Not a real "athlete" by any means. Neither am I. But into it. And when we came back east and I got into Harry's Rules, she got into that, too. We do it together, not every day but a lot. And I cannot tell you how much better that is.

Think about it: six o'clock on a winter morning . . . dark out . . . time to struggle off to that wretched gym. It's so much easier if there are two of you. You go out together, you do it together, you come home together soaked in sweat in the freezing air. To the coffee and the paper. And you both feel great . . . pump each other up. Nice.

Or this summer at the lake in New Hampshire, where I've always done a bit of rowing. Two years ago, Hilary suddenly got into it. We go off, side by side, in matching single sculls these days. At dawn, usually, with the loons laughing at us, in still water before it gets hot. Sometimes I go farther, sometimes she does, but mostly we do it together, and I can't tell you how nice that is. Biking these days . . . same deal. No one would have predicted that ten years ago.

Give it a shot. It'll be good for the exercise program and good for the marriage. And if you can get Fred to be serious about leading the good life, it may cut down a bit on that five- to ten-year stretch of your being alone at the end. Or at least shorten the period when he's gaga and you're wiping the goo off his face.

That's a little blunt about the goo, sorry, but it does happen and the best thing you can do (apart from dumping him, I guess) is to get him up on his pins right now. You truly don't want that long, grim slide into aging we talked about in the first chapter. You want a long, great life . . . then over the falls, *boom*! So make him *do* something.

Here's a hopeful bit. In a way, marriage in the Next Third is easier. It's like farm couples in olden times: less divorce and less angst because both players, husband and wife, had such important roles, keeping the farm going. Same here: you both have such important roles keeping your new lives going that, intuitively, you're going to show each other more respect, pay more attention, simply care more about each other than you have in the past. And by the way, that nutcase flood of testosterone, which made him such a jerk sometimes, ebbs a bit. That helps.

One last notion. Teach Fred to be independent. That sounds odd because the theory has been that the men have been the independent ones and the women the reverse. It's interesting how that gets twisted around when Fred doesn't have a job to fall back on. The fact is that there is a significant risk that, upon retirement, Old Fred is going to try to rely too much on you for support, at least in the early stages. Men are a bit dumb about preparing for retirement; we go into denial and stay there. So, when the day does come, an embarrassing number of us turn, with something like tears in our eyes, and expect the women in our lives to take up the whole burden of keeping us interested, loved, hated, amused. And you can't do that. Even if you want to (and I hope you are coming into a stage of your life when that's the last thing you want to do), you simply cannot. You cannot and should not bear that burden. Let's say you're nuts about him (quite the little assumption), you still cannot shoulder that huge load and you shouldn't have to. You're entitled to your independence; he's going to have to learn about his.

He's going to have to work at connecting and committing to other people, other groups, to make his own life work. Without an enormous, automatic structure, like his old job, pointing the way. He's going to have to learn to be flexible and creative and to connect. Just as you've been doing for so much of your life. Interesting switch, isn't it? Think of all the times he hollered about your being on the phone to your friends. Turns out, that was a genius thing to do. He should be so lucky, these days, to have that gift . . . have those friends. You may have to take the lead in this whole area but, in general, the more broadly and variously you can both manage to connect and engage with others, before or during retirement, the better off you'll be.

The Drafting Model

Here's a weird notion that comes from the world of bike racing. All cyclists know that a group of riders (or only two riders) will go much faster—perhaps as much as 25 percent faster—if you "draft." That is, if you take turns leading, while the non-leader crouches out of the wind behind the leader. When you draft, you swap the lead back and forth, and *both* of you cover the overall distance much faster and with less effort. When you watch the Tour de France, that's what goes on between team members. With social biking, it works the same way. And the expression, when you go to the front, is "Okay, I'll pull for a while." Because that's what it feels like . . . as if the leader is actually pulling.

Well, there may come a time when it makes sense for you to tell your husband (or whoever it is you're spending your time with these days) that you'll "pull" for a while.

Maybe he pulled most of the way, maybe not. But swapping back and forth still makes sense and is in your mutual interest. You both do better.

I picked up this idea at bike camp in Idaho, when I was talking to a recently retired CEO (and strong biker) whose wife has lately turned into a bit of a rocket ship. At sixty-two, not only has she become a deadly serious biker, but she's also taken a bigger part in running both their lives, socially and otherwise. Let me be clear: This guy is most assuredly no sissy. But his wife has just hit this streak in her life when she's *huge.* He's remarkably calm and, I think, wise about it. He welcomes the shift in power and is happy to let her pull for a while. And he fly-fishes. They're both having more fun.

This is not isolated weirdness. I know a number of couples where this pattern is emerging. Partly it's a matter of timing. A close pal was a leading lawyer forever, and now he wants to retire. His wife got her MBA late—at about forty—because she'd been rearing children. Now he wants to cut back and she's coming into a particularly hot part of her life as a senior executive. You can see her energy increasing, too, even though they're about the same age. So she's running more and more of their life, even though she also works much longer hours. It's her turn. Drafting. Nice.

So, if there comes a time when Old Fred starts to fade, don't be so sure that it's time for you to quit. He may just be drafting.

Okay, enough. The black-letter rule for this particular chapter is this: Get in touch with your husband. Or wife or significant other or best friend or whatever you've got. Recalibrate, restructure, and strengthen your deal. And head into the Next Third as full partners . . . homesteaders in tough, sometimes hostile new country. You'll have much better luck and more fun doing it together. Start with this book. Ask your partner to read it (or the guy's version) and talk it over. Use Harry's insights into evolutionary biology to trick your bodies and minds into staying strong for the next thirty years.

You're a couple of kids in an old Western, and you're going to knock over the Darwinian Casino together . . . live on the loot forever. You'll be waiting with the horses down by the river. Or he will be. And you're both going to ride for your lives. It's a romantic story . . . surprising after all these years . . . and you're in it together.

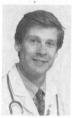

CHAPTER THREE

The New Science of Aging

A while back, when I had been in practice as a general internist for ten years, I sat down and took stock. Things were going well. I loved my job, I loved my patients, and I had wonderful colleagues, but there was a problem. Many of the patients who had been with me from the beginning were coming into their late fifties, sixties, and seventies, and things were happening. Some had become friends as well as patients, but most I saw only occasionally— once a year for their physicals and from time to time as problems came up. The annual checkups were like time-lapse photography, and in those jerky pictures I saw women and men I cared about getting old at an alarming clip. Many were sedentary, but even those who were moderately active were becoming increasingly overweight, out of shape, and apathetic. And some were getting seriously sick. They were having strokes, heart attacks, bad falls, and bad injuries. A number had died, and the timing did not seem to make sense.

One of the hardest things about medicine is delivering

bad news: "We'll need to do some more tests" . . . "This looks suspicious" . . . "Why don't you sit down so we can talk?" All the euphemisms we use to say that life has suddenly—and irreversibly—taken a bad turn. I became increasingly aware that most of these conversations were happening long before they should have, and for reasons that were clear and avoidable.

It was not that I had missed a diagnosis or failed to spot something on an X-ray. I had done what doctors do well in this country, which is to treat people when they come in with a disease. My patients had had good medical care but not, I began to think, great *health* care. For most, their declines, their illnesses, were thirty-year problems of lifestyle, not disease. I, like most doctors in America, had been doing the wrong job well. Modern medicine does not concern itself with lifestyle problems. Doctors don't treat them, medical schools don't teach them, and insurers don't pay to solve them. I began to think that this was indefensible. I had always spent time on these issues, but I had not made them a primary focus. And far too many of my patients— including some very smart and able women—were having lousy lives. Some were dying.

I had some further thoughts at that ten-year review. Most modern medicine is what lawyers and bankers call transactional: a one-shot deal. You hurt your knee, you have a heart attack, and you see a specialist. A short, intensive period of repair follows, and the parties go their separate ways, probably forever. I realized that my practice was entirely different. I was likely to have long relationships with people . . . twenty, thirty years. That's one of the best things about being an internist. But that privileged, long-term look into patients' lives has put me on a different footing from that of the specialists. I am "on notice" of how my patients are living, and of how they are dying. I am "on notice" that the normal American way of life—and especially the American way of aging—is dangerous and sometimes lethal. I am "on notice" that, no matter how great our medical care, we all need great health care too—and very few of us get it.

It is inexplicable that our society, plagued by soaring medical costs and epidemics of obesity, heart disease, osteoporosis, and cancer, cares so little about these things. The simple fact is that we know perfectly well what to do. *Some 70 percent of premature death and aging is lifestyle-related.* Heart attacks, strokes, the common cancers, diabetes, brittle bones, most falls, fractures and serious injuries, and many more illnesses are primarily caused by the way we live. *If we had the will to do it, we could eliminate more than half of all disease in women and men over fifty. Not delay it, eliminate it.* That is a readily attainable goal, but we are not moving toward it. Instead, we have made these problems invisible by making them part of the "normal" landscape of aging. As in "Oh, that's a normal part of growing older."

"Normal Aging" Isn't Normal

The more I looked at the science, the more it became clear that such ailments and deterioration are *not* a normal part of growing old. They are an outrage. An outrage that we have simply gotten used to because we set the bar so shamefully low. A lot of people unconsciously assume that they will get-old-and-die: one phrase, almost one word, and certainly one seamless concept. That when they get old and infirm, they will die soon after, so a deteriorating quality of life does not matter. *That is a deeply mistaken idea and a dangerous premise for planning your life.* In fact, you will probably *get-old-and-live.* You can get decrepit, if you like, but you are not likely to die; you are likely to live like that for a long, long time. Most American women today will live into their mid-eighties or early nineties, whether they're in great shape or shuffling around on walkers. Every day I sit down with patients after their checkups—smart, reasonably healthy women in their sixties and seventies—and point out that they are statistically likely to live another twenty or thirty years. Although there are some who light up at the prospect, by far the most frequent response is "Oh, I'm not sure I want that." Which misses the point entirely. The point is that you are likely to live that long *whether you want to or not.* Statistical longevity is simply a fact of life today.

So let me say that again: You may well live into your nineties, *whether you like it or not.* But *how* you live those years, on the other hand, is largely under your control. Which is good reason to make the Last Third of your life terrific—and not a dreary panoply of obesity, sore joints and apathy. "Normal aging" is intolerable and avoidable. You can skip most of it and grow old, not just gracefully but with real joy.

This was my epiphany. I thought, "I cannot, as a doctor, sit here and watch people I care for, and care about, go down a road that is leading them to an awful place without doing something. It is not enough to wait for the car to crash and then do a good job of treating the injured and dying." If 70 percent of the serious illness I see is preventable, then it's my job to prevent it. The good news on this front is that you do not need to wait for a presidential commission or a national health initiative to do something. This fight can be led, fought, and won one person at a time. Starting with you.

As I have looked at the steady stream of people coming in for their first visit over the years since that epiphany, I have been struck by just how many of them suffer the downright bad health that seems to be the American lot these days. Not just older people, either; the horrendous effects of idleness and a rotten diet show younger and younger. With each new patient, I have the same talk I had with Chris, and if the patient is at all responsive, a new collaboration begins. The great news is that most people get it, and a lot of them have gone down the path toward getting younger.

Change on the Cellular Level

We are in the midst of a revolution in the science of aging. It is part of a larger revolution in our understanding of how our bodies work at the cellular level, and it has opened the door to healthy aging. The science behind this revolution is vast and extraordinary, covering fields as diverse as cell physiology, protein structure, biochemistry, evolutionary biology, exercise physiology, anthropology, experimental psychology, ecology, and comparative neuroanatomy. Definitive conclusions from this research are still emerging, but the basic lines are clear enough that women and men from forty to ninety should act on them now. If they do, they can live radically better, happier, *healthier* lives than their parents, grandparents or anyone else in all of biological time.

Let's back up. Ten years ago, the basic science of health was unknown territory—the huge blank space on the map. But we have finally learned enough from studying disease to understand health. As it turns out, health is biologically more complicated than disease. In disease, the train has gone off the tracks and the laws of physics take over. The crash is terrifying and destructive, but the science is simple. Health is the reverse. It has carefully designed control mechanisms to keep the train *on the tracks*. The science of those mechanisms—the blueprint for our bodies—is phenomenally complex. Luckily for us, the controls are simple to operate. You need to understand only two basic, background points about the evolution of your biology to take charge of your health.

The first is that the human body is not a neatly integrated design package. The wonderful but wacky biological commune you call your body was cobbled together by nature from parts that evolved in different species millions, even billions, of years apart. Your opposable thumb, wiggling down there at the end of your arm, and a couple of extra pounds of brain are the only parts of you that are distinctly "human." Everything else is from another species. And don't think chimps here. We are talking bacteria, dinosaurs, birds, worms, gazelles, lions—the list goes on for pages. Your body, created with great optimism and fanfare by your parents in 1950, or 1930, or whenever, is mostly made up of cells whose basic structure and operation were developed by bacteria billions of years ago. The messages that run these cells are not the conscious thoughts that gave rise to the Renaissance or constitutional government. They are not thoughts at all. They are primitive electrical and chemical impulses that predate the dawn of consciousness by many aeons.

The second point is that you can control your deeply primitive cells with your miraculous, Renaissance-creating brain, but not in the way you would expect. You have to talk to your body in code and follow certain immutable rules. We're here to give you the code and explain the rules.

Not our rules, by the way. Nature's rules, and you can't get around them.

Some Good News . . . With a Catch

You inherited a biological fortune. You have a stunningly good body, whether you think so or not, and a truly amazing brain. As a matter of fact, you actually have three *separate* truly amazing brains, from three very different stages of evolution, all working together. In simple terms, you have a *physical* brain, an *emotional* brain and a *thinking* brain. Although they are chemically and anatomically distinct (neurosurgeons can separate them like sections of an orange) and have different purposes, all three are densely wired together to get you through your day.

But here's the catch. Your body and brains are perfect for their natural purposes, but none of them was designed for modern life: fast food, TV, or retirement. They were designed for life in nature, where only the fittest survived. Most of your body parts have as little business in a mall as a saber-toothed tiger. Left to their own devices, your body and brains will consistently and without fail misinterpret the signals of the twenty-first century.

Decay Is Optional

There's a critical distinction between aging and decay that you need to keep in mind from here on in. Aging is inevitable, but it's biologically programmed to be a slow process. Most of what we call aging, and most of what we dread about getting older, is actually decay. That's critically important because we are stuck with real aging, but *decay is optional.* Which means that most of *functional* aging is optional as well.

There is an immutable biology of aging, and you can't do anything about it: hair gets gray, gravity takes its toll, and movies go to half price. Your maximum heart rate declines steadily over time, regardless of how active you are. That's big. Your skin degenerates, too, regardless of lifestyle. So you will *look* old, no matter what. But you do not have to *act* old or *feel* old. That's what counts. We haven't figured out a way to last forever, but aging can be a slow, minimal, and surprisingly graceful process. And even on the appearances front, there is a huge difference between a great-looking, healthy older person and one who has let go.

Nature balances growth with decay by setting your body up with an innate tendency toward decay. The signals are not powerful, but they are continuous, they never stop, and they get a little stronger each year. Chris refers to this as the relentless tide, which is a good metaphor. Whatever you call it, in our forties and fifties our bodies switch into a "default to decay" mode and the free ride of youth is over. In the absence of signals to grow, the body and brain decay and we "age." We may not like that arrangement today, but we are certainly not going to change it. What we can do, with surprising ease, is override those default signals, swim against the tide and change decay back into growth.

So how do we keep ourselves from decaying? By changing the signals we send to our bodies. The keys to overriding the decay code are daily exercise, emotional commitment, reasonable nutrition, and a real engagement with living. But it starts with exercise.

You have to exercise all the time because it's who you are. More importantly, it's also who you *were*. What you came from, hundreds of millions of years ago. Your body is a gift from trillions of ancestors, and the fact that you're here means that every single one of them survived. Each one of them got it right; each one passed on a little more strength, speed, and smarts to the next generation.

Our bodies and minds are precision instruments designed for succeeding in harmony with the natural environment. We are literally constructed to grow in good times—to be alert, to hunt, to explore, to work together, to build, to laugh, to play, to run, to heal, to love . . . and to survive. To do all this, we need our bodies and minds to be strong, active, and completely in sync.

On the other side of the biological equation, however, we must allow decay to occur when necessary, because every ounce of body structure takes energy to maintain. Every muscle fiber, every scrap of bone and cartilage, every brain connection, every skin cell, and even every thought consumes its share of fuel. Each has to contribute to survival and reproduction or it decreases the odds of genetic success. So in bad times, in stressful times, in drought, famine, or winter, we are built to shut down, to hibernate, to retreat—to atrophy and decay as quickly as possible. From the point of view of the species, once the years of childbearing and rearing were done, this may have been a good way to age. In that mode, less food is used and, of course, death comes sooner to make room at the trough for the next generation. That's the Darwinian code for aging. That's how nature designed your body, and it's why decay becomes a little more insistent each year. It's circle-of-life stuff. Sound good to you as you head into those years?

Perhaps not. From an individual's point of view—from your point of view—there are problems. This is an appalling way to live, for one thing, and it does not make sense, for another. We live in temperature-controlled houses, not in an ice age, and most of us have far too much to eat, not too little. In the absence of paralyzing cold or famine, you might think our bodies would begin to adapt away from the semihibernation defense. But it was only a hundred years ago that we escaped those pressures—a staggering event in human development but a nonevent in evolutionary time. Our physical mechanisms have not adapted at all to the modern world of retirement, and they are not going to. Indeed, they have not changed one bit from the systems that were devised, over millions of years, to function in a knife-edge world where there was never enough to eat and always a surfeit of danger. Evolutionary change may happen, but not for many millions of years, so you may want to make other arrangements. You may want to come to grips with your old, Darwinian body right now . . . see what you can do to force some adaptation in your own lifetime. Remember, without your input, your body will constantly misinterpret the signals of today's world. It will trigger the "default to decay" setting. You'll start to deteriorate, to die. To understand why, we need to look at both the good times and bad times in nature, and how our ancestors adapted to them using the mechanisms and signals that are still part of us today.

Springtime on the Savannah

Let's start with the signals to grow, to get younger. It's springtime on the African savannah . . . a time of plenty in the place where we grew up. The rains have come, the grass is lush and the water holes are full. Predators are relatively few, and not a major threat. They demand alertness and respect, but not anxiety. Prey abounds, but the antelope, nuts, and berries are scattered over a wide area, so hunting and gathering require hours of walking every day. Even today, women of the Kalahari walk eight to ten miles every day, foraging for food. *That exercise—the physical work of hunting and foraging in the spring—has always been the single most powerful signal we can send that life is good; that it's spring and time to live and grow.*

In response to the chemical signals sent by that exercise, your body becomes lean, powerful, and efficient. Excess fat becomes superfluous because the energy supply is fairly constant. Your body keeps a modest fat reserve to guard against hard times, but more than this is just a liability because lugging it around takes energy and slows your reaction time. Bone strength and joint health increase to handle the repetitive shock loading of the travel. Your heart and circulatory functions increase to supply the blood and oxygen to your muscles. The muscles themselves become strong, supple, and more coordinated. Immune function increases to repair the ongoing wear and tear—the sprains, cuts, bruises, and minor infections that accompany active outdoor life.

Your brain changes, too. As it gets these consistent physical signals from your body, it develops a chemistry of optimism: the ideal mood for hunting and foraging. Lab animals in similar exercise environments demonstrate actual physical and chemical brain changes that lead to increased curiosity and energy, an increased willingness to explore, increased interactions with other group members, increased alertness, and what looks for all the world like increased optimism.

Lean, fit, happy, optimistic, energetic, brimming with vim and vigor: these were nature's design specifications for you in the ideal environment—what you were built to be in the spring. This is the good life, and it's out there waiting for you. A life characterized by strong, aerobically fit muscles, a healthy heart, lean body, good bones, good immune system, high sex drive, and an alert, inquisitive, optimistic mind geared toward working well in groups and building strong social networks.

We'll show you how to get there, but before we do, let's look at the dark side, at the way we live now. Let's look at our modern lifestyle, with junk food, too much TV, long commutes, job stress, marital stress, family stress, poor sleep, artificial light and noise, and perhaps worst of all, no exercise. Springtime on the savannah? Not hardly. In nature, this lifestyle sends signals of deadly peril, and your body and brain make deadly changes in response.

In a paradox that you absolutely have to understand, endless calories and lack of exercise signal your body that you're heading into a famine that you may well not survive, and in response your body and brain head into a low-grade form of depression. Ironically, in nature, depression is normal. It's a critical survival strategy. Let's look at real nature for a moment . . . not the beautiful sunsets, the songbirds trilling in the garden, and Bambi and Thumper playing tag in the glade, but the killing fields. The nature where 50 percent of antelope foals are torn apart by coyotes in the first two weeks of life. Where kill or be killed is not a metaphor, but deadly real, every day. The nature where there is no margin for error. Not a small margin, but *none*. Adapting to good times is easy; adapting to bad times—to drought, winter, or danger—is critical. Dead animals don't reproduce.

So, winter comes to the tundra. Darkness falls. Temperatures plummet to twenty below zero. Blizzards howling down from the north bring sleet, then snow— drifting to ten feet, burying food, driving prey into burrows, making it impossible to move. Most of what little food you get is burned up shivering just to stay alive. You start the long starvation of winter. As the months drag on, you wear down to skin and bone. The fat you built up over the fall steadily melts off as you battle cold and famine. You are locked in a slow race with death as you wait for spring.

What is hard for us to grasp today is that this was a regular, *normal* part of our human experience, and that depression-as-ultimate-defense lies deep within our bones. We used it every winter, and in every time of drought or famine. We survived by getting depressed. Not clinically depressed, or Prozac depressed, but survival depressed, as in let's slow down the metabolism, build up the fat stores, withdraw, turn inward, hibernate, cut everything back to bare minimum. Shut down and survive by letting all but the most critical systems atrophy and decay.

In fact, *all chronic stress works the same way.* Chronic stress, whether physical or mental, tells your body that the environment has changed for the worse and that you're in for a long-haul survival challenge. Low-grade depression combined with physical decay is your body's preferred state of health for this situation. The thing is, the signals for this particular state of health are pretty much the lifestyle of standard American aging: being sedentary, withdrawing from social contact, and eating everything you can get your hands on. These are the primary signals of famine or winter, and your body will respond. With the unerring certainty born of billions of years of survival, it will respond to your behavior.

Being sedentary is the most important signal for decay. Your body watches what you do, your physical behavior, every day, like a hawk. In nature, there is no reason to be sedentary except lack of food. Remember that we grew up in Africa. No matter how plentiful the game, it rotted in hours. No refrigerators, no convenience stores, no microwave popcorn. You had to get up and hunt or forage for hours every single day. The *only* reason not to was famine. Regardless of how much food you eat, that's what you tell your body every day you don't exercise. And on those days, you're telling your body that it's time to get old. To rot. To get survival depressed — low energy, apathy. To store every scrap of excess food as fat, dump the immune system, melt off the muscle, and let the joints decay. Time to find a cave, huddle in the corner, and start shivering.

And this all starts in a heartbeat, because the decay signals get sent continuously, no matter what you do. That's the tide Chris talks about. Your body tissues and neural circuits are *always* trying to decay. Muscle, bone, brain: always trying to melt, like ice-cream cones in the sun. The good news is that the decay signals, though constant, are weak. If you don't send any signals to grow, decay will win, but even a modest signal to grow — a decent workout, even a good, stiff walk — will drown out the noise. Thing is, you need to do something every day to tell your body it's springtime. That's the key to this book. It isn't complicated, but you have to work at it every day.

Keep in mind that decay is not biological aging. Decay is the dry rot caused by our modern, sedentary lifestyle. Decay comes from turning on the TV when the sun is out. From every drive to a fast-food place to get a supersize order of fries or a soft drink full of sugar and caffeine. From riding around the golf course in an electric cart. From sitting home alone.

Decay comes from giving up on life and failing to engage. But decay can be stopped — or radically slowed — by using the Darwinian mechanisms we've talked about. Aging is up to nature, but decay is up to you.

The Brain Chemistry of Growth

L et's say you've decided to choose a "springtime" state of health. How do you get your body to comprehend your choice? Some of it happens automatically in your muscles and other tissues as you exercise, but a critical component is controlled by your brain. Not your thinking brain, but your physical brain—the one that came to you from millions of years back.

This brain is deaf, dumb, and blind. Literally. Apart from smell, it has no direct connection to the world. Inside your skull, it is always dark, wet, a little salty, and 98.6 degrees. Your physical brain knows only what you tell it by the way you live your life. Your physical brain and body evolved in a harsh world, with no second chances, and their mechanisms are as fundamental as the orbit of the earth around the sun. Until the day you die, they will believe, with relentless certainty, that you still live in nature. That's why the way you choose to live your daily life determines your state of health—good or bad, whether you like it or not. Health is your physical brain's *perfect* adaptation of your body to the world it *thinks* you live in. This is not about disease, that's different. No one chooses disease. It's just plain bad luck, though often piled on top of bad health. But *you* choose your state of health. You can see this as a burden or a privilege, a gift or a curse, but you can't put it down and you can't get away from it. That's great news, if you understand the rules, because it's not that hard to take over the controls.

Taking charge starts with a look at how the whole system was designed, and that takes us back to the beginning. The first stirrings of life began 3.5 *billion* years ago, with our direct ancestors—algae, yeast, and then bacteria.

That pedigree is not humiliating, it's awe-inspiring, and we should be grateful for it. We do ourselves a great disservice by thinking we can divorce ourselves from evolution. Your family tree goes back 3.5 billion years, and every second of it was spent perfecting the body and brains you inherited. Not one second of wasted time, mind you, but 3.5 billion years of making you perfect.

The Information Age

About half of your basic metabolic machinery comes directly from bacteria, unchanged, ticking along perfectly for millennia. These single-cell ancestors, together with yeast and algae, lived in a constant street fight where every cell competed for itself alone. All advanced organisms, from worm to human, have organized multiple cells that work together. The whole *is* greater than the parts, for the same reason that organizations are often more successful than individuals: communication.

Simple organisms communicate by leaking chemicals directly between cells. It's the origin of your sense of smell, which is your most primitive sense: the way the smell of coffee and bacon in the morning wakes up your whole body is a good example of how well it works. In general, however, the more cells in a body, the more information needed to make it all work, and as we evolved larger bodies with more sophisticated tissues, we developed primitive nervous systems, along with the blood-borne chemical signals we call hormones. As we continued to evolve, the neural and hormonal systems became ever more complex and adaptable, and allowed us to explore an ever-expanding range of biological possibilities.

Today, you are awash in information. You have billions of cells, and each one is constantly signaling its neighbors with highly nuanced chemical messages. Every scrap of tissue has a rich network of nerve connections and hormonal receptors, and millions of their signals fly around your body all the time. All the traffic on the Internet and all the phone calls around the world are dwarfed by the information traffic in your body.

That's not a metaphor. You send *trillions* of internal signals all day, every day, from the moment of your conception until you die. You talk to your body all the time in a constant stream of chatter, day and night, year in and year out. You won't, and indeed you can't, shut up. And all your tissues, every single part of your body and your brain—they listen to you, all the time. They hang on your every word, obey your every command. But they don't speak English. They read the language of your body. And you will shudder when you learn what you've been telling them.

The Language of Nature

Five hundred million years ago, give or take, our early invertebrate ancestors (snails and jellyfish and such) developed most of the neural hormones and brain chemicals we use today—chemicals very similar to Valium, adrenaline, cocaine, and morphine. We didn't invent any of this stuff when we came along; we just bought it off the rack as we moved up the evolutionary ladder. It's true. Worms and snails run their bodies and nervous systems with the same chemicals and hormones you're using right now as you read these words.

It took another couple of hundred million years to get

from worms to the first brain, but finally the fish figured it out. Salmon have the same basic physical brain you do, or, more accurately, you have theirs. The fish passed it on to the amphibians, who spun off dinosaurs, reptiles, and birds (more ancestors: it's getting crowded on the family tree), and they all kept refining that physical brain. Structurally, it sits right at the top of the spinal cord, sorting millions of inputs every second and coordinating the output to match.

We split off from reptiles two hundred million years ago, but we carried their gift, the physical brain, with us, largely unchanged, and it runs our bodies today. It's your purely physical brain, but what a brain it is! No feelings, and no true thoughts, but phenomenally complex physical reactions. It's a work of art, a miracle in its own right, an absolute treasure. Think of a marlin leaping out of the water or a hawk swooping down on its prey. The sheer athletic poetry of motion is a function of this brain. So put aside all your conceptions of fish, reptiles, and birds as lower life-forms. There is not a single bird alive that you can match for physical grace and coordination.

Neuroscientists label this brain the reptilian brain, the hindbrain, or the primitive brain. Each label carries with it the dismissive suggestion that this is some crude piece of machinery along the road to the perfection of our human neocortex. The reverse is far more accurate. The physical brain runs our bodies, and it does so with near seamless perfection. Try to use your thinking brain to ride a bike and you'll end up surfing the pavement on your face. Then watch old footage of Greg Louganis, spinning and tumbling through space in a perfectly coordinated free fall and entering the water without a trace. Or Nadia Comaneci in the incredible routines that earned her not one but *seven* perfect 10s. That's all completely automatic, not a thought to be found. It's the physical brain, and yours is innately as powerful as theirs.

Your physical brain also runs your metabolism, ceaselessly gearing every organ, tissue, and cell to the immediate energy demands of the moment. Automatically monitoring every conceivable aspect of your physical being and keeping your whole body in a supreme harmony. That's why exercise is the master signal for growth, because it's the language of your physical brain. Celebrate this brain, and understand that it operates on some miraculous autopilot level every moment of every day. This is the brain that does *exactly* what you tell it to every second. This is your body's master control center.

You need to reconnect directly to your physical brain. You've shut it in the closet long enough. After days spent indoors, and nights in front of the TV, this miracle machine is waiting for you to take it out for a spin. To *not* do this is a dangerous waste. Because there is also a dark side; there is also decay.

Life is energy. That's all that matters to nature. For 3.5 billion years, life has walked a razor-thin edge between energy and exertion. Biologically, there is no such thing as retirement, or even aging. There is only growth or decay. And your body looks to you to choose between them. Fast food, sedentary lifestyles, modern stress, loneliness, retirement, and old age have no evolutionary basis. Your physical brain does, and it is ancient and primal beyond anything you can imagine. Billions of years of life, but especially of death, have honed it to shut down nonessential functions with the ruthless efficiency of the shark from which it came. And like the cold, dead eyes of the shark, this brain has no care for your happiness, no thought about your aging. It is a ceaseless machine, in relentless pursuit of the perfect match between input and output—between growth and decay. It does its job every second of every day, whether you like it or not, whether you know it or not, and whether you take charge of it or not. With that in mind, think about what your physical brain learned from the way you lived today, and think about whether it told your body to grow or decay.

Stepping Out of the Crucible

The game has changed for us because we have luxuries and choices in our modern lives that have no parallel in our biology. In a remarkable triumph of ego over intellect, we simply assume that we were "made" for this life; that we were purpose-built for life in the twenty-first century. That is a deeply mistaken view, and one we must get over.

Unique among all the generations of living creatures that have wandered this earth for more than three billion years, we have stepped out of the crucible of evolution. We simply stood up and walked out of nature. Most of us are not likely to face starvation. We are not hunting or hunted. Life for us is not the razor-thin line between famine and plenty. From the point of view of shaping our species, death by starvation or cold has gone away. For the first time ever, there is enough to eat and no one capable of eating us. It is impossible to overstate the importance of that development or the depth of the change. Almost incomprehensibly, the great problem of our time is surfeit. And idleness. Our ancestors ran for their lives for hundreds of millions of years, desperately searching for food, storing it up in their bodies against the certainty of drought, ice, and starvation. And then, in a twinkling, all that was gone and a fundamental law of creation ceased to apply. This is arguably the most profound shift, ever, in the way the world works.

Understandably, our Darwinian bodies and primitive brains are not going to catch up with this astonishing state of affairs. We live, in this new safety, in this new time of plenty, like drunken sailors freshly delivered from terrible peril. And sure enough, we have become ill. We forget our roots, forget our past, forget how our bodies and our minds were made, and we contract terrible and weird new sicknesses. Our bodies do not know how to "read" this plenty, and we eat ourselves to death. Our minds do not know how to "read" the absence of danger, the absence of the need to hunt or gather—the idleness. And we soften to death. Our amazingly effective hearts start to fail us in epidemic numbers, and in ways that have no parallel in nature.

In short, we have adopted a lifestyle which—for people designed as we were designed—is nothing less than a disease. Think about that. Our lifestyle—especially as we age, especially in this wonderful country—is a disease more deadly than cancer, war or plague. We live longer because of modern medicine, but many of us live wretchedly and many of us die much younger than we should. The point of this book is that we have to learn to cure ourselves, or, in the midst of all this plenty, we will live and prematurely die in unnecessary pain—in bodies that believe they are in the grip of famine.

So how do we choose between decay and growth, between older and younger? We are not going to become hunter/gatherers again. Or even farmers the way farmers lived a hundred years ago, by the sweat of their brows. So, instead, we have to simulate a little of life in the survivalist world. We have to play on the physical stage in order to take control of our Darwinian bodies, and our minds, too—since they are so intimately wired together that it is useless to think of the well-being of the one without the other.

The take-home message is simple. Everything you do physically, everything you eat, everything you think and feel, every emotion and experience changes your body and your brain in physical ways that were set in stone millions or billions of years ago. Physical exercise and involvement in life trigger great waves of "grow" messages throughout your body and mind. If you send the right messages, you have several billion years of evolution and trillions of ancestors on your side, sending out primitive messages by the billions, making you stronger, more agile, smarter . . . better able to take hard knocks. Exercise is the only way to engage your body and your physical brain, but if you do it, you will get "younger." Not completely, but to an astonishing degree.

The physical messages you send by being consciously and steadily active, and the emotional messages you send by being engaged in the great hunt of life, *can override the default message.* With relatively little effort, you can mimic a younger woman in her prime — exercising, interacting, making love — and your body will go along. Remember, the tide is relentless, but it is not that strong. If you are relentless yourself, if you are active and engaged *every day,* you can resist and even swim against the tide into very old age. It takes work, routine, and a fair amount of juggling to keep your priorities straight day after day, but that's familiar territory. It's what you've done so well for years on end. Bring those gifts and that discipline to bear on this new set of problems, and you can set the *realistic* goal of living like fifty until you're eighty and beyond.

CHAPTER FOUR

Swimming Against the Tide

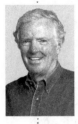

When Harry and I started this project, we thought it was all going to be pretty simple. Which it is, ultimately, but it gets a little complicated in places. Which is why we think it's a good idea to set out one simple rule at this point. A rule to follow when all else fails, to follow when you're going to hell, to follow when you've forgotten the dog's name. Call it Harry's First Rule.

It goes like this: *Exercise six days a week for the rest of your life.* Sorry, but that's it. No negotiations. No give. No excuses. Six days, serious exercise, until you die. And do not kid yourself that this is a lad's law that doesn't apply to women. If anything, it applies with more urgency. It is *the* great lifesaver and life enhancer for women, even more than for men. So just do it. If you're still in your forties and stretched to the breaking point with work and kids, commuting, soccer games, and your own aging parents, we can talk about four or five days, but six is much better even then. And after age fifty, six is mandatory. By then the tide is starting to pick up and you need help staying off the rocks. In fact, my version of the rule would have been "Exercise *hard* six days a week," but Harry convinced me that that would scare the horses.

This is not an exercise book for old girls. It's not an exercise book at all. And it is possible that Harry's First Rule is not our most important piece of advice. But this is where you begin. Do this and all else follows. It really does. Sounds weird, but it's absolutely true. Following this rule, and seeing the early results, spins your head around. It opens you up to seeing the Next Third of your life differently.

Tell you a story. I had a wonderful aunt, Katherine Butler Hathaway, who was a hunchback and a dwarf and who wrote an astonishing book in 1942 called *The Little Locksmith,* about magic and transformation. She believed in magic and courage and iron determination as agents to transform your life. As she, amazingly, transformed hers. She had "an island in the palm of [her] hand," a magic loop in the fate line that she clutched to herself, a magic amulet, all through an appalling and agonizing childhood. And, in her thirties, it worked and her life was utterly transformed. She went off to Paris, wrote books, fell in love (which she had been told was out of the question), married and had an intense if foreshortened life. She died at fifty—in agony, I'm afraid—just as she finished the book. It was an extraordinary, posthumous success.

It is called *The Little Locksmith* because there was a locksmith in Salem, Massachusetts, who came to the house from time to time when Aunt Kitty was a little girl, to silently fix the locks. He was a figure of fascination and dread to her all during the *nine years* when she was literally strapped to a special bed (with a five-pound weight attached to her head), in a long, painful and ultimately fruitless effort to save her. Save her from becoming what the locksmith had always been . . . a hunchback and a dwarf.

You've heard the old line, which she quotes, "Love laughs at locksmiths." Love laughed at my Aunt Kitty for a very long time . . . until she transformed herself. *The Little Locksmith* is a beautiful and compelling book and of course a family treasure. It is still in print; if you read it, the little girls are my sisters and Lurana is my mother. It may explain why we are all such profound believers in magic and transformation. We have seen it.

All right, back to business. *Exercise is magic.* I'm absolutely serious. It gives you the strength, the optimism, the flexibility to do the rest. It is the amulet you squeeze in your palm to change yourself from the apathetic, crippled, and exhausted creature you might otherwise become into something quite different. Someone *transformed.*

This sounds like craziness, but it's not. There is craziness in our lives—that tide, those Darwinian imperatives that have nothing to do with modern life—but exercise is the opposite of crazy. It is the thing you use to drive the craziness away. Think about it again. Here is this nutty tide, right inside your own precious body, that wants you to get old and fat and sick and stupid. Wants you to fall down, talk nonsense, break your hip . . . get the sniffles, get the blues. Wants to sweep you up on the beach, where the gulls and the crabs are waiting to eat your guts. That's what's crazy. Doing something about it is sane. Exercise is sane. Better than sane . . . it's magic.

Some guy—probably a jerk—told me that women, more than men, like the idea of pills, potions, and gadgets to cure all ills. All right, think of exercise as a one-a-day pill. A feel-good pill that ought to be illegal but isn't. You take it every single day, and it makes you feel absolutely great.

Right away. No matter how crappy and self-pitying you felt when you took it. There are no side effects except good ones. And it always, always works. You can pop 'em for years and years and never grow immune, never need to up the dosage to dangerous levels. And if you get addicted—as you almost certainly will—you'll be lucky. How about that?

If you want to be a little more scientific, think of doing exercise as sending a constant "grow" message to override that crazy tide. Think of it as telling your body to get stronger, more limber, functionally younger, in the only language your body understands. Because that is exactly what it does. And it works. It is the only thing that works.

Harry and I are not dopes. We do not think you're going to slap the book down at this point and run out the door to the gym. But we think eventually you'll do exactly that, which is why we are now going to tell you a couple of things that will help get you thinking the right way. In later chapters we're going to tell you exactly what kind of exercise to do, and how much, and how to use your heart monitor, for heaven's sake— more detail than you can bear. But forget that for now. For now we want to set you up so that you at least have a shot at starting what we recognize is a revolutionary regimen . . . a wild change in the way you live your life. Read this next bit on spec. Before long, you may want to take a serious stab at the life we're peddling, and this will be helpful.

Exercise, Mood, and Depression

This next bit is fascinating, if tricky, stuff. The information is preliminary and anecdotal, but there begin to be indications that real exercise can be a *significant* help to some people who are dealing with depression. No one argues that steady, serious exercise doesn't improve your mood, not just in the short term but over time. But the news may be better than that. I backed into this subject when a friend told me that a depressed relative of hers was part of a medical school study of exercise and depression and that exercise seemed to be working. Then, oddly enough, a close friend wrote me a note that same week that looked, at first, like an ordinary "fan letter." Except that she is not an ordinary person and this was not an ordinary letter. It was about depression.

Smart, able, and accomplished, this woman has wrestled with grave depression for all of the twenty-five years that she and her husband and I have been friends. And hers has not been just "I'm-blue-and-not-having-a-nice-time" depression. It's been "I've-got-this-rock-on-my-chest-and-cannot-get-out-of-bed-for-weeks" depression. Serious business. She had tried absolutely everything—therapy, the full panoply of drugs, what have you—and had had a certain amount of luck. But the results were uneven. She was still tormented much of the time and incapacitated some of the time. Then she took up a really serious exercise regimen. After reading *Younger Next Year,* interestingly enough . . . hence the letter. She had been a standout athlete as a girl but had been inactive since she was nineteen, so it was a huge undertaking. (Here's an interesting sidelight: she did not take up one of the normal regimens we suggest. She started hiking the Appalachian Trail. Like a lunatic. It changed her life, and now it's spin class, biking, a whole range of other exercise activity.) Within a couple of months, she had what she and her husband both see as a major turnaround—the best luck she's had with any single approach in twenty-five years of trying. They don't know if it will last, but for now they are talking "miracles."

Incidentally, she has lost twenty pounds and looks

terrific, but it goes way beyond that. To an outside observer, she is simply a different woman. Her husband e-mailed me yesterday to say she had casually asked him that morning if he wanted to do a quick twenty-mile bike loop before church. That is an absolutely astonishing, tear-inducing bit of news. She would no more have suggested that a year ago than she would have suggested that the two of them fly around the house for an hour. A transformation.

Caveat! This is just a story, not news of some cure. If you suffer from medical depression, for God's sake, stay with your doctor, stay with your meds and don't go traipsing after this as if it were some panacea. It is not. This is an anecdote, not "evidence" of anything. My pal still swears by her meds, which brought her to the threshold of what she is doing now. Be cautious.

But here's some great, safe advice. Regardless of how the scientific inquiry turns out, try exercise anyway. It can only help. If it does not "cure" your depression, fine. It will still make you feel a hell of a lot better and it will radically improve your physical health. Think of it as an untested drug that some people *think* may have an effect on depression. The only thing they *know* is that it has no side effects. Except good ones. Gotta love that. So . . . don't drop your meds or whatever your doctor has you doing. But talk to her or to him about exercise. And give it a shot.

Make It Your New Job

We urge you *not* to start gradually. It is far better to make a sharp break with the past and a serious commitment to the future. If you're not working or if you're at or near retirement, we urge you as strongly as we can to make this your new job. Your single most important job. If you're working like crazy—and the kids are still around and retirement is a ways off—think of it as your first priority after work and kids and do the best you can. But remember, as you get older, steady exercise rises on the priority list because the tide is rising, too. The tide has its priorities, and you must have yours. Or you'll be swept away.

There is one thing people learn in their work lives that is enormously useful at this point. They learn to go to work. Without thinking much about it, they learn a skill that children and heiresses do not have. They learn to go to work and do their job. That simple knack is one of the most powerful organizing forces in life, and you have it, etched deep in your conscious and unconscious mind, no matter what kind of work you've done, or whether you've done it in an office or at home. Nice going. Now use it in your new life.

One of the terrific things about the go-to-work, honor-your-commitments habit is that it's a great prioritizer. Work trumps everything except serious illness or family. Daily exercise should be treated the same way. If you're going to have success with this excellent new life, you're going to have to give regular exercise that priority. Which may be hard. Some people have trouble thinking that exercise is "serious." They feel vaguely guilty about it, because it's too much like play. Or self-indulgent. All we can say is, get over it, because that's nuts. Nothing you are doing in the Next Third is as important as daily exercise. As important to you, to Old Fred, to the kids, to the ones who have to take care of you if things go south. If exercise feels like play, great; you're one of the lucky ones. But it's deadly serious, because it will keep you from becoming a pathetic, dependent old fool. You think there's something more important than that? Get over it!

Harry and I are always asked, "Why six days? Why is that so important? What's wrong with three days? Or two? Or one? Isn't anything better than nothing?"

No, you silly twit! It's not better than nothing! Or, in any case, it's so much worse than six days for women over fifty that we don't even want you to think about it. It will sap your strength and drain your resolve. It will put you on the beach. It's six days because it has to be. Don't argue. Please! Actually, it should be seven. The tide is seven, and it's a boa constrictor. People think boa constrictors squeeze, but they don't. They just wrap around you and wait. You let out a breath . . . they take up the slack. Do it again . . . they take up the slack again. Until you're dead. The tide is like that. You relax . . . and it takes up the slack. So, no slacking. You're lucky that only an hour a day works so well.

May I say that I have not reached my seventies without learning a thing or two about human frailty and its corollary, the pathetic excuse. There will be days when, armed with a pathetic excuse, you will insist that you are unable to exercise. Fine. That will happen. But do not conclude that it's time to change Harry's First Rule. It's not. The rule stands. Try to get back in sync with it as soon as possible.

Do not try to get the rule in sync with you. That would be dumb.

Jump-Start Your Life

The best way to get into this new life is to take a deep breath, make a profound resolution, and jump in, full tilt, for life. Do it as dramatically and with as much fanfare as you can muster. Get your partner on board. Tell everyone you know. Open a great bottle of wine. Whatever it takes. Because, let's face it, this is not easy. It's the most important thing you can do, but it's not easy. So improve your chances by making the beginning as big, as joyful, as solemn as you can. Don't decide to "try it for a few days." That won't work. Think about it hard for as long as you need and then jump in for the rest of your life. With ruffles and flourishes.

It's interesting, since most men aren't worrying about such things, but I think women wonder, "Well, what about Fred? Will Fred want to do this with me?" A reasonable question, and it is certainly true that this stuff is more fun (and more likely to succeed) if your partner does it, too. So give him a shot at it.

But don't wait for Fred! He wouldn't have *thought* about waiting for you. And this is that great, come-and-get-it stage in your life when the focus ought to be sharply on what *you* want. You've been deeply trained to wonder and worry all the time about the kids, about the dog . . . about Old Fred. It's deep in your bones now, if it wasn't in your DNA from the beginning. But it is also true, as I mentioned, that for an awful lot of lucky women the grip of that instinct loosens some with menopause. Which, we respectfully submit, is absolutely wonderful. Invite Old Fred to save his life, too. Urge him to join you. But if he won't get up out of the La-Z-Boy, the hell with him. You do it. On your own.

Here's a nice story. I came home just three days before I went to work on this chapter, and there was this attractive woman of about fifty, working in a sleeveless T-shirt, painting the new bookshelves in the living room. I introduced myself, and she said, "Oh, you wrote that book! Your wife lent it to me last week, and I love it. I love the part about how you may have to age but you don't have to *rot.*" She hit the word *rot* hard, as if she meant it. We got to talking,

We're Moving the Middle of the Road

Here's another thing we hear all the time: "Yeah, but you guys are athletes. And this is nothing but another exercise craze. I'm no athlete. And I hate exercise. So this is not for me."

Oh, yes it is. Neither Harry nor I amounted to much as athletes when we were kids. We've gotten into it, thank God, so it's become fun, but that's not the point. The point is that steady exercise is *a coded message to your body*—and your mind—telling you not to turn into a busted-down old crone. Serious exercise, six days a week, is not extreme; it's the middle of the road. They just haven't moved the road yet. That's what we're doing, together. We're moving the road.

Early on, Harry said something that grabbed me: "In twenty years, failure to exercise six days a week will seem as self-destructive as smoking two packs of cigarettes a day." Two packs a day was normal when I was a kid. They finally moved that road, and we're going to move this one. You're going to lead the way.

and she said, "I got separated eight months ago, because my husband's decided to rot. And I'm not going to. I was up nights with that book. I've already lost forty pounds since we split up, and now I'm gonna keep on going." She grinned as if it were Christmas. And showed me her triceps, proud as punch. She was emotionally *big* . . . she was in her fifties and she was getting *big*. I was nuts about her. In her case, it did not make sense to wait for Old Fred.

Okay, with or without Fred, you might think about a

"Jump-Start Vacation"—a trip where exercise is the central activity. For example, take a week off, you and Fred—or a friend if he won't play. The "girls' trip" is a great institution . . . increasingly important at this stage in your life. And a trip like this can be a wonderful annual event. Go on a bike tour in New England. Or Ohio. Or Europe, if you've got the dough. If you've really let yourself go to hell in recent years, you'll have to work out some just to be able to take such a trip. But no matter where you are on the fitness scale, you can probably find a trip that will be right for you.

As you will have begun to sense, one of our little agenda items here is to urge women to accelerate what we think is a natural tendency toward much greater strength and independence in the Next Third. A trip like this—with the girls or not—can be a significant step down that sunny and pleasant road. You'll love it. It will be great for your body. And your mind. And your spirit. Not bad.

And don't think you have to spend a lot of money. You can bike somewhere near home. Or you can rent or borrow a cottage on a lake or the ocean and get a pair of sea kayaks (don't do that one alone) . . . do that every day for four hours or so, and you'll really get a nice jump. Or hike in the Rockies or the Appalachians. Or go to one of the hundreds of cross-country ski houses; they're pretty reasonable and there is no better exercise or fun on earth. Or go to a spa . . . or a "boot camp." The magazines are full of ads for these places. But don't go to one where the emphasis is all herbal wraps, manicures, and touchy-feely talk. There are lots of men and women who want to con you into thinking you can save your immortal soul and your body by humming some mantra or popping a supplement. That's nonsense. Saving souls—and bodies—is hard work. Worthwhile work but hard. Just *do it* and don't give way to feel-good horseshit.

For example, find a spa with serious workouts and diets. Sniff around and find a good one. Then go. And work at it. We're saving souls here.

A downhill skiing trip counts, too. There's a gutsy, brave thing that will work wonders. I have a lot of female pals who

"Do not delay because you do not happen to have a bath . . ."

If it turns out you don't have the money to take a jump-start trip anytime soon, forget about it. Just begin. It's too important to let it slide, and it would be pathetic to use the jump-start thing as an excuse. Worse than letting Fred sideline you.

I came across a marvelous book in the funky 1890s camp where I worked a lot on this project, on a tiny island in Lake Winnipesaukee up in New Hampshire. Written in 1905, it's a Danish exercise book that was purchased by one of my grandfathers—an English professor by trade, but a bit of an exercise buff by inclination. It's terrific stuff, heavy on Indian clubs, photos of the mustachioed Dane in his undies, elaborate advice about the tremendous importance of baths. For some reason, the author was adamant about baths. Toward the end, he makes this excellent point: "Whether you are weak or strong, young or old, I advise you to begin with these exercises at once and rather today than tomorrow. . . . Do not delay because you do not happen to have a bath; you can buy one when convenient, and in the meantime be content to rub yourself all over with a wet towel."

So don't fool around just because you don't have the time or dough for a fancy bike trip. Just rub yourself all over with a wet towel and get going.

now do women's ski trips routinely and thrive on them. With the girls or with Fred or alone, go out west or up to New England and ski for a week. Or two weeks, if you can. A month, if you can afford it. That's what I did when I turned forty, a thousand years ago. Took a whole month off from a frantic law practice and learned to ski, almost from scratch, at an age when most people are quitting. A little extreme, but it gave me one of my core pleasures, especially in retirement.

Incidentally, there's a lot of talk about skiing in this book, just because Harry and I both happen to do it. Don't be put off if you don't ski; most people don't. It's just a metaphor for vigorous sport. Anyhow, skiing counts, and you can learn it in a few weeks, whether you're forty or sixty. (You can learn cross-country in a day.) Try it. It'll be fun, and it will put your feet on a path you can travel with delight for the rest of your life.

One last thought about jump-start trips. These are the prelims, not the main event. The main event is the rest of your life. Take this book along. You and Fred, if you can get him into it, can read to each other back in that cozy room at night. And swap ideas about what you're going to do when you get home. Plan. Scheme. Write stuff down. Start a notebook. Figure out which one of you is the planner and which the inspirer ... divide up the tasks.

But get ready for what you're going to do when you get home. That's the point.

Join a Gym

A lot of people fight me on this one, but you have to join a gym. Though women seem to be more open to it than men, thank God, a lot of 'em hate the idea, too. Get over it. It doesn't have to be fancy—the Y is fine—but there's a structure to having a gym that nothing else provides. If you think outdoor exercise is ten times as pleasant and healthy as indoor exercise, fine. Join a gym anyway. You need it for rainy days. For winter. For the group classes and the weight machines. And to find the brute who's going to show you how to do weight training. You need a place to go, every day. You may do non-gym things a lot of days . . . bike, run or ski. But there will be days when, no matter what, you will just have to drag your butt out of bed and go to the gym.

One of the great things about the gym is that you do stuff with other people. Women, for the most part, have a natural taste for that. Which is perhaps why more women than men join them. Whatever, but the instinct is sound. It's good to do this stuff in packs. You're more apt to keep it up, more likely to *go for it,* more likely to succeed. That's what working in packs has been all about since the dawn of history: it's more fun and it works better.

If you live in a small town with one gym, go there. But if you live in New York or Chicago or L.A., with a gym every few blocks, consider your choice carefully. First consideration? Probably money. Some of these places can cost an absolute fortune; if you don't have it, don't spend it. The simple places almost always have everything you need. Which is to say, a few aerobics machines and some weights, whether stationary or free, and an adequate, clean space in which to use them.

But remember, this is a priority in your life now. Bear that in mind when you decide what you can afford. Don't pick someplace nasty just because it's cheap and then quit because you don't want to walk on the locker room floor. That is false economy. Proximity counts for a lot, too. Getting there is more than half the battle. But it isn't the only thing. These places have their own peculiar ethos, their own atmosphere, just like companies or colleges, and it's important to find one that feels right. There's a beautiful gym almost on our block in New York, but for some reason it draws a petulant and depressed crowd. Better to walk a few blocks and go someplace fun. My general preference is for a place where there's a mix of ages and interests, with a slight emphasis on younger and cute. That's just me. You decide.

Hilary and I joined a place a while ago where everyone else is in their twenties or thirties. The facilities are remarkable, but let me tell you, even though I'm in decent shape these days, I still felt odd for a while, down in the locker room with all those young hardbodies. There's an edginess among young athletes that isn't relaxing if you're deep into your middle years. I've gotten over it, but I still think the ideal gym for women and men in their fifties and sixties is a place with a decent number of young people and some people one's own age. Not so easy for me, because I'm so incredibly old. I hope this book will draw out gangs of people; I need the company.

But if you look so horrible that you can't bear to go to a place with lots of kids and gym rats . . . that's no excuse! There are plenty of places that cater to older people, and even more that do one-on-one training, if you have that kind of dough. Me, I'd get over it and go to a regular gym, but tastes vary. The big thing is to *go*.

We'll talk more about trainers in a later chapter, but get a trainer, too. Find one whom you like but who's a real motivator. My friend Tina says that's the key. She and her husband found a woman in Colorado who's a former triathlete: "tough, no-nonsense, and fun. I *want* to work hard for her and I like her praise. Every woman should have one in her life . . . a friend, a trainer, *anyone* who makes you want to *work* at it." As Tina points out, too many of her pals slack off after menopause or retirement, as if they should take it easy on themselves now that they're frail or something. Which is precisely what *not to do*. Don't just "do the tread-mill" for fifteen minutes or take a walk and call it exercise. Go for it, for God's sake. That's what works. And don't kid yourself, *please*.

But if you're in the early stages, don't think you have to go nuts or not at all. You have to start somewhere. Maybe you'd like a women-only place. My youngest sister, Petie, who's eighty, beautiful, and about as much fun as anyone you've ever met, swears by a place like that.

Even more important than the age mix or sex mix at a gym is its spirit. Try to figure out if the trainers and staff are cordial to one another . . . say hello and stuff like that. The place should feel good. It's bad enough to have to go at all; it's impossible if the people aren't pleasant. Of course, you also want a place that has the right activities. Spin class, yoga, swimming, or whatever gets you going.

So shop carefully, if you have a choice. And remember, a lot of these places will insist on your signing up for a num-ber of potentially expensive months, so read the fine print. Special point for retired folk: If you're going to be away for months at a time, be sure to check the gym's policies for suspending your membership. There are some ripoffs in this area. Last thing: Be sure the joint is clean and the towels are decent. Gotta have good towels.

Excellent Tip: Try a Class

Classes or group activities are great motivators. My own favorite, which I don't recommend for everyone, is spin class. This is a group of crazies on stationary bikes who race to loud music and manic exhortations from a class leader. Lots of women love it, oddly enough. Not for you? What about step class or aerobic dance? Take your pick. One of the best, especially for women, is yoga class. There's something about it that speaks to women more than to most men. But it's superb exercise if you don't get tangled up with some young yoga nazi who is clueless about being over forty and may cause you injury. But good, temperate yoga is great. Give it a shot. Some of the most beautiful bodies you'll ever see—men or women, young or old—are the ones you'll see in yoga class. This stuff obviously works. Pilates is good, too. Some of our closest (and fittest) pals are Pilates nuts.

Whether yoga, Pilates, or something else, try some kind of class or group activity. First, you're more likely to go because there's a set time for class and that creates a certain discipline. Second, you're far less likely to dog it once you get there. (It's way too easy to dog it when you're alone.) So look around. What you want eventually, it seems to me, is a solid exercise habit, supported by a structured class, at a pleasant gym or yoga studio.

Second Tip: Pick a Time to Go to Work

One of the luxuries of my life and not having a regular job is that I can do this stuff whenever I like. But you know what? Whether you're working or not, it's a lot easier to exercise if you have a regular time. A time when you change your duds and head off to the gym. Or the track. Or the water. Same time every day, so there's not a new decision every time. For me, early in the morning is best. I can't sleep anyway, because I'm an old person.

At six o'clock, I get out of bed and go straight off to class. Try it.

Harry can work out at the end of the day but not early in the morning. But give him credit—in a very busy life he is pretty regular. Noontime works for some. Instead of that big, fat lunch. But no matter what, pick a time. The only real trick is to have a schedule and a habit. No one has the character to make the fresh decision every day to go to the gym. Go on "automatic" or you'll quit.

My Third Tip: Tap into a Passion

f you're lucky enough to have an athletic passion (most people don't), by all means tap into it as a support for your exercise program. If it's an aerobic sport, you can make it your core activity. Running, cross-country, swimming . . . just do it. But even if it's not an aerobic sport, you can build your routine around it to give it focus and make it more fun. Don't miss a single chance to make this fun and close to what you enjoy.

Personally, I have the great good luck to enjoy a number of sports these days (ironic, when you think what a mess of an athlete I was as a kid). I love to ski, bike, sail, row, windsurf, and God knows what. When I sit on the hateful quadriceps machine, in pain, pushing that stack of weights up the ramp, I think of skiing the bumps at Aspen or the steep pitches at Stowe. Sure, this is hell, but the payoff will be on those magic hills. And it will be worth anything. Pleasantly enough, a serious program of aerobics and weight training will absolutely revolutionize your ability to do other sports. The thought of that can keep you going.

Same with the biking. I sit in that darkened room full

of spinning men and women, blazing with teenage music that makes my head hurt, pumping my heart out. And in my mind's eye I am biking along a pine-scented road, between stone walls up at the lake in northern New Hampshire, getting ready to climb a mighty hill. It doubles my pleasure. It keeps me going. Tap into your passion, if you have one. It helps.

So, you're asking, how serious is this serious exercise? Suffice it to say for now that you have to exercise hard enough, after the first days, to take up the slack. You will want to sweat. You will want to strain. You will want to feel your body getting traction. Not a casual walk . . . not a round of golf . . . not an hour in the garden. Don't worry about the details for now. Just know that you have to put a strain on the lines of your life so that your anchor will hold in that tide we talked about.

The Best People Hate Exercise

Some of the people Harry and I like best hate exercise. People who live a life of the mind. Bookish folk . . . lunatic professionals . . . artists . . . teachers . . . gardeners. People like my sisters who love to eat and drink and talk. And who read in the privacy of their very own homes. They hate sports, hate exercise, hated school because of sports and exercise. And hate people like us who try to tell them how great it all is. They are never going to change.

Well, yes they are, if they can hear a couple of things. Like: There is no "life of the mind." Mind and body really are one, just as the dear old Romans said. A sound mind in a healthy body or however the old wheeze goes.

Besides which, from a Darwinian perspective, you most

assuredly are an athlete. Never mind that you were a skinny little thing (or not!) in junior high school. Never mind that your hand-eye coordination was a painful joke and that you'd rather read or shop than almost anything. You were still designed to hunt. In packs. You ignore that basic fact at your peril. You may not like exercise, but do it anyway. For your heart, for your mind, for your immortal soul. And for the rest of us. We want your company.

CHAPTER FIVE

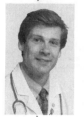

The Biology of Growth and Decay: Things That Go Bump in the Night

Biologically, there is no such thing as retirement, or even aging. There is only growth or decay, and your body looks to you to choose between them. So, this is the place where we take you backstage to look at that process—at the actual mechanisms of the new biology that has forever changed our thinking about aging. If things get mildly complicated, just remember that we are always talking about growth and decay. Come back to that simple point, and the details will fall into place.

First off, you may think your body is a "thing," like the Empire State Building or a car, but it's not. It's made of meat, sinew, and fat and many other parts that break down over time and have to be constantly renewed. The muscle cells in your thigh are completely replaced, one at a time, day and night, about every four months. Brand-new muscles, three times a year. The solid leg you've stood on so securely since childhood is mostly new since last summer. Your blood cells are replaced every three months, your platelets every ten days, your bones every couple of years. Your taste buds are replaced every day.

This is not a passive process. You don't wait for a part to wear out or break. You destroy it at the end of its planned life span and replace it with a new one.

Stop for a moment, because that's a whole new concept. Biologists now believe that most cells in your body are designed to fall apart after relatively short life spans, partly to let you adapt to new circumstances and partly because older cells tend to get cancer, making immortal cells not such a great idea. The net result is that you are actively destroying large parts of your body all the time. On purpose! Throwing out truckloads of perfectly good body to make room for new growth. Your spleen's major job is to destroy your blood cells. You have armies of special cells whose only job is to dissolve your bones so other cells can build them up again, like pruning in autumn to make room for growth in the spring.

The trick, of course, is to grow more than you throw out, and this is where exercise comes in. It turns out that your muscles control the chemistry of growth throughout your whole body. The nerve impulse to contract a muscle also sends a tiny signal to build it up, creating a moment-to-moment chemical balance between growth and decay within the muscle. Those two same signals are then sent to the rest of your body. If enough of the growth signals are sent at once, they overwhelm the signals to atrophy, and your body turns on the machinery to build up the muscles, heart, capillaries, tendons, bones, joints, coordination, and so on.

So exercise is the master signaler, the agent that sets hundreds of chemical cascades in motion each time you get on that treadmill and start to sweat. It's what sets off the cycles of strengthening and repair within the muscles and joints. It's the foundation of positive brain chemistry. And it leads directly to the younger life we are promising, with its heightened immune system; its better sleep; its weight loss, insulin regulation and fat burning; its improved sexuality; its dramatic resistance to heart attack, stroke, hypertension, Alzheimer's disease, arthritis, osteoporosis, diabetes, high cholesterol, and depression. All that comes from exercise. But let your muscles sit idle and decay takes over again.

Exercise Is Healthy Stress

When you exercise fairly hard, you stress your muscles. You drain them of energy stores, and you actually injure them slightly. The stress of exercise is good, because it tears you down to build you back up a little stronger. You wear out little bits that need to be replaced after each use, requiring lots of fine tuning and minor repairs. This type of injury is called *adaptive microtrauma,* and it's critical to your growth and health. It's the signal to your body that it needs to repair the damage — and then some. It needs to make the muscle just a little stronger. To store just a little more energy for tomorrow. To build a few more tiny blood vessels inside the muscle. To get a little younger.

The way it works is that enzymes and proteins from the exercised muscle leak into your bloodstream, where they start a powerful chain reaction of inflammation. White blood cells are drawn to the scene to begin the demolition process. These cells are the wrecking crew, the team brought in when you start renovating your house. The guys with sledgehammers, crowbars, wheelbarrows, and dumpsters who tear down the old plaster and rip the walls apart to take your house back to its healthy foundation.

Since white blood cells are part of your immune system, you may think they exist primarily to protect you against infection and cancer. Well, that's part of the story, but your immune system's other job is to demolish big chunks of your body every day so you can grow. White cells are killer cells programmed to destroy bacteria, viruses, and cancer cells by dissolving them in a toxic, caustic brew, like paint stripper. But they also use these same mechanisms to demolish the millions of cells that die their natural deaths every day.

With the short-term stress of exercise, this works well. Once the demolition is done, growth and repair take over. In a healthy body, the demolition actually triggers the repair process. That's a key point. The inflammation itself automatically triggers repair. Decay triggers growth. When the demolition is done, the plumber, electrician, and master carpenter come in. New pipes, new wires, and new walls go in where needed. The old stuff that's worth saving, the infrastructure and the detail work, is polished and sanded back to its original state.

Just remember two things. One: Decay triggers growth. And two: Exercise turns on inflammation, which automatically turns on repair. There's a carefully timed delay to give inflammation time to do its work, and that's when the demolition crews pick up the phone and call the carpenters directly: "We're all done, it's your turn now." Inflammation and repair, demolition and renovation, decay and growth— they're all ineluctably joined together in an automatic cycle.

The challenge for your body is to regulate inflammation in order to keep decay in a healthy balance with growth. If the stress is short-term, the decay triggers further growth. But if the stress is chronic, decay remains firmly in charge.

Designed in our most primitive ancestors, way before brains were around to run the show, it's a simple arrangement that works beautifully out there in nature. The right amount of inflammation automatically produces growth. But too little, or too much, turns off growth . . . leaving only the background decay.

A Closer Look: The Messengers of Change

You have two information superhighways in your body: your nervous system and your circulatory system. It may come as a surprise that your bloodstream carries information, but it does. Plasma, in particular, is a complex, living river of thousands of chemicals and proteins signaling and controlling virtually every aspect of your body: growth, decay, mood, immune function, cancer surveillance, fat metabolism, sexuality, joint health . . . and it all operates through inflammation and repair.

Here's how it works: When your cells sense damage, say, from exercise, they automatically release chemicals to start the inflammation—to set the stage for repair. A few of those chemicals leak into the bloodstream, and those few molecules draw white blood cells to the injured area the way blood in the water draws sharks from miles around. After the inflammatory cycle has done its demolition work, the white blood cells go away, leaving behind a clean, fresh surface so the construction crews can get to work on the growth part of the cycle.

This chemistry is at the core of the new science we talk about in this book, so let's go into more detail here. The proteins that control inflammation are called cytokines, and they regulate every aspect of your biology. Cytokines are messenger molecules. They turn on or off virtually all the metabolic pathways in each tissue and cell in your body. Each tissue has its own specific cytokines, but they cross-react to coordinate growth or decay throughout your body.

Hundreds, perhaps even thousands, of cytokines are at work in your body, regulating growth and decay down to the most microscopic level. For the purposes of this book, however, imagine that there are only two cytokines in your whole body—two master chemicals that control growth or decay in every tissue and cell. It's a massive simplification, but surprisingly accurate. We'll call these chemicals cytokine-6 and cytokine-10, after the specific cytokines called interleukins 6 and 10 that control growth and decay in your muscles.

Cytokine-6, or C-6 for short, is the master chemical for inflammation (decay), and cytokine-10, or C-10, is the master chemical for repair and growth. C-6 is produced in both the muscle cells and the bloodstream in response to exercise, and C-10 is produced in response to C-6. This is your body's brilliant mechanism for coupling decay and growth. C-6 actually *triggers* the production of C-10. Decay triggers growth.

Now let's take a fresh look at the power of exercise to change your whole body in light of this new information. You have 660 muscles, which make up almost 50 percent of your lean body weight. Those 60 or 70 pounds of muscle are a massive reservoir of C-6 and C-10, a massive reservoir of potential youth if you do your part. Exercise triggers repair, renewal, and growth by producing C-6. All forms of aerobic exercise produce C-6 in logarithmic proportion to both the duration and the intensity of exercise. In marathon runners, the level of C-6 rises a hundredfold by the end of the race. It is an *automatic* measure of how much exercise you do, how much inflammation you cause, and how much growth you will experience. In other words, how much C-10 will be released.

C-10 is key, because growth is the magic you are after. But growth is too complicated for neat description. Demolition is easy to describe, because, while it's important that you don't hit a gas main or anything, it's basically sledgehammers and dumpsters. But growth is blueprints, and master carpenters, and electricians, all controlled by C-10. We're not going to go into the fine details of how the cytokines actually do this because, frankly, it's too complex to fit in this book, but you will see C-10's effect as you build your stronger, healthier, younger body. The most important thing to understand about C-10 is that it is automatically turned on by C-6. Inflammation controls growth; that's the critical concept. C-6 peaks right after the marathon and turns on the cytokines that control repair, which peak an hour or so later and which stay at higher levels for hours after exercise, repairing your body.

At rest, only 20 percent of your blood flow moves through your muscles; in a trained athlete, that rises, with exercise, to 80 percent. Picture it: torrents, rivers of blood flooding through your muscles with exercise, picking up the cytokines, the messages of inflammation and repair, of growth and healing, and taking them to every corner of your body. From the top of your head to the tips of your toes. From your heart to your hands, fingers to knees. Every joint, every bone, every organ, every tiny part of your magnificent brain gets its bath of C-6, and then the wonderful, rejuvenating C-10 each time you sweat. That's the right balance, good decay triggering growth.

Play the Music

This is important: Not all decay is good, and cytokine-6 does not always trigger the production of cytokine-10. When we are sedentary, the devil does indeed find work for idle muscles. There is a steady slow drip of inflammation, *but not enough to turn on C-10*. That explosion of growth comes only with the surge of C-6 you get with exercise.

Remember the old days, when you fell asleep with the stereo on and woke in the middle of the night to the needle going round and round at the end of the record? That faint *hiss-bump, hiss-bump,* filling the background silence? Almost but not quite inaudible? That's the C-6, playing in the background. The steady trickle of C-6 to every nook and cranny of your body all the time. No C-10, no repair, no growth, just decay. *Hiss-bump* in the middle of the night.

Another depressing point: You secrete more background C-6 as you age, no matter what you do. Dust in the grooves. Sad, but true. The tide sets against you. *Hiss-bump, hiss-bump* in the middle of the night.

Your brain is part of this, too. Chronic emotional stress also produces a trickle of background C-6. Loneliness, boredom, apathy, worry—*hiss-bump.* You can change this by being fit, or filling up your life, or both. Both is better by a lot, but let's stick with exercise for the moment. When you exercise, you get a high enough level of C-6 to trigger the C-10. You get to play the music of growth. It's not hard, you just need to become a daily C-10 woman. Exercise every day, at least enough to sweat, and you'll be fit, guaranteed. You'll be able to hike up a mountain at eighty, dance all night at seventy, and outrun your kids at fifty, but more than that, you'll be healthy, more relaxed, more optimistic. Why?

Because C-10 will automatically flood your body an hour after exercise like a sprinkler coming on at sundown.

C-6 and C-10 are shorthand for chemical cascades involving hundreds of proteins in a dance of such complexity that we are only beginning to understand the details. Cell biologists will also tell you that inflammation is just cleaning up the debris caused by programmed erosion. Since the fine details of the mechanisms that regulate this may take fifty years to understand fully, we've used C-6 and C-10 as metaphors for the broader concept.

Stress on the Savannah

Stress, either physical or emotional, triggers a flood of fight-or-flight chemicals from your automatic, primal brain. When the lioness jumps out from behind the bush (yes, it's usually a lioness that's doing the heavy lifting), adrenaline floods your bloodstream and, through it, every corner of your body. The adrenaline triggers every member of the C-6 family and hundreds of other chemicals, too, in a surge that changes the activity and biology of virtually every organ and muscle. Two things happen. Your emergency powers—physical strength, visual acuity and mental focus—jump to their maximum intensity. The more interesting phenomenon is that all nonessential powers shut down to let your body focus on the danger. Your stomach, intestines, and kidneys shut down. The liver stops cleaning your blood and dumps its sugar reserves straight into your bloodstream to give you that extra edge. Your immune system stops all background surveillance activity (say, for cancer cells) and gets ready to deal with the impending massive trauma. Your brain abandons long-term thinking and the development of long-term memory or higher cognitive function and focuses exclusively on the present. All muscle construction stops, bone construction stops, blood vessel construction stops, blood vessel repair stops. In short, in life-or-death situations, every scrap of energy and effort swings from long-term to immediate, from infrastructure to survival.

In nature, the bounce-back from this kind of stress is more vigorous than the decay was. (In other words, the surge of C-6 triggers a bigger surge of C-10.) So you grow a little stronger, a little faster, a little smarter, a little more alert.

In nature, life-or-death situations last only a few seconds. The lioness either catches the antelope in a frenetic sprint or fails in the attempt. After thirty seconds of effort, the antelope is home free or dead. It doesn't matter whether you're the lioness or the antelope in that scenario—the chemistry is the same—but think of yourself as the antelope for a moment. As long as you got away, that was good stress. The shock told your body that there were predators, and that it was important to stay fast and strong, so when the adrenaline went away, and your body turned back to growth and repair, it did so with a renewed vigor and purpose. The same holds true for the lioness. She may charge the antelope herd ten times a day, and go hungry more days than not, but the adrenaline of a failed charge tells her body that it needs to grow faster and stronger.

Our bodies *like* that. They crave the bursts of speed, the long trots to new grazing, the foraging, the roaming. Lots of alert but low-stress time, punctuated by bursts of excitement, and with a little danger thrown in. It's why we all crave a little bit of excitement. Daily variety. Adrenaline and C-10, perfect together.

But this positive message—grow a little better, a little stronger—depends on *daily* swings in chemistry. There is a chemistry of foraging and grazing, a chemistry of hunting, a chemistry of escape or capture. These are *daily* chemistries, the daily rhythms of life, and the messages are cumulative. Day in and day out, the messages accumulate, and every day that C-10 predominates, you grow.

Now we're ready to look at stress in our modern "advanced" lives. We have given up on swings in daily chemistry. No exercise, 70-degree climate control, too much to eat day in and day out, artificial light, but especially no exercise. So what are you left with? Endless carpooling followed by equally endless commuting. Stress at work, stress at home. No time for exercise, no time to sit down and talk, or watch the sun set. We don't go back to foraging anymore, we just run from the lioness over and over again, and that creates a novel, modern chemistry of chronic stress.

Animals are rarely hunted into chronic stress. Changes in the environment do that . . . changes like drought, famine, or winter with chronic C-6 and little C-10. And the stress of modern life sends those same steady signals for decay. Indeed, the levels of key chemicals found in our bodies today, such as cortisol, adrenaline, and testosterone, are similar to those found in people who suffer starvation, depression, war, domestic abuse, post-traumatic stress disorder, chronic illness, and other conditions where the *environment* is dangerous, or perceived to be dangerous, over long periods of time.

With the chronic stress of modern life, the chemistry of inflammation persists but the renovation never gets started. Decay becomes a career path for your body, and your blood itself becomes an inflammatory, caustic stew of C-6, carrying decay throughout. Not chronic stress as in two months of drought or four months of winter, but chronic stress as in decades of emotional strain, decades of being sedentary and overweight, decades of living in isolation. The tide is set against you. *Hiss-bump, hiss-bump* in the middle of the night, forever.

You can control the cycle. Commuting, loneliness, emotional stress, not enough sleep, apathy, too much alcohol, and TV all trigger the inflammatory part of the cycle. But daily exercise, joy, play, engagement, challenge, and closeness all trigger the crucial repair. And that's why the fittest women have one-fifth the mortality rate of the most sedentary women.

Face the Facts: How Women Die

magine that you're sitting in a restaurant and someone at the table next to you collapses on the floor with a heart attack. You call 911 and immediately start CPR, but in vain. The paramedics cover the body with a tablecloth, and you drive home silently, thinking of the suddenness of it all.

In your mind, reading that paragraph, did you picture the victim as a man or a woman? Most people picture a man, but statistically it was a woman who collapsed and died at the next table, because heart disease kills more women than men. Heart disease, for all the images of the guy clutching his chest, is a woman's disease.

We all have our secret dreads, the illnesses we fear on a visceral level. Many women fear breast cancer the most, followed by ovarian cancer. But the number one killer of women, *by a huge margin,* is heart disease. Fear of specific illnesses is universal, based on our individual life experiences, but it's important to plan—and live—your life based on what is *most* likely to kill you, rather than on what you're most afraid of.

More women die of heart disease each year than of *all* cancers combined. *Ten times* as many women die of heart disease as breast cancer. In fact, cardiovascular diseases (heart disease and stroke) kill more women than the next *seven* causes of death combined.

For reasons that are still unclear, women are relatively protected from cardiovascular disease before menopause, but catch up quickly and then surpass men in the decade after menopause. Two-thirds of strokes happen in women. *Hiss-bump.* And that two-thirds number keeps on rolling. Two-thirds of women have no warning symptoms before their first heart attack. Two-thirds of women never recover full function after a heart attack. Two-thirds of women who survive strokes suffer significant disability for the rest of their lives.

But the extraordinarily good news is that most cardio-vascular disease is *preventable.* The number varies with different researchers, but 70 to 80 percent of heart attacks and strokes are caused by *lifestyle.* By the long-term sum of the choices we make every day. Which means that making different choices—starting with exercise—will change your life.

Researchers gave stress tests to 3,000 women to see how fit they were, and then followed the women for an average of eight years. Over that time, the most sedentary women were *five times more likely to die* than the fittest women. The progression was stepwise, so each rung up the fitness ladder put women a corresponding rung up on the survival ladder, with the death rate being reduced for cardiovascular disease *and* for cancer. Exercise both reduces the risk and increases survival for breast cancer, colon cancer, ovarian cancer, and uterine cancer. And not by small numbers. The increased survival for breast cancer, for instance, has been as much as 50 percent in some studies. So be sure to get your mammogram, but keep in mind that showing up at the gym (and continuing to show up) is *ten times* more likely to save your life, partly by reducing the risk of breast and other cancers, but mostly because, contrary to the image we have in our heads, it is cardiovascular disease that kills women.

It's All About Circulation

About sixty million Americans have some form of cardiovascular disease. Most of them don't know it, because it's preclinical, but it's there. That's the vast majority of American women over fifty. It's been the leading cause of death every year since 1918, even during World War II. Being sedentary is formally classified as a major cardiovascular risk factor, increasing risk more than smoking or high cholesterol. Vigorous exercise, the real thing, is the most powerful way we know of cutting down your risk of heart attack.

Let's talk about the biology of heart attacks for a moment. It has almost nothing to do with our hearts, and everything to do with our circulation. Hearts don't fail; coronary arteries do. Arteries get blocked, they clot, and we die.

Our arteries are the one part of our body exposed to the cytokine-6 in our blood all the time. In nature, arteries never wear out; they never harden, they never clog, and they never burst. In modern life, however, our arteries are exposed to the chemistry of inflammation, of decay, for decades on end—a steady bath of C-6 for fifty years.

In response, they become weak and inflamed. White blood cells invade the walls of our blood vessels and sit inside, pulling down the walls, ripping out the old plumbing and, as an afterthought, absorbing cholesterol. That's what kills you, the afterthought. The absorbing cholesterol part.

Biologically, the cholesterol buildup is a mere footnote, a bizarre accident. Chronic stress alone won't kill you. It will melt big chunks of you, but it won't kill you. We, however, have taken it a step further, because we've coupled chronic stress with cheese and butter and red meat and sugar and chips and French fries. In nature, chronic stress is always coupled with starvation. The blood is caustic, but carries no fat. In the wild, there is no cholesterol to be absorbed. You are under chronic stress because you are starving to death.

C-6 draws white blood cells right into the walls of your arteries, and when you combine chronic stress with our rotten diet, the white cells turn into vacuum cleaners sucking fat out of your bloodstream. They grow to obscene proportions. They absorb so much fat that the actual cellular machinery of your arterial walls becomes invisible, buried under a mountain of goop. We don't even call them white blood cells anymore; we call them foam cells. In a renovation project run amok, the walls of your blood vessels fill up with all the junk of random demolition, held fast in a glue of fat and cholesterol. Over decades, this turns into the stuff called plaque, and plaque kills at least half of us.

Now let's talk about your heart. Your heart pumps blood out through a huge pipe, about an inch in diameter, called the aorta. The pumping has nothing to do with heart attacks. Your heart is also a muscle, which needs its own blood supply. That's where heart attacks happen: in the blood supply to your heart muscle, not in the rivers of blood it pumps out to your body. Blood comes into the heart muscle through two little arteries that come off the aorta. These arteries have even tinier branches, each about the size of a single strand of hollow spaghetti, that bring blood to your heart muscle. Shut off one of those spaghetti strands, and a piece of your heart muscle dies. You've had a heart attack. Shut it off high up, and it's a massive heart attack; you either die, or live as what we call a cardiac cripple.

Biologically, your heart is a *simple* piece of machinery: four chambers, four valves, and a little pacemaker. That's it, the whole thing. It's not the engine; it's just the fuel pump. $39.95 plus installation. It was perfected aeons ago, and it hasn't needed any refinement since. If your immune system didn't reject foreign tissue, we could replace yours with a dog, cow, deer, or baboon heart tomorrow. For the average sedentary American, a cocker spaniel's heart would proba-bly be big enough.

So what does exercise do for the heart? The answer is, not much. But it does wonders for your circulation. And it's your circulation that can kill you.

The Athletic Heart

Your heart will beat roughly four billion times over your life without a break. Not one minute of rest or recovery. You start out with your maximum car-diac capacity, and it's there waiting for you your whole life. It's your circulatory capacity—the ability to get blood and oxygen deep into your muscles—that changes dramati-cally. Your heart muscle is still virtually perfect today, a few billion beats down your life's road, despite your sins. But those small arteries are not. Even the arteries of "healthy" fifty-year-old women are coated with plaque that looks just like the topping on a cheese pizza. Medical students invariably swear off pizza after their first autopsy . . . for about a month.

Let's assume that you don't have anything about to pop right now, but let's also assume, without waiting for your autopsy, that your arteries have their share of pizza topping, a slight, subclinical blockage. Your stress test will be normal, but you won't be able to send quite enough blood to every part of the heart muscle that needs it. Nothing dramatic here, not true heart disease yet, just slightly less blood flow than the heart needs. Steady, low-grade secretion of C-6, but no C-10, and the plaque grows slowly larger. Pizza topping at autopsy, *hiss-bump* in the middle of the night.

If you ever have occasion to watch your own angiogram, you'll be astounded at how boundingly athletic your heart is. When it's full of blood, at the beginning of a beat, it's the size of a small grapefruit. With each beat, it collapses violently down to the size of your fist. The coronary arteries, those little strands of spaghetti, are embedded on the outer surface of your heart, so they go along for the ride. They are coiled, twisted and kinked into half their original length, and then snapped back to full stretch about eighty times a minute. And this happens four billion times over your life.

The arteries are remarkably flexible and robust, but their walls become brittle as cholesterol plaque grows and stiffens over time. ("Hardening of the arteries" is a literal term.) At some point, as the blockages get larger and stiffer, one of the cholesterol plaques in the artery cracks. It's just a microscopic little nick on the inner wall of the artery, like the nick on your ankle bone from shaving with a blade that's past its prime. But it's still a nick, a tiny cut, and a little ooze of blood and rancid, inflammatory cholesterol leaks into your bloodstream from inside the plaque. The funny thing is that even though it's the inside wall of an artery, it's still a cut and your body thinks it has to stop the bleeding, so a clot forms right in the middle of your bloodstream. The clot grows to fill up the spaghetti strand, the blood flow to that part of your heart muscle stops, and you have a heart attack. Decades of toxic lifestyle have caught up with you, literally in a heartbeat. That piece of your heart muscle dies within a few hours. The more inflamed your blood, the more the plaque is likely to crack and the bigger the clot is likely to be.

Strokes happen the same way, but since the clots form in the wall of the large carotid artery to your brain rather than the small arteries to your heart, they don't block it off at that point. Instead, a piece of the clot breaks off and floats up into your brain until it reaches an artery small enough to plug. That part of your brain dies, and that's a stroke.

There are two ways out of this deadly situation. The first is to starve the plaque of cholesterol with diet or medication. The inflammation remains, but it's much less deadly. You get old and weak, but you aren't nearly as likely to die.

The second escape route is to change the biology from inflammation to repair. Either exercise or joyful living will do it, but they work best together. This is the exercise chapter, but remember this biology when we start talking about how you live. Remember always that exercise and mood share the same chemistry. They work on each other and through each other. Exercise has been shown to fight depression, anxiety, and insomnia. The "runner's high" is real, and it's both physical and mental. The chemicals of mood, arousal, excitement, fear, anxiety, optimism, lust, and challenge are dumped into the bloodstream from the brain above, and the chemicals of local inflammation and repair are dumped into your bloodstream from the muscles below.

Calling Off the Double Whammy

Overall mortality falls with exercise. That is not a surprise when you consider that it's wounded blood vessels that kill you and that exercise heals wounded blood vessels. Blood vessels go to every corner of your body, and every one of them shares the chemical bath of inflammation or repair. Plaque in the arteries to your brain: stroke and dementia. Your kidneys: hypertension and, worst case, dialysis. Your retina: blindness. And the list goes on. None of this is hyperbole; it's modern aging, and it's getting worse, not better. Of course, genetics and things like smoking and diabetes can accelerate the process, but underneath is the double whammy of sedentary, stressful lifestyle and dietary fat. They are the real killers.

Exercise changes all this because if, and only if, you exercise regularly, the chemistry of your blood changes. The chronic inflammatory signals of sedentary life get replaced by signals to grow, to heal, to recover. C-6 gives way to C-10. Remember, half your body is muscle, releasing floods of C-10 into your blood for hours after exercising, and your blood goes everywhere.

That's the biology of growth or decay. Heart attack gives way to health, death to life. And the bottom line? Exercise reverses the chemistry of decay. You swim against the tide.

CHAPTER SIX

Life Is an Endurance Event: Train for It

M an! C-6 and C-10, the Weird Sisters of growth and decay, coursing through your body, doing their mysterious work. Idleness as a powerful signal to decay ... yikes! Exercise as the one great signal to grow ... to live well. Wow.

All right, with this surprising knowledge in your brainpan, you're ready to start thinking about Harry's Second Rule, which goes like this: *Do serious aerobic exercise four days a week for the rest of your life.* The first rule still applies, of course. You still have to exercise six days a week. It's just that four of the six have to be devoted to aerobic exercise, no matter what. (We'll talk later about strength training on the other days.) Aerobic exercise, as you doubtless know, is the steady exercise that gets your heart rate up and keeps it up: biking, jogging, hitting the treadmill, speed walking, and the like. It does not include doubles tennis and golf—wonderful sports and wonderful for you, but not aerobic.

We're talking about steady, endurance activity that elevates your heart rate and keeps it elevated.

Eventually, most of you will be doing four days a week of aerobic training (at different levels) and two days of strength (or weight) training. But for the first few weeks or months it's going to be six days a week of aerobics. Most of that will be at fairly low levels, where you're sweating but can still talk with comparative ease. This is what we call "long and slow" aerobics, during which your heart will be beating at 60 to 65 percent of your maximum heart rate. (Don't worry about the details now . . . just take it easy.)

The reason for starting off with six days a week of long and slow aerobics is that most of us need, as a first step, to improve our ability to circulate blood around our bodies. More than any other single thing, circulation is the key to good health and to doing stuff. It controls our capacity to get fuel and oxygen to the muscles, where they are burned to create the power that keeps us moving. And—a matter of surprising urgency—it takes away the debris from the burning process. When you pant for air during exercise, this doesn't mean your body is desperate for more oxygen; it's desperate to get rid of the waste. Ditto the pain in your muscles: it's not from torn or stressed muscle fibers, but from the buildup of "ashes" in the form of lactic acid. Finally, circulation brings the blessed tides of C-6 and C-10 to prevent heart attacks and strokes, generate great mood, and all the other wonders Harry talks about.

I don't know how you feel at this point, but I would guess you either want to close the book and watch TV or tear out the door and crank out a quick fifty miles on your bike. I wouldn't do either. The best move right now—and Harry agrees passionately with this—is to make a realistic assessment of the shape you're in today and then make a start that fits your condition. Start too easy and you'll get bored. Start too hard and you'll quit or hurt yourself. To help you position yourself, you might want to think about the early experiences of three very different people who started or continued exercise programs at Harry's suggestion.

The Man Who Couldn't Walk to the Mailbox

S tart with my favorite, John, a patient of Harry's who retired at sixty-five. (Don't be put off because he's a man; it's a unisex story. I know it got my sister Petie to realize that all this stuff was for her . . . got her started.) Anyway, at his checkup, just before he stopped working, John was a hundred pounds overweight. He had dangerously high cholesterol, high blood pressure, low energy, and he was eating mountains of garbage. He was under a lot of stress at work and at home, and he was sick with anxiety about retirement, even though he was not mad for his job. He was in dreadful shape, and he was depressed. In other words, he was like a lot of Americans of his age and station in life. Not typical, maybe, but damn close.

John and his wife were moving to Florida and got a place a block from the beach. Harry was worried about him and started talking about exercise. John wasn't having it. No, he said almost angrily, he was not an athlete, never had been one and had no plans to start now. Harry, in his understated way, said, "Fine, but there's a good chance you will die soon if you don't do something." John reluctantly agreed to walk on the beach once a day, six days a week, for a while.

The first day, he walked about a half a mile and felt pretty good. The next morning, he felt as if he'd been hit by a truck. Everything ached, and he could barely get out of bed. But here's the thing. He showed up the next day. Tottered out of bed, God bless him, took a couple of Advil, and went to the beach again. He walked about a hundred yards this time and went home exhausted. The next day, he did the same thing. And for several days thereafter. Soon he was walking a couple of hundred yards; then more. He felt like a dope, waddling along the beach out of breath, but every day he got up and did his job. In a few months, he was walking a mile in that soft sand, and he was feeling significantly better. He had better energy, took more interest in decent food, and felt more enthusiastic and optimistic about starting life over down there in Florida. That daily bath of C-10 was working its magic.

A year later, John returned to New York to see Harry for his annual checkup. He reported that he was walking five miles a day on the beach, seven days a week. He had lost sixty pounds. His cholesterol and blood pressure were within normal ranges, and he looked ten years younger. He felt great. He feels great today.

Here's the obvious point: Don't feel like an idiot if you can barely stay on the treadmill for fifteen minutes at low speed the first day. That's serious for you, and your feet are already on a sacred path. It is not *struggling* on the first day or the thirtieth or sixtieth that's going to work. It's *showing up* every day and doing something. Do *something* every day for a week, and at week's end you'll be doing twenty minutes. Or thirty. Whatever. Push yourself a little, but don't push yourself over the edge. You get full credit if you change into your workout duds, go to the gym (or out on the road), and do some aerobic activity. The tide runs every day. So do you, if you want to stay young. Before too long, you should get up to doing forty-five minutes a day of aerobic exercise.

Throughout the book, when we talk about doing a day of this or that, we mean at least forty-five minutes of actual exercise unless we say otherwise.

The Master Athlete

At the other end of the spectrum, consider my pal Patricia. She has been a pretty good athlete all her life, but she decided to crank it up in her late fifties. She had had some health problems along the way and wondered if she could really go for it at that age. She checked with her doctor, and he said, You bet. Go for it. Which she conspicuously did.

For her, that meant a carefully structured exercise program, focused on a series of seniors' bike races, which had her doing an average of two hours a day of heavy biking and other aerobics—often with her own trainer—and some serious strength training. And it worked fine. This summer, at sixty-two, she got a silver in a big seniors' bike race out west. Next year, or the year after, she's going for the gold. It will happen; she is a solid athlete, she works like crazy at it, and she loves it. She is one of the fittest women I've ever met of any age, never mind sixty-two. This book is not designed for women like Patricia—they don't need it. But keep her in mind when you worry that maybe you're doing too much. You've probably got a little room yet, before you catch up with her. I promise you I do. I don't intend to try.

Incidentally, it may be worth stressing that even good athletes like Patricia occasionally have some serious illnesses. You may ask, How come? How come they get sick if exercise is such a cure-all? The answer is that there is a randomness to disease and death, just as there is a randomness to life. There's genetics, which matters much less than people think, but still matters some. And then there's rotten luck. But the point is, following the regimen that we're pushing enormously improves the chances of good health and a great life. I mean improves them by 70 percent. You don't get a guarantee—you still have a chance of picking up a fatal case of this or that—but 70 percent is not bad. There is not a pill or a course of treatment in all of medicine that comes anywhere near that.

Chris in the Middle

When I first talked to Harry, I was in much better shape than John, in better shape than most of Harry's patients, but not on the same planet with real athletes like Patricia. In response to Harry's urging, I took up spinning, which means joining a class of twenty to thirty people pumping away on stationary bikes to the accompaniment of music and the exhortations of a leader. I already liked to bike, and I had heard spinning was great exercise. Also, if I was going to follow Harry's Rules, I had to find something I could do every day in a manageable chunk of time. I thought spin class might be it.

So here I go. I am at the gym. I have signed up for a year at shocking cost, and I have gotten the spin class schedule. It's six-thirty in the morning, and I am feeling very, very shy. Because I am very old, I am forty pounds overweight, and I do not look becoming in my biking costume. The instructor, an alarmingly pretty woman with a slight Euro accent, sees me looking helpless; she comes over to my bike and shows me what to do. The bike has a huge flywheel in front with a brake-like thing that can make it easier or harder to pedal.

Don't Skip This Box

You're going to get this twice, once from me and once from Harry. It is not pro forma advice, it is real. *See your doctor before you embark on any of this.* It is possible, at your age, that you have a condition you're totally unaware of that could make a sudden, new exercise program a grave threat. Don't take the chance. By now, you should be seeing your doctor once a year anyway. Do it before you start a serious exercise regimen.

In the same vein, let me join Harry in urging you not to overdo it on the first day. I did, but I am a bit of a wackadoo and have to take extreme measures not to be bored. Harry has a lot of war stories about people who went nuts on the first day and were knocked out for a week. Or never went back. Remember, we're talking about being *younger next year,* not *younger tomorrow.* Feel your way. You are a slightly old girl now. You have Blacky Carbon and Gummy Sludge in your circulatory system. And your muscles and joints are not ready to go full bore. Take it easy. Sounds banal, but it's good advice.

It's hard to get it started and really hard to slow it down. I feel as if I could wreck my ankle if I got off wrong. Maybe break a leg.

The room fills with beautiful creatures in their twenties and thirties. One or two old numeros, but no one as old as I am. The music starts . . . a din with a heavy, compulsive beat. The instructor has a mike, and she starts telling us how to pedal . . . how fast and with how much resistance. My hearing has gone to hell, but I follow as best I can. Speed up, slow down. Tighten or ease the resistance with a knob on the frame. I do not fall off, but I feel as if I could. And I do not break my leg trying to slow the damn flywheel, but I *know* I could do that.

"Out of the saddle!" the instructor shouts, and everyone stands up, pumping like crazy.

"Resistance!" she shouts, and everyone takes a turn to the right on the resistance knob. My quadriceps, which I thought were strong, start to scream. How many seconds can this go on? Actually, it goes on for about three minutes, but I don't. Did I mention that the walls are all mirrors? Well, they are, and I have just caught sight of my own face. I am so frightened that I sit down. (The instructors often urge novices not to stand for long.) My face is purple, a bad purple, and I am sweating in a way that suggests the onset of serious illness, not good health.

After that, I only do some of the things the instructor says to do. But I hang, man. I stay there until the end, all forty-five minutes of it. There are stretching exercises when it's finally over. My color is still peculiar. As I totter out of the room at the end, the instructor comes up and says, "Nice going. First time?"

"How could you tell?" I give her a wan smile.

She just nods and says again, "Nice going." I stumble home, bathe, and go to bed. It is now 7:45 a.m., and my day is over. It is good that I'm retired; I could not go to work like this.

Okay, spin class was a bit intense, but the beauty of it—for a person of my ridiculous temperament—is that it caught my attention. It was *hard.* It was interesting. It was a challenge. And, with a touch of dread, I went back the next day. And every day for a long time after that. I was there this morning. And yesterday. And the day before. I've been doing it for years now, and I still get a kick out of it. And I'm in very, very good shape, at least for a guy who loves to eat and drink and is congenitally unathletic. I sometimes feel guilty for not doing more, but from Harry's more rational perspective I am one of the success stories. He says I've probably achieved about 70 percent of my potential fitness (as opposed to Patricia, who is 85 or 90 percent, or the gods of sport, who are 100 percent), but that's fine. That's as far as I'm going. I can do everything I want to, and I feel great almost all the time. Gotta love that.

In the long run, too, you want to push yourself but not go completely nuts. Patricia has the character and temperament to stay at her present, hectic level for years. But a lot of people burn out. A happy problem, you may say, but a real one for some. Our modest advice: Find the right level for you. I do not urge you to go out and push yourself to the point of purple on the first day, and Harry is appalled by the idea. But I do urge you to get into pretty heavy aerobics eventually. Remember, that walk in the sand in Florida was heavy for John. You have to do what's heavy for you. My early spin regimen would have been too easy for Patricia, too hard for most Americans in their sixties, and near-fatal for John.

Harry and I are now of one mind on how to start. Start slow. Slower than feels good. But hold at that level only until you get your feet under you. Take it up as you get more comfortable. Feel your way, but eventually give yourself a little push. Don't go so slow that you get bored. Get heavy for *you*, but only after you've been at it for a few weeks and feel comfortable. You'll know.

But just in case, here's some good advice from someone who is, finally, old enough to know better. Set a sensible fitness goal. Get there. And be happy. Don't make yourself crazy thinking, "Gee, that was easier than I thought. I bet I could . . ." And so on. Don't do it. Don't wreck and abandon what you've achieved with a huge effort for something that's not that much better. This is not competition, this is not athletics, this is lifestyle. This is feeling good. All the time.

I exercise six days a week. Always. I exercise pretty hard (60 to 75 percent of my maximum heart rate every day, 80 to 100 percent a lot of days). I am pretty good about the stinky weights. As a result, I can do all the stuff I like to do. I can walk around without pain. And can ski like a mildly gifted fifty-year-old. And ride the amazing Serotta bike that I gave myself this spring, high into the Rockies. Row my single scull in pretty waters. And I feel great more or less all the time. My legs are probably stronger than Old Fred's, and I am in better aerobic shape than most fifty-year-old men, all of which is astonishing and way more than I had dared to hope when I started.

But I am still ten pounds overweight. My arms are weak, and I have these little wattles under my chin, which is not a good look. And every Masters athlete in the country is better at whatever he or she does than I am. My thought is this: Fine.

This is good enough for me. Much better than I expected and plenty good enough. Although way below what a real athlete like Patricia would want. There is a point where the lines cross: effort and time on the one hand, condition and feeling good on the other. Forty-five minutes to an hour and a half a day is about right for me. I could go beyond that, and I do sometimes. But that's about enough for me. There are times when I get the bit in my teeth and want to train for a marathon or the Triple Bypass Bike Ride in the Rockies. And I may, if I feel like it. But probably not. This is the level, I believe, which I can keep up for the rest of my life. I'm stopping here. So I won't stop completely.

My advice to you: Do all this stuff for a year. Maybe two. And then think hard about where you want to be and how much effort you're capable of putting in. And decide when to say, enough. Intensity reaps great and sudden rewards; I love the feeling after a 70-mile bike ride. Or a hellish climb. But please remember this: Consistency trumps intensity every single time. It is far, far more important to find a good level for you—and stay there for the rest of your life—than to dip too deep into the intensity experience.

This is getting a little elaborate, but here's some good related advice. Inevitably, there are going to be cycles in your training and in your passion for it. You will crank it up in the spring, say, as you head into summer. Or slack off in mud season in the fall. I think that's a positive, a good thing. Too consistent and you'll go nuts. But remember: No matter where you are in the intensity swing, work out six days a week. You may default, more days than not, to Long and Slow rather than sprints. Okay. But do some damn thing every day, six days a week. And always for at least forty-five minutes (once you get started). You can dog it some of the time by just loping along at 60 percent for forty-five minutes. But never quit early. And never stay home. Ever. Or you'll start to slack off completely. And turn into that little old lady you struggled so hard to leave behind.

So, What Kind of Aerobic Exercise?

The menu of aerobic activities is long and pleasant, and it doesn't make any difference at all which ones you choose, as long as you like them. Or can bear them.

If you have some favorites, start with those. If not, here are some thoughts.

A surprising number of women like the endurance machines at the gym . . . the treadmills, elliptical machines, stair-climbers, skiing machines and the like. This may make sense. They're easy to use, it's easy to regulate the "dosage" and the process is bearable for most. You can wear headphones and listen to music or watch TV, which helps a lot of people. The best one for me is the elliptical machine, with moving arms as well as feet, so I get both upper- and lower-body exercise.

The simple treadmill seems to be the most popular, but here's a hint: I think you do best to crank the *angle* of the treadmill up a ways and get your exercise by "walking up a steep hill," rather than trying to trot or run on the flat. Better workout for your leg muscles, less jarring on your joints, and you get a serious cardio workout much sooner. Rowing machines are great, and I do see more women than men on them. But only about seven women in the country have the sterling character necessary to keep them up long enough to do any good. If you're one of the magnificent seven, excellent. Same thing on cross-country ski machines: NordicTrack is a great workout for the people who can keep it up (including the endlessly virtuous Harry), but I cannot, even though I love cross-country.

Running is fine if you're up to it. Most people my age tell me their joints cannot take it, but there are plenty of lucky exceptions. If you try it after years away, go at it carefully to improve your chances. Do as little as fifteen minutes the first day. Hurting your knees or your shins or ankles at this stage is the work of minutes, but the consequences last for months or years. I hurt my Achilles tendon riding on a damaged bike in 1982 when I was forty-seven. It took me a year to get back into biking, and I couldn't run until 2004. Tendons are a slow heal. Being bored is much better than getting banged up and quitting. Run every other day. Or even every third day. Do something else in between. And continue to go slower than feels natural. This is not to say you should dog it forever. Eventually, you'll want to get a heart monitor and make sure you're doing it hard enough. But not the first week or two.

Take Up One of the Healing Sports

Let me give a brief, heartfelt plug at this point to the blessed ... the heavenly ... the *healing* sports. Some sports, like tennis, pull you apart because they're centrifugal. Others, like running, beat on your joints remorselessly. But a few actually knit you together. Your muscles and especially your joints feel *better* when you're done than when you began. Biking is peculiarly like that. Swimming, cross-country skiing, and rowing, too. They are the healing sports, and you ought to have at least one of them in your repertoire.

There is no machine more beautiful, more perfect in the form-follows-function line, more ideally suited to your purpose than the bicycle. In my thirties, after getting divorced, I kept my bike on the mantelpiece, the only piece of art in a dismal little apartment ... a symbol of virtue and beauty in a chaotic life. New bikes—the composite/titanium beauties—are miraculously improved over the models of only fifteen or twenty years ago. If you're rich, run right out the door now and get one. For five thousand bucks. Maybe ten! But you most certainly don't have to. You can get a super road bike, with modern gearing and brakes, for a few hundred bucks. If you're more or less a beginner, you may want to get a "combination" bike; it's more comfortable and doesn't cost much, either.

In fact, if you haven't biked seriously for a while, or ever, give some serious thought to a combi, a bike with slightly fatter tires and an easier ride. I took a ride last weekend with my son Tim, who is about to turn fifty. He's a serious aerobic athlete, but he hadn't biked for a while and he astonished me by saying that modern racing bikes, with clip-on pedals and shoes, are *hard to ride*. I've been at it so long that I had forgotten this simple and obvious truth. They are delicate, they take some balance and they're a little ditzy . . . they dance around a little bit, compared to their stodgy brethren. It doesn't take long to get used to them. Not like a pair of hot skis. But it takes a while.

A Word About Bikes and Safety

If you haven't biked for a while, you may want to remind yourself that you are forty or fifty or sixty, not twenty, and that you have to be a hair more cautious. Wear a helmet all the time. I still bike in New York City traffic, but frankly, it's starting to scare me and I don't think it's a great idea. In fact, if you're just getting back into the sport, I'd start someplace pretty calm and bucolic. And, as with skiing or any "movement" sport, look around a lot more than you used to. Most important in biking and skiing: Be predictable. Go in predictable lines, and don't veer off without making damn sure there is no one behind you. You want to have fun, but you want to come home, too.

So don't hesitate to begin with a more user-friendly combi for a few hundred bucks. They still have great gearing and brakes, and they will give you more exercise, if anything. And graduate into the stunning road bike when you're a little further along and can appreciate it. But not on day one.

Oh, and get a comfortable women's seat. There's a period, early on, when women—and a lot of men—experience some discomfort, as they say, on a bike seat. There's a certain amount of bunching or some damn thing down there, and women do not like it. And they do not have to have it. Some of that discomfort goes away with familiarity, but the hell with it. Get a good women's saddle on day one. If you find it's not working out later on, you can get one of those little skinny-minnies some women like, but not to begin with.

In the same vein, get a decent pair of biking shorts with the right seat (with some extra padding built in). Maybe bib-top shorts. They make a huge difference from the very beginning. Lycra bib-tops are super comfortable, and they act just a teeny bit like the girdles my sisters were wearing in World War II . . . you'll appear to drop an instant eight pounds and bike better, too. Gotta like that.

Three other biking points: 1) You already know how to do it. 2) It's wildly good for you. 3) It's great for your legs. Later on, we make the point that building up your legs is particularly important in the Next Third. Failing legs are what can put you in the walker or in the chair. When in doubt, default to exercise that helps your legs. Like bicycling.

Or go swimming. It's cheap and easy to do. And if you go at it with some energy, it's great aerobic exercise. Swim fans often say it's the perfect exercise, and we can see why. You use almost every muscle in your body, it's aerobically demanding, and it also stretches you out in a healthy way,

Start Out Long and Slow

In the next two chapters, we'll crank it up a bit, but for now just stick with "long and slow"—the pace at which you're breathing pretty heavily and sweating some but not killing yourself. You can talk while you're doing it, and you can keep it up almost indefinitely, once you're in decent shape. Pick your activity and go do it for twenty or thirty or forty-five minutes a day for a week or so. Or a month. However long it takes to feel okay.

like yoga. You see swimmers' bodies and think, hey, that's perfect . . . just what I want for the Next Third. My son Tim, who was once a bit of a triathlete, used to combine a weights workout with a half-hour swim. He says a half-hour swim is a very serious aerobic workout, all by itself, and the combination is ideal. If you really get into it, there are Masters race organizations all over the country. And the equipment consists of a tank suit and a pair of goggles. If you don't think you look so great in the suit, just keep your goggles on.

If you're anywhere near snow, do not miss cross-country skiing. Even if you've never done it before. For one thing, it's bone-easy. After exactly one day, you'll be doing fine. It is a species of walking, after all. And once you get the hang of it, you can give yourself a massive dose of the very best aerobic exercise there is in some of the most beautiful places in the world. There is nothing better on earth than sliding gracefully along, under trees heavily laden with fresh snow, up a rise in the Rockies . . . down a country road in Vermont . . . over the golf course in your hometown. The only sound the hiss of your own sweet skis. Sneak off alone and try it. You will thank me for the rest of your days.

Of course, that first trip to the gym may not be a congenial one. After all, you're probably not in sensational shape. And it is at least possible that you are more overweight than you'd like. You may not look your best in gym clothes. (I weighed a slobbery 200 when I really got into all this and looked nasty.) And, of course, you are slightly old. This may be your "new job," as Harry and I insist, but the gym sure doesn't look like the office. You don't know your way around, you don't know how to behave, and you're probably a bit clueless by local standards, whatever the hell they are. One thing's for sure, almost everyone at the gym is younger than you. And some of them are absolute gym rats . . . in great shape and proud as peacocks. You have the strong feeling that they're looking at you funny. Or with contempt.

Well, the hell with 'em. You are here to save your life, not to make pals with a bunch of weirdo hardbodies. *So suck it up, be strong, and do your job.* Think about John on the beach the first day and where he is now. This works so much faster than you can believe when you're beginning. Just tough it out for a couple of weeks and you'll be fine.

Lying, Self-Abuse, and Related Problems

One of the great barriers to success in this business is lying. People lie to themselves about what they're doing. They are absolutely delusional. They insist that their endless minutes walking to the john or whatever are all the workout anyone needs. Some women tell me of the many, wonderful hours they spend with their dear friends on the golf course, sometimes even working up a bit of a sweat, God bless them. Well, that's nonsense. Golf is wonderful, but it is not aerobic. Gardening is wonderful, but it's not aerobic. Quit lying to yourself and sweat. You've got to get out there and do stuff.

I talk to women about this book all the time, and the single constant in all those conversations—actually, with men or women, young or old—is that almost at once the person I'm talking to starts to tell me about her own exercise regimen and how wonderful it and she is. It's ridiculous. They all tell me that they agree entirely about exercise and are already hard at it. Well, that is nonsense! Outrageous nonsense! Please, please, please, whatever you tell me, whatever you tell your partner, whatever you tell your God . . . *quit lying to yourself!* You are not doing anywhere near enough if you're significantly overweight. If you're short of breath. Do not lie! You are getting in your own way.

Here's an interesting aside from Harry on that delicate point. For years, there was this neat little anomaly in how hard people said they worked out and their mortality. In surveys, there was a clear correlation between how much *men* said they worked out and how early they died. The results were: Work out more, die later. Makes perfect sense. But for *women* there was no correlation at all. Weird. So they did tests to correlate actual fitness, as measured by stress tests, and mortality. This time, there was a near perfect correlation for men and women. How come? Women lied more about how much they worked out.

Men lied some. Women lied a lot. Just tuck that away, ladies, and listen to me later when I tell you to go get a heart monitor.

A Word to the Weak and Uncoordinated

The message of this book is probably least agreeable to people who, like me, were skinny and weak as kids or had the wrong body types to be good at sports. Or older women who predated Title IX and the surge in women's sports. None of you are old enough for this next bit, but there was a time in this nation when there was a serious body of thought that exercise was bad for women. My very own mother experienced it. One day, up there in bucolic Danvers, Massachusetts, perhaps in 1900 or 1902, when mother was six or eight, she came home to this serious scene. Her mother and an acquaintance were waiting for her in the formal parlor of the Conant Street house. Because, as the man had told my grandmother, "I saw Lurana *running* this morning." He thought my grandmother ought to know. She was told not to do it anymore. In the fifty years I knew her, I never saw her do a single athletic thing. Not one. Pa, either, come to think of it.

Anyhow, I have a huge soft spot for people like you and me who never cared much for sports or weren't any good at them or whatever. And some heartening news. In a funny way, people like us have an easier time with this regimen than the athletic gods of our childhood. There are two reasons. First, it's surprisingly hard for real athletes to come to grips with the fact that they are nowhere near as good as they were at twenty or whatever. They sulk. They refuse to play. They go to hell. I don't know what it's all about; it's not my problem. Or yours, probably. If you were not athletic as a kid, you don't have to get over yourself. Just doing it is fine. Congratulations.

Second, if you were not an athlete as a girl, there is every reason to anticipate that your Personal Best is still ahead and that you have years and years of getting Younger Every Year. A personal story: I am seventy-one years old, and I have never skied better in my life. Literally. I was not much of a skier at twenty-eight, to be sure, but now I am a god. Better than, say, 60 percent of the people on a serious mountain on a given day. Do you have any idea what fun that is? To come sweeping down those hills with a turn of speed and a touch of grace at this late stage in the day? I grin for the pleasure of it. Ridiculous old fool? You bet. Shamefully behind people who can really ski? You bet. And I love it. Race you to the bottom!

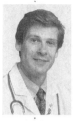

CHAPTER SEVEN

The Biology of Exercise

B illions of years ago, life on earth divided into two great kingdoms: animals, which move, and plants, which do not. Our ancestors chose movement, and that basic biology hasn't changed since. When you get in shape, when you exercise, when you dance, you are sharing the ancient chemistry of movement with every other animal on the planet.

We can move because we have muscles that contract. Our muscles are sophisticated machines that use oxygen to burn fat or glucose (blood sugar) in millions of tiny engines called mitochondria, which then produce the energy for contraction. It's straightforward internal combustion, just like your car but without a flame. The mitochondria are the key to muscle contraction and to the evolution of movement on earth.

Bacteria developed mitochondria two billion years ago to burn oxygen. Not to produce energy, but to get rid of the oxygen that was just then creeping into the atmosphere and that turned out to be highly toxic stuff, both then and now. It's toxic because it's explosive on a molecular level. That's why fires burn when you add oxygen and why they go out when you remove it. The ability to burn oxygen inside cells is what gives animals the power to move, but free oxygen is dangerous; it burns holes in our DNA, leading to cell death and ultimately to things like heart disease and cancer. Since storing and handling oxygen is such risky business, we have elaborate oxygen detoxification systems that work around the clock to protect us. The antioxidants in the fruits and vegetables we eat soak up the remaining free oxygen (so eat a lot of them), and with all these systems working hard, we get by pretty well. Bacteria didn't have any of this. Instead they used the oxygen to burn sugar in their mitochondria, producing harmless water and carbon dioxide as exhaust.

Five hundred million years ago, bacterial mitochondria somehow moved inside the cells of our primitive ancestors, who harnessed them to their muscles and gave birth to aerobic metabolism. It was access to the unlimited supply of cheap, oxygen-based energy that fueled the explosion of higher life-forms from then on. Bacterial mitochondria make all higher animal life possible, and they live in every muscle cell of every animal on the planet today, including yours. All animal motion is fueled by the mitochondria inherited from bacteria—the energy you use to walk in the park, run a marathon, scratch your nose or swim a lap. The DNA in your mitochondria is still bacterial, not human. You inherited it like some ancient, permanent trust fund. Incidentally, plants inherited photosynthesis from algae the same way we stole mitochondria from bacteria, so all life energy on earth today comes from machinery developed by either algae or bacteria.

Pathways to Higher Energy

With that brief look at the last few billion years to put things in perspective, let's talk about getting in shape. Aerobic fitness is all about making more energy in the muscles. That means building more mitochondria and bringing them more fuel and oxygen. Mitochondria can burn either fat or glucose. It's like having a car that can run on either diesel (fat) or gasoline (glucose), depending on your needs: diesel for long-haul road trips, high-octane gasoline for speed and acceleration. Your muscles prefer to burn fat most of the time, because it's a more efficient fuel, but for hard exercise—for speed and power—you burn glucose.

At rest, and with *light* exercise, you burn 95 percent fat and 5 percent glucose. Most fat isn't stored in your muscles; it's stored around your belly and hips and in a few other prime locations. Your body has to bring it to your muscles through your circulation. That's harder than it seems, because your blood is largely water and fat doesn't dissolve in water. Fat has to be carried in special molecules called triglycerides, which your doctor probably mentioned during your last checkup. The trouble with this, from your muscles' perspective, is that your capillaries can handle only a few triglyceride molecules at a time. So each capillary can deliver only a trickle of fat to your mitochondria. With consistent aerobic training, your body builds vast new networks of capillaries to bring more fat to your muscles. Eventually, however, you are delivering as much fat as you possibly can, and if you want to go faster, or harder, you need to start bringing glucose to the mitochondria to use as a second fuel.

With *harder* exercise you keep burning fat in the background, but all the extra energy comes from burning glucose.

Most of the glucose is stored in your muscles ahead of time, but your circulation gets a double workout, first bringing in more glucose and the oxygen necessary to burn it, then carrying away the exhaust, especially the carbon dioxide.

Any way you look at it, circulation is the basic infrastructure of exercise. Steady aerobic exercise, over months and years, produces dramatic improvements in your circulatory system, which is one of the ways exercise saves your life. Exercise stresses your muscles, and they release enough C-6 to trigger C-10. The C-10 released by the adaptive micro-trauma of exercise drives the creation of new mitochondria, the storage of more glucose in the muscle cells, and the growth of new capillaries to feed them. Your muscles get hard as you get in shape because they're stuffed full of all the new mitochondria, capillaries, and extra glucose. It's a fun image—that newly hardened muscle full of all the stuff you grew by exercising.

The Metabolisms of Hunting and Gathering

Any form of regular, hard aerobic exercise will do the trick, but you can get more mileage out of your exercise if you understand the difference between burning fat and burning glucose. That's the key to really effective aerobic exercise, because different exercise intensities trigger different biological changes throughout your body.

You have two natural aerobic paces, easy and hard, and they depend on two very different muscle metabolisms, which are determined by the fuel you use. Low-intensity, light aerobic exercise burns fat, while high-intensity, hard aerobic exercise burns glucose. It's a critical difference, because these two paces trigger the two distinct metabolisms of foraging and hunting, which are our essential physical rhythms. That's a key point. Those two activities consumed most of our waking hours in nature, and each one called for distinctly different body and brain functions: highly coordinated and specific patterns of thought, mood, energy, digestion, immune function, and muscle metabolism. Our bodies and brains geared themselves to our daily environment based largely on our exercise patterns, and that's still how it works today. Never mind that you're walking through the park rather than foraging, or at spin class rather than hunting: light and hard aerobics are still the master control signals for C-6, C-10, and countless other physical and chemical rhythms throughout your body, including your basic brain patterns of behavior and mood.

One natural question is whether women are more physically geared to foraging and men to hunting. The answer is no. It does appear that women did more of the foraging in human society, and men more of the hunting, and there are slight differences in our makeup as a result. But these are tiny, superficial variations on the themes. Our underlying biology predates this specialization by millennia, and any difference is about as significant to our performance as the color you choose for a sports car. Look at the Olympics, where women compete every bit as hard as men do; if you control for the gender-specific differences in muscle mass, we all perform equally. It comes as a surprise because men run faster and lift heavier weights, but that's just because we carry proportionally more muscle mass on our skeletons. Pound for pound, female muscle equals male muscle. In fact, all mammalian muscle is identical. In the lab, scientists can't tell human muscle from rat muscle from whale muscle without a label. If you don't believe me, go take a spin class with Chris. Talk about high-intensity aerobics; the pure biology of hunting! And then note that the vast majority of the other people in the room will be women. Hunting in spandex.

To be clear, sex roles in exercise are nonsense. We are all hunters and foragers. None of this is modern. It's deeply rooted in the mists of evolutionary time, and the point is that you can choose between the biologies by how you exercise.

That's why Chris is going to urge you to buy a heart rate monitor. You need to know how hard you can go burning fat and how hard you can go burning glucose, because that controls health and fitness throughout your body. Your heart rate is the only way to know for sure which metabolism is at work and which signals you're sending. Your heart delivers more and more blood to your muscles the faster it pumps, and your muscles can extract more and more fat from that blood until you reach about 65 percent of your peak heart rate. Chris will give you formulas for this in the next chapter, but for an average fifty-year-old woman, that's a heart rate of 110 beats per minute. If you're sixty-five, it's about 100 beats per minute. That's a good, stiff walking pace for most of us, and it's the limit of your first gear in nature.

As soon as you push your body a little harder, you start burning glucose in addition to fat, and you need more oxygen to do this. That means bringing more blood to the muscles, so your heart rate goes up. Any heart rate north of 65 percent means that you're burning glucose and that you've moved into a different metabolism. You've shifted into second gear.

Your body starts drawing on the glucose stored in your

muscles, feeding it into your mitochondria to produce the extra energy you need to run and hunt. At some point, however, the glucose metabolism also has an upper limit. You can bring loads of oxygen into the blood and carry away a lot of carbon dioxide, but above a certain level of exertion, the chemicals just can't move between blood and muscle, or within the muscle, fast enough to keep up with the demand. That happens at a heart rate of around 80 percent of maximum. For the fifty-year-old, that's a heart rate of 136 per minute; at sixty-five, it's 124. If you go above your number, your muscles become starved of oxygen and the glucose can't burn all the way down to carbon dioxide. Instead, you build up a sludge called lactate, which is incompletely burned sugar and which shuts down your muscle function after a few seconds of exercise at peak levels (like sprinting the length of a football field). As with the switch from fat to glucose, the switch into "anaerobic" metabolism, where there isn't enough oxygen, has ripple effects throughout your body.

The only way to tell when you reach and cross these thresholds is with a heart rate monitor. You can't do it by how you feel. Even Olympic athletes, training six hours a day for years, can't do it by how they feel. You can certainly get in shape without a heart rate monitor, but you'll waste a fair amount of your time and effort.

Light Aerobic Exercise: Distance, Not Speed

The concept that exercise intensity is a master signal that regulates chemistry throughout your body and brain is so important that it's worth a closer look, starting with light exercise. Light aerobic exercise is long and slow exercise at an easy pace—up to 65 percent of your peak heart rate. At this level, your muscles burn mostly fat, so it's your most fuel-efficient pace, the one you can keep up all day. It's the pace you once used for foraging and now use for walking miles—for those times when speed doesn't count, but mileage does. You might think it's a waste of time to exercise in this zone, but it's a wonderful pace. This is the metabolic zone where your body and brain heal and grow. It's the zone where steady, low-grade C-10 drives the slow, consistent growth of infrastructure: blood vessels and mitochondria in your muscles; repair and health throughout your body. You become more fit with harder exercise, but you gain more endurance and general healthiness with prolonged light exercise. Do this outdoors with your heart rate monitor and you'll love it. Learn what it's doing for you inside and you'll become an addict.

Let's go for a walk on the beach and talk about this some more. When you first wake in the morning, your body is still asleep and your muscles are in hibernation, running on a trickle of blood and burning fat in the metabolic equivalent of a pilot light. As you stretch and greet the day, the changes begin. Simply opening your eyes activates large parts of your brain, releases adrenaline and increases blood flow to your muscles. Your heart rate rises a few beats as you roll out of bed. You start to move, to walk and shower, and your heart speeds up, pumping out more blood with each stroke. Arteries dilate throughout your legs, forcing oxygen-rich blood deep into the muscle fibers, sending the chemical signals that bring your body to life. Your knees and hips pump their lubricating fluid around, and the stiffness slowly leaves your joints. Have a light breakfast, finish your coffee, and head out the door to the beach, where another beautiful day has started.

Sand between your toes, early morning sun coming off the water. Give yourself five minutes of slow, relaxed strolling to warm up, then ease into a good, stiff walk. You could keep this up for miles. And you feel that way for the first twenty minutes of the walk. You're taking it easy, and your muscles are burning fat over a low flame. As you loosen up and start to hit your stride, the fat burns hotter and faster. When you hit about 65 percent of your heart's maximum output, your leg muscles are working at the upper limit of their low aerobic zone. ("Aerobic" means your muscles have all the oxygen they need.) This is as fast as you can go burning fat. It's like diesel: great mileage but low torque. You can go all day, but you can't go fast.

Well, it turns out you don't have to, because you've walked steadily into C-10 territory. Think of growth and repair in terms of a public works project: building an interstate takes time, and new capillaries don't sprout up all at once after the first day at the gym. Your body thinks about it for a while, plans the route, and organizes the materials before it starts construction. Your body also doesn't trust you, or, more accurately, it doesn't trust nature. If you fall off track for a little while, even for a distressingly short interval of sloth, construction stops. The real benefits of exercise come with months and years of sustained, steady growth. Short-term gains in fitness are fun but misleading. They depend on surges of C-10—metabolic tricks your body uses to forage during the January thaw, ready to hibernate the moment the cold snap hits again. Months and years of exercise are different. They produce the slow, deep currents of C-10 that sustain the steady engagement of your infrastructure in long-term growth.

This all happens automatically through a carefully choreographed chemical dance within your bloodstream and body. The C-10 pattern of long, slow exercise regulates literally dozens of chemical signals in your body and brain. Names you might recognize, like growth hormone, adrenaline, and serotonin, and names you don't, like endothelial growth factor, tumor necrosis factor, and platelet-derived growth factor. The point is that long, slow exercise builds your muscles, heart, and circulation, mobilizes your fat stores, and then goes beyond that to let your body heal. Long, slow exercise is the opposite of the chronic inflammation of modern living. It's the tide of youth.

With training, you can easily double the circulatory and mitochondrial capacity you had before you started. Several months of long, slow exercise will turn you into a happy, Zen-like powerhouse of aerobic capacity. Zen-like because your brain does not know you're walking on the treadmill. It thinks you're foraging, and it moves automatically into the chemical state where your mind is engaged but relaxed. Your thinking is clear; your mood is calmer and more alive than it was at rest. Your brain wave patterns on an EEG are similar to meditation states, and for good reason—this is the pace you used in nature when the threat was low.

What's interesting is that the actual pathways of relaxation and focus in your brain become stronger with use. Long-term memory improves with regular exercise, and the risk of Alzheimer's drops. Long hikes and long, easy bike rides are the kinds of low aerobics Chris and I prefer, because frankly it's pretty tedious walking slowly on the treadmill for an hour or more. Besides, it makes sense to try to put the mental and physical sides of foraging back together. Hiking five miles into the forest with your friends to bird-watch is perfect foraging, and biking twenty miles on a weekend morning is pure heaven.

Hard Aerobics: Pushing the Herd

Exercising hard enough to push your heart rate above 65 percent calls for a new fuel. You need more power than you can get from fat alone, so your muscles start to burn glucose. This shift into high gear changes your metabolism because harder exercise is the automatic signal that you've started to hunt.

Here's how it works. Animals in nature *never* move out of their low aerobic zone unless they're hunting, being hunted, or playing (rehearsal for the first two). Glucose is powerful but expensive fuel. Your body knows that you would *never* move fast enough to burn glucose while foraging. That would be a waste of energy, which is to say that it would be biologically insane. If you're burning glucose, you must be hunting, which triggers a major metabolic shift that affects your muscles, brain, gut, immune system, kidneys, liver, heart, and lungs.

Picture this: Prey is in sight. Adrenaline surges, C-6 surges, nonessentials shut down, and blood floods your active muscles. You become engaged and alert. You notice more; your step has more bounce. In the lab, with harder exercise, whole new areas of your brain light up on functional MRI scans; you process visual information faster and do calculations more quickly; your attention goes outward, your reflexes sharpen, and your salivary flow increases. Back on the beach, this means you're warmed up, fully engaged, and ready to run. As you hit your stride, your head comes up, your nostrils flare, and your pupils dilate. You feel more alive, clearheaded, and younger. Not because of anything conscious, but because you've automatically turned on a whole series of complex control mechanisms by exercising harder.

Your arms swing freely, you breathe more deeply and your legs start to really work. You feel a surge of energy as your heart rate climbs steadily past 65 percent. Welcome to the high aerobic zone. You have just started to burn glucose—your high-octane gasoline equivalent. Not such great mileage, but a lot more power. You keep burning that low level of fat in the background, but all the extra fuel from this point on up is glucose.

All those days of long, slow exercise you did earlier built you a bigger engine. Now, with glucose added, those extra mitochondria and blood vessels are running on rocket fuel. This is the benefit of low aerobic training. It's a trick nature invented so you could catch the antelope, and it's why every athlete in the world does long and slow to build the base fitness for harder aerobics. Every Olympic hopeful, every world record holder, does it, and so should you. Remember Bonnie Blair? Her sport was the 500-meter speed-skating sprint—38 seconds of all-out speed and power, 30 mph on ice. And her training program rested on a rock-solid base of endurance training. Bonnie Blair became the most decorated Winter Olympics athlete in U.S. history—man or woman—but the stakes are actually higher for you. Olympic athletes are merely chasing gold; you are chasing youth.

And it gets better, because as important as long and slow is, adding hard aerobics makes your body faster and more powerful still. It drives your body to store more glucose right in the muscles, making them ready for sustained, hard exercise.

Nature's perspective on hard aerobic exercise is that you are designed to be an endurance predator, able to work with your pack to run down antelopes on the savannah. You may not feel much like an endurance predator, but you are. You are designed to be able to circle the antelope herd for hours, running them hard enough to find out which are the weak and old. A person in good shape has enough glucose in his muscles for about two hours of hard exercise. Not full out, but a pretty good effort. Two hours of pushing the herd.

This is also why exercise kicks your brain into high gear. Not to write *Pride and Prejudice,* but to eat. Think about tracking hundreds of caribou for hours across the tundra, picking out individuals, assessing their fitness, watching them run, marking and remembering your prey. That's the brain function you turn on with high aerobic exercise. The intense concentration, excitement, physical power, challenge, and opportunity of hunting is automatic, it's healthy, and it's fun. And the more you hunt, the better your brain gets at this.

Hard aerobics, working up a good sweat, is our favorite exercise rhythm because hunting brings out our youngest and best biology: strong, fast, energetic, and optimistic all day long. That's why you should do low aerobic exercise a couple of days a week to build your base, and then go out and play hard on the high-aerobic fields the other days. Tell your body it's springtime, and remember that Title IX has always existed in nature. Female wolves run and hunt just as hard as males, lionesses do most of the hunting, and female dolphins hunt in bursts of speed up to 45 mph. Women are meant to run hard, to swim hard, to dance hard, and to sweat hard. Sex does not matter in this. All that counts is how often you show up and how hard you work.

Anaerobic Exercise: The Lactate Burn

One of the nice things about stepping out of nature is that most of us no longer need to kill to eat or worry about being killed. But when we did, we had an extra gear to call on—ten seconds of raw power for what wildlife biologists call "escape or capture" moments.

You can push the glucose pace all the way up to about 85 percent of your maximum heart rate, where you hit the limit of your high aerobic capacity. That's the fastest pace you can sustain, but for a few seconds you can go faster still. In a burst of youthful enthusiasm at the beach, you can sprint 100 yards to the top of a dune. You double your power output for those last 300 feet. Your heart is putting out 400 percent of its resting capacity, and still you go way beyond its ability to deliver blood and oxygen. You kick in the afterburners for that burst of power, dumping energy into your muscles in a controlled chemical explosion. You have gone anaerobic, your third metabolic gear, the realm beyond oxygen. Sand is flying, your arms are pumping, your heart is pounding, legs burning, you can't keep it up any longer—and suddenly you're standing on top of the dune, winded but fully alive.

That's not aerobic exercise, it's not endurance training, and it's not something you should do every day, but it's fun to play with. It's anaerobic exercise, where there's no oxygen in your muscles. It's also your oldest metabolic pathway, dating back to the days when there was no oxygen on earth, before the bacteria invented mitochondria. It's more primitive than aerobic metabolism: less efficient and less biochemically elegant, but far more powerful over short distances and a critical gear to have in the evolutionary transmission. It saved your ancestors' lives, or let them end someone else's, countless times over the past few billion years.

Playing at anaerobic levels is a great way to get in peak shape. It's the ultimate hunting signal. It doesn't do anything for longevity, or probably for overall health, but it's great for vim, vigor, and pure fitness. Don't bother with it until you get into pretty good basic shape, then add in interval training a couple of times a week. It's not the key to the rest of your life, but a little bit of escape/capture is important once you're back in predator mode. It's the climax of the hunt, standing victorious on top of the dune.

Make It Happen

Exercise is the friendly trick you play on nature. Your body expects you to walk ten miles a day, with an hour or two of hunting and some sprinting and heavy labor thrown in, but fortunately it's not that smart. You can convince it that spring has come to the savannah with just under an hour a day of exercise . . . less than an hour a day to be lean, fit, alert, energetic, healthy, and optimistic for decades to come.

Nature is not a treadmill at the gym. It's an ever-changing physical environment, so it should come as no surprise that a variety of different exercises and intensities do more good than a single, unvarying routine. Practically speaking, most people also burn out on any given exercise program over time, so we suggest incorporating a lot of variety over the next thirty years. Nature's rule is simple: *Do something real every day.* Ignore all that talk out there about exercising three or four days a week. Ignore it! Like our national cholesterol guidelines, it's a bare minimum, a desperate plea from the medical profession to a nation of couch potatoes. Remember, your body craves the *daily* chemistry of exercise. Whether the exercise is long, slow, and steady (an hour or two of good, hard walking) or shorter and more intense (running, swimming, or using the exercise machines at the gym) is a lot less important than the "dailyness" of it, six days a week. So experiment with a variety of different aerobic exercises at the gym, and work hard to find some outdoor sports that you like: biking, kayaking, downhill or cross-country skiing, or stiff hiking. Keep your heart rate in the high aerobic zone at the gym and in the low aerobic zone while exercising outside, and you'll get great results. Remember that the whole point is to give your body and brain the sustained signals that tell them to grow younger. It's not important whether you get younger quickly or slowly; you have plenty of time. What is important is to keep moving in the right direction.

Showing Up

People don't fall off track because they do the wrong exercises at the gym. They fall off track because they stop going, just for a day or two, and then never go back. I've worked on this with thousands of patients, and it's the *habit and routine* of exercise that lead to success.

And that's not so easy. We are hardwired to eat, to make love, and to sit down and rest whenever we can, because in nature it was not clear when—or whether—the opportunity would come again. Now, in times of plenty and ease, those instincts are disastrous, but they are never going to go away.

Luckily, you can rewire your brain with structure and routine. Just take that amazing life skill you started building the first day you showed up for kindergarten and turn it to a new purpose. Show up at the gym. Think of it as a great job, which it is. It will change your life, slowly but surely, because once you show up you are virtually certain to do some meaningful exercise. *And even if you don't, you will show up again tomorrow.* That's the key—showing up again tomorrow for the rest of your life.

It makes sense to think of this as a job, because once you pass the age of fifty, exercise is no longer optional. You have to exercise or get old. Chris doesn't wake up and think about whether or not to go to the gym every day, any more than he woke up and thought about whether or not to go to work when he was a lawyer. No matter how he feels, he gets out of bed and he goes. It's easier that way, and he is much, much younger as a result.

The earlier you start, the bigger the payoff, which brings us to the decade before menopause and the decade or so after—to the challenge of exercising while your life is still full to overflowing. It may seem exhausting to fit exercise into your crazy schedule, but that's looking at it backwards. We are not tired at the end of the day because we get too much exercise. We are tired because we do not get *enough* exercise. We are mentally, emotionally, and physically drained from being sedentary. Being exhausted by seven o'clock each night is not living; it is merely surviving large stretches of the only life we're likely to have. Besides, study after study shows that we are more productive and happier—on less sleep—when we're fit. If you put any value at all on your quality of life, the time you spend exercising becomes a bargain. The reality is that your life is so full in these years that you can't afford *not* to exercise. The only real issue is that it's tough to keep up the motivation to exercise when life is crowded with obligations and stress. So rely on structure more than motivation. Carve out the time to exercise, make it "protected time," and guard it fiercely against intrusion.

Getting Started

The jump-in-at-the-deep-end strategy happened to work for Chris, but the risk of injury is relatively high if you're out of shape. Start out by pushing yourself hard enough to sweat, but at a level that matches your current fitness. The worse shape you're in and the older you are, the more important it is to keep each day's exercise well within your limits. This means keeping the intensity low and building up the duration. Remember the chemistry of inflammation? Well, for decades all those C-6 chemicals in your bloodstream have been telling your joints to decay. Arthritis is largely an inflammatory disease of sedentary societies: it's a disease of C-6. So after a few decades of decay your joints are *old*—older than your heart, your arteries, your lungs, your brain, and older than your muscles by decades. If you make this into a contest between your muscles and your joints, your joints will lose. Show up every day, but take it at your own pace as you settle into harness. Finally, no matter how fit you are, check with your doctor before you start any of this, and ask if you need a stress test.

There Are No Limits

Getting into great shape is fun and wonderful if you're healthy, but it's essential if you're not. Even if you're in truly lousy shape now, or if something really bad happens to you down the road, take heart—everyone can do this. I have patients who didn't come to regular exercise until *after* strokes, cancer, heart attacks, or hip fractures, but once they did, their lives improved dramatically. Arthritis, strokes, heart attacks, brain tumors, broken bones, and a host of other woes may put limits on what *kind* of exercise you do, but none of them can stop you.

I walk to work through New York City's Central Park (one of the world's great commutes), and for at least a decade I've watched an old guy running there. He must have had a major stroke, because he has the strangest, floppiest gait I've ever seen. Apparently, he can only really run with the good half of his body and just throws the other half forward in an act of faith with each step. The stroke probably affected his temperature regulation as well, because he never wears a shirt. But he's out there—skinny old chest, shirt off in 20-degree snowstorms, looking prehistoric and, as far as I can tell, living the hell out of his life. There is something enormously appealing about seeing this guy appear out of a snowstorm, half naked, with his queer, lopsided gait, but so *alive*. It doesn't matter who he is, he's facing a lot more than you, Chris, or me, and he is triumphant because he shows up day after day, year after year. Remember this guy when you think you can't exercise. He had a stroke and can barely walk, so he *really* can't exercise. But he does, and I bet he loves it. You will, too.

CHAPTER EIGHT

The Heart of the Matter: Aerobics

T hink of that ... we can burn either diesel or gasoline, at a whim, whenever we want. That's amazing. There isn't a car on the road that can do that. And we can burn stuff without using oxygen at all. A miracle. May we respectfully suggest that the least you can do to show your appreciation for this marvelous machine is to keep it in something like working order? And not just out of gratitude. If you let it get mucked up with Blacky Carbon and Gummy Sludge, it will blow up. And kill you dead. Well, maybe not dead, but open-heart surgery. Did Harry have a chance to talk about open-heart surgery? I didn't think so. Consider it for a minute, to strengthen your appetite for this slightly pedestrian chapter. Open-heart surgery is hugely popular these days, apparently because so many people prefer it to reading about aerobics and working out.

The surgery's not really that tricky anymore. All the surgeons have to do is cut open your chest with a knife, then crack your sternum like the shell of a lobster with a huge pair of shears. Snip, snip, snip. And then the team—don't worry, they've done this a thousand times—cranks the bones back so the doc can reach in and . . . Hey, you don't want to hear about open-heart surgery, do you? You think it's scary and disgusting. Fine. Some patients say it's not as bad as it sounds but that it's, well, intrusive. Quite the little scar, too. Exercise is intrusive as well . . . takes up almost an hour a day, which is a lot. You can skip it if you like, along with this chapter. But you may eventually have to learn that skin-the-lobster trick. My recommendation? I'd read a little further, but that's just me. By the way, even if you skim this chapter, first time through, don't miss "Powder Rules Apply" at the end; it's nice.

Long-Term Goals

Let's assume you feel queasy about open-heart surgery. What to do? Endurance exercise, of course. Send those critical signals to your cells. And the best way to do that is to set long-term goals and get to work on them. The most important one is this: A year from now, you should be able to do long and slow aerobics (that's breathing hard but still able to talk; it's 60–65 percent of your maximum heart rate) for, say, three hours without getting exhausted. You should be able to do that in your sixties, seventies, and eighties . . . and a variation of it in your nineties. That's an all-morning bike ride or a hike at a firm but not punishing pace. You should do something like that, oh, once a month. Two hours is okay some months, but three is better; make it a real outing, a real commitment. Make it a focus of your training, while reminding yourself that this is what it's all about. If you can get to that level of fitness, and stay there, life will be good and you can probably keep the lobsterman at bay where he belongs. But we think you should do more. You should certainly add strength training, discussed in Chapters Ten and Eleven, because that addresses a whole different set of issues. You should also do aerobics at higher levels so that you can get other fuel systems involved. But remember John on the beach down there in Florida. He never got beyond long and slow, and he's one of our heroes.

Let's keep going. For a second endurance goal, you should be able to do high-endurance aerobics for an hour (that's a serious clip where you can no longer talk, other than a few panted words; it's 70–85 percent of your maximum heart rate). If you can maintain this pace for two hours, that's wonderful. But watch it, you may be turning into an athlete. An hour at this clip is a lot, and it's not easy. Reach that goal and you'll be in super shape.

Finally and least urgently, you should be able to do real hell-for-leather sprints or some other flat-out activity at anaerobic levels (that's everything you've got until you *have* to stop) for a minute or two. This is the least important goal, but it's worth considering. As you know, it uses a different fuel and combustion system (the super-turbo, no-oxygen gear that works so well and makes such a mess afterwards), and it's nice to have all three systems in working order. It's also nice to know that your ancient "fight or flight" mechanism is there if you need it. I like to ring this bell once a week, but tastes vary. Judging only from what I see at the gym and in spin class, I suspect that more men have a taste for this flat-out exercise than women, but there clearly are women who go for it, too. As I say, it is not the most important thing in this little program; follow your own taste for it. Pretty good fun, though.

The Utter Necessity of Getting a Heart Monitor

N ow that you have some goals, how do you get there? The first step is an odd one. You buy a heart monitor. If you haven't been in training for a while, all those references to "percent of your maximum heart rate" in the last section may strike you as arcane and not very useful. How many people know their maximum heart rate or the percentage they're using? The answer is, everyone who is at all serious about endurance training. All modern endurance athletes know precisely what level they're working out at, *all the time,* and you should, too. Again, just based on my own observation in spin classes, more women than men use heart monitors. And they're right to. Modern training is always cast in terms of going at different levels of intensity (different percentages of maximum heart rate) for different periods of time and for different purposes. The heart monitor is the tool that lets you build and maintain a strong aerobic base. It works better than anything else you can afford, and it makes the whole business of endurance training a lot more interesting.

A heart monitor is a simple device that tells you how many times a minute your heart beats. That's it. You can get one that analyzes your spit and remembers your mother's maiden name, but you don't need all that. Of the existing models, the simple versions are fine. But you can't do without one; a heart monitor is as important to your training as a decent pair of sneakers.

People resist this advice like crazy. Maybe because it's new. Or a little bit creepy. You *do* have to put this black strap around your chest which is a little odd. And it *is* a computer . . . a few folks still resist that. Most important and

Figuring Out Your Target Heart Rate

L et's take some baby steps, because this is important. First, subtract your age from 220. If you're sixty, you'll get 160. That's your theoretical max. Now take 60 percent of that. (You don't need a pencil and paper: 60 percent of 100 is 60. Okay? And 60 percent of 60 is 36. Add 'em up. Sixty percent of your max is 96. There you go. Now do it for 70 percent. Do it for 80 and 90 percent, too. Memorize those numbers. Or do the math again in your head, you clever girl. Fight Alzheimer's.) The three paces, as you should know by now, are long and slow (60–65 percent of max), high endurance (70–85 percent of max), and anaerobic (85–100 percent of max). Know your personal beats-per-minute for those three ranges.

unpleasant, it gets in the way of your endless lying about how hard you work out. You may find other reasons for not doing it. Well, fine! It's your miserable body. But you should know this: *Every single soul who cares about training swears by the heart monitor.* Every single one, from the gods of sport right down to me. It is the device that defines the terms for everyone's workouts. Including yours.

A heart monitor is a two-piece gizmo: One piece is like a wristwatch and the other is the band you put around your chest. Simplest thing in the world. The band picks up your heartbeat and radios the news to the watch. Tells you how many beats per minute (bpm), instantaneously and constantly. Not bad for sixty bucks, which is about what the simple versions go for in discount places.

Read the directions (they're obvious) and put it on . . . try working out with it on for a couple of days. See what you see. Figure out your theoretical maximum heart rate using this simple formula: 220 minus your age. That gives a rough maximum heart rate number. Pretty soon, you'll want something more accurate, but this is fine for now. Then just go through your normal workout and look down once in a while; see what percentage of your max you're working at. Do not try to go to your theoretical max until you're in really great shape, if ever.

At some fairly early point, you might also want to know your resting heart rate. There are hip communities where people talk about their resting heart rate at cocktail parties; you might as well be ready. Your resting heart rate is a vague index of the kind of shape you're in. More importantly, *changes* in your resting heart rate are a pretty good indicator of your own relative condition from day to day. The way you get it is like this: Put the gadget on the bedside table when you go to bed. When you wake up the next morning, put on the strap and put the watch on your pillow where you can see it. Go back to sleep. Almost. When you're drowsy and can barely open your eyes, sneak a peek at the monitor. What does it say? Is it around 50 . . . 60 . . . 70? Good. That's your resting heart rate. Tell everyone about it. Over time, as you get in better shape, your resting heart rate should go down some. And if you wake up some morning and it's abnormally high, that may be a sign that you're coming down with a cold. Or you're hungover. Or you're overtraining. Or your heart is going to stop later in the day (just kidding). If your resting heart rate is high, back off on the intensity of your workouts for a while, until your resting heart rate comes back down.

Harry thinks that knowing your resting heart rate is the cat's whiskers. If you agree, you'll want to check it every morning without the monitor. (We're weird, but we do not suggest keeping your monitor as a bedside companion for the rest of your life.) Just check it the old way—with a finger to your throat or wrist. Keep your eye on a second hand and start counting. Do it for ten seconds, multiply by six and there you go. Easy-peasy. That system is too slow and cumbersome to use on the road or on your bike, but it's fine for this once-a-day test.

This next bit is much more important. Once you're in decent shape, you'll want to figure out your *real* maximum heart rate, which is probably higher than the one you get with the simple formula. If you use the wrong max, all the percentages—and all of our excellent advice—become useless.

The way to get your real max is to work out pretty damn hard. Once you're in great shape, crank it up until you're doing, say, 90 percent of your theoretical max. How do you feel? Do you have another 10 percent in you before you fall on your face? Try it out. Sniff around your theoretical max, if you feel pretty good. Go beyond it, if you can. Remember, your real max is the real-world peak—the pace you can maintain for only sixty seconds or so, going flat out. Don't try to get to your actual max unless you're in fabulous shape (and you've had that physical we told you to get), but get up into the neighborhood and assume that that's 90 or 95 percent of your actual max. Recalculate your numbers, based on the new assumption. It's worth going through all this. My theoretical max, for example, is 150. My actual max is 170. That's a huge difference, and if I were not aware of it, my workouts would get all messed up.

You might think that another good way to find out your real max would be a stress test. I mean, there you are, working out like a lunatic, with a nice heart doctor right at your side to save your life if you go over the line. But it doesn't work out that way. Turns out that the docs who give stress tests just aren't interested in your maximum heart rate. They don't need it for what they do; it takes longer and they're just not into it. So you probably have to grope around on your own.

Recovery Rate

Want another neat number you can boast about? Try your recovery rate—the speed with which your heart rate drops in the sixty seconds after you've gone from peak exertion to a walk. This is the best, most readily available indicator of your aerobic fitness.

Let's say you're thrashing along on your stationary bike at 130 beats per minute, which is, maybe, 80 percent of your max. Now just pedal easily and watch both the monitor and the second hand on a watch. The instant your heart rate drops one beat (be sure to wait for it to go down one tick before you start timing; it often goes up when you first slow down), start timing. See how many beats per minute your heart rate drops in sixty seconds. Anything over 20 bpm is satisfactory; more is better. If it drops less than 20, you need a lot more work on your aerobic base. If your recovery rate goes to 30 or 40, tell absolutely everyone you know. It will bore them stupid. The day it hits 50, please call Harry and tell him. I would like to know, too, but I will probably be busy that day.

A One-Hour Hike in the Mountains

And now for a live demonstration of the heart monitor at work . . . it may give you a better idea of how it functions and why it's worth fooling with. This part of the book was written during a work/ski vacation in Aspen, where we lived for a while. Most mornings I'd work out for an hour or so before sitting down to the computer. Here's one of those workouts.

It's the fourth day of our stay. I'm used to the altitude, but I'm still on New York time so I'm up at five. It's dark out, even after breakfast, but I can see that it snowed several inches last night. I dress warmly in layers, grab the dog, and drive to the bottom of the Smuggler Mine Trail. Aengus, the Weimaraner, is ten years old, but he's doing 360s in the snow while I lace up my boots. He loves this stuff, and so do I. Old boys at play.

Smuggler is a steep Jeep trail that rises from about 7,800 feet to some 9,000 feet, all of it affording stunning views of the little town and the ski mountains. I can do the round trip in about an hour in heavy boots in the snow. Local kids probably do it in half that time. At the bottom, I look at my watch and my heart monitor. Resting heart rate: 65. That's great.

I know the climb well and use the monitor to regulate my pace. Warm up at 100–105 bpm (60 percent of my personal maximum heart rate) for the first five minutes. Then up to about 120 bpm (70 percent) for another five minutes. I feel as if I'm walking pretty hard, so I look down at the monitor to check. Oops: 112. I take a deep breath and pick up the cadence. It's amazing how often you *think* you're working out at a certain level but are actually doing less. Gotta have that heart monitor. A third of the way up, I want to get into the mid-130s (high endurance, or 70–85 percent) for ten or fifteen minutes as the road gets steeper and the air a little thinner. There's a telephone pole two-thirds of the way up ... a steep patch. I want to be at 140 (82 percent) when I get there. I speed up slightly and hit 140 just at the pole. Good.

Good views, too. I can see the Sno-Cats working on a race course on the big mountain. Buses and cars full of workmen, coming in from down valley. Breathtaking scenery all around. This is high-endurance aerobics at the high end.

Okay, a little steeper here, and I hold the cadence ... maybe lengthen the stride a bit and get into the upper 140s. My personal maximum heart rate is 170, so 145 is about 85 percent, a serious effort. I want to have an anaerobic rush at the end ... get up into the low 150s, or 90 percent for me. If you're in shape, you're not going to blow a head valve at 90 percent, even at altitude, but it does clear your pipes. We're rounding the last, long switchback. I'm huffing, and my glasses are steamed. Tip back my fur hat ... try to cool down a little.

Still in the mid-140s, I push a bit and break into a very slow jog ... careful on the snow and ice. Pounding along now, pulling like a train, around the last turn and up to the little platform at the top. Bingo! Okay, it took twenty-eight minutes, which is good for me with this footing. And, more important, my heart rate is peaking at 157 bpm, or about 92 percent. Excellent. I can only do a few minutes at this anaerobic level, but that's fine. I have given myself a serious aerobic workout—tougher than I would have managed without a heart monitor—and amused myself, too. That counts.

Now recovery. I immediately check my watch and the

monitor and time myself for sixty seconds from the first instant my pulse starts to go down from 157. Time! Good. It has dropped to 120, or 37 bpm, in sixty seconds. That's terrific. A strong assurance that I'm in pretty good aerobic shape. I may ski into a tree this afternoon, but I probably won't have a heart attack. No guarantees—the heart's a joker—but probably not. I head down the hill at a serious clip, but I can barely hold my heart rate at 60 percent of max. If the footing weren't so slippery, I'd run to keep it a little higher, but I don't want to break my neck. Very important not to bust anything. A couple of times we stop because Aengus has ice stuck between his paws; he still gets to the car ahead of me. We've been gone an hour. Like endurance predators everywhere, we stop to pick up the local paper, get another cup of coffee, and head home. No one else is awake yet; we have stolen a march on the day. And beaten back the tide. All with the help of a little gadget that costs less than sixty bucks.

A Basic Program of Aerobics

Okay, back to basics. We keep protesting that this is not an exercise book, and that's true, but it's going to look an awful lot like one for the next few pages. The reason is that many of Harry's patients and other pals of ours ask for a simple exercise program to get them through the first weeks and months of working out. So we have put together a one-size-fits-all, three-level regimen. Remember, of course, that one size does *not* fit all in this business, so you'll have to tune it to suit yourself. For example, some people—perhaps many—will spend a long time at Levels One and Two, regardless of how fit they get. We think that every woman really must add weight training as early as possible—that's Level Two. But once you've done that, you can stay at the long-and-slow level forever, if you prefer, even though we think there's a lot to be said for getting into high-endurance and anaerobic exercise. Your choice. Our only caveat is this: Don't kid yourself. Start where you should start and stay there until you're really ready to move on. Consistency trumps intensity every time.

If you're already in great shape, you may be off our exercise charts from the beginning. That's fine. Make your own way with your own trainer or with one of the books on serious endurance training referred to in the Author Notes. But there's one thing that does apply to you, no matter how fit you are, and that is the *mix* of different kinds of exercise we're recommending (eventually aerobic exercise at different levels four days a week and at least two days a week of strength training). That mix is as important to everyone. If you concentrate only on one sport or activity, you inevitably ignore some muscle systems. As you get older, your body will get less and less tolerant of that kind of concentration. The systems and muscle groups that you're ignoring will atrophy and raise hell with the rest of your body. That's what cross-training is all about, and it's important.

It may help to walk you through it in some detail. First, whether you're pretty fit or in god-awful shape, put on your workout duds and your heart monitor, go to the gym or out on the road, *and warm up*! Temperamentally, I am not the warm-up type, but even I have become a true believer. At my age, I can feel the difference. And whether it's happened to you or not, sometime in your fifties or sixties you'll realize that it takes much longer for your blood to start moving and for your muscles and joints to warm up. I need five minutes these days and sometimes more like fifteen. Feel your own way, but don't skimp just because you're in a hurry or feeling great. Even $10 million athletes are forced to warm up so they won't get hurt. The same applies to you.

Here's another thing: A good warm-up is *the* great antidote to injury, and the risk of getting hurt is different as you get older. First, it's easier to get hurt. Second, it's harder to recover. So, warm up.

After the warm-up, slowly increase the intensity of your biking or jogging or whatever you're doing, and get your heart rate up to 60–65 percent of your max and level off. Keep it up for ten or fifteen or twenty minutes that first day, whatever is comfortable. Cool down for a few minutes. Maybe do some stretches. Go home. You have just started the sacred process of building your aerobic base . . . adding a few mitochondria, stringing a few new capillaries, sending some new signals to your whole body. Giving yourself that all-important squirt of C-10. Nice work. Very nice work.

Next day, do the same thing. If the first day knocked you sideways, do less. If you feel pretty good, do more. Keep inching along at the long-and-slow level—with your heart rate at 60–65 percent of max—for all of the first week and maybe for much longer. Your goal is to go long and slow for forty-five minutes without getting wrecked. (Ultimately, of course, you want to be able to do two or three hours of this.) If, at the end of the first week or the second or the third, you still cannot go at 60–65 percent for forty-five minutes, that's fine; just keep on keeping on. It's the very best thing you can do. There's no rush. Building your aerobic base is the most important aspect of this regimen. It is also one of the most important things you will ever do for your body . . . absolutely critical. If you don't get anything else out of this book, learn about your aerobic base and the utter importance of building it up and keeping it strong. Big stuff, ladies. Big stuff for those heart attacks and strokes and lots of those nasty cancers. Building up your aerobic base is a lifesaver. And it makes you feel great.

One of the tip-offs that you are not ready to move on is something you can only get from your heart monitor. If you're tooling along on your treadmill or your bike at 65 percent of your max and your heart rate suddenly spikes up ten or fifteen points, even though you're not working any harder, you've reached your temporary wall for the day. Slow down or, more likely, quit. Resume long and slow the next day.

I'm talking about a spike, not a "drift" upward of five or six beats a minute. Everyone, no matter how fit, experiences some upward drift after working out for a while. Just this morning, I was having an extended long-and-slow day—an easy all-morning bike ride at 60–65 percent of my max. Toward the end, I was biking at about the same clip but my heart rate had gone up to 70 percent. That's drift, not a spike. No reason to slow down or stop. But if it goes to 75–80 percent of max, slow down, or quit and come back tomorrow. If you're just beginning to work out after a long layoff, you may hit that wall in ten minutes, not two hours.

At some point, you must add weights and go to Level Two. We talk about that in Chapters Ten and Eleven, but I mention it here so you can have a complete sense of the program. Read the chapters on strength training before you start, but add weights at some point. Earlier is better.

Eventually, a workout should last forty-five minutes to an hour, including the warm-up and cool-down. That's true of both aerobic and strength training. You can add more time eventually, but forty-five minutes to an hour, six days a week, is plenty. We are not trying to turn ourselves into athletes here; we are trying to live the good life.

You Are an Endurance Predator: Act Like One

Once you can do forty-five minutes of long and slow, it's time to mix in some high-endurance aerobics. That's the next level, the one at which you get to 70–85 percent of your max. It's not absolutely essential that you get to that level, but it sure is a good idea. First, because you use a whole different fuel system and it's sensible to keep all your systems working. Second, you get a great high from all the yummy C-10, which high-endurance exercise generates in massive doses.

You might eventually decide that high endurance is not to your taste, but give it a try. Take a spin with that excellent glucose-burning system; see if you like it. No sense having it, really, if you're not going to use it.

A high-endurance day should go something like this. Warm up, of course; that never changes. Then up to 60–65 percent of your max for five or ten minutes. Then crank it up to 70–75 percent and hold at that level for five or ten minutes. Feel your way. That's intense enough for your high-endurance work in the early stages and maybe forever. Then back down for recovery at 60–65 percent. Over time, be sure to amuse yourself with variations. Make it hard enough to be interesting, but not so hard that you're knocked out. Eventually, you should be able to hold at 70–75 percent for twenty minutes without much strain. After a while, as you know, you should be able to hold it at 70–85 percent of max for an hour or two without flying apart.

If you have trouble getting up to the 70–85 percent level, think about aerobics classes of some kind. I often find it hard to make myself go to high endurance all alone, even though I know it's great for me and that it will feel good. I feel a terrible temptation to dog along at 60–65 percent. But in spin class I *always* get up in the high-endurance range; indeed, that's what spinning is all about. Other types of classes do the same thing.

Or consider a demanding bike ride or hike, like the hike I described taking in Colorado. Most of us don't have a serious hiking opportunity in the backyard, but there are lots of ways to skin the high-endurance cat, and not all of them involve sucking in someone else's exhaust and being yelled at in the gym.

Fight or Flight: Dodging Traffic

The final aerobic stage—adding some real sprints or doing intervals to go to the anaerobic level (85–100 percent of your max)—is completely optional, though pretty good fun if you're in shape. You can't get that special endorphin rush any other way. Or the pleasant knowledge that you won't necessarily be dead meat if you get the ancient "fight or flight" call some dark and stormy night. Going anaerobic is not to be undertaken lightly or unadvisedly, however. It's barely mentioned in our exercise program, because a lot of women of a certain age shouldn't go there. If you do decide to go for it, wait until you're in really good shape and be sure to check with your doctor first.

Okay, the way you get there is this. You go for it. Which probably means doing something along these lines. First, as ever, you warm up. Maybe a little longer than usual, so you won't be as likely to hurt yourself when you really hit it. Then go to, say, 75 percent of your max. On an anaerobic (or "sprint" or "intervals") day, 75 percent is going to be the base you go back to for rest. After ten minutes or so at 75 percent, crank it up to 80–85 percent for a five- or six-minute stretch. Drop back to recovery level (75 percent) for a couple of minutes, then hit it with everything you've got for two minutes. Maybe only one. The object is to get to 85–90 percent of your max at this stage. Now relax and rest at, say, 75 percent of your max for two minutes. Then hit it again, for one minute, as hard as you can. You should be up in the 90th percentile now. Relax for sixty seconds and hit it again. These are "intervals," designed to get your heart rate way up there. You should definitely be in the 90s by this time. You may or may not do a third or fourth interval, but pretty soon it's going to be time for a longer rest, first at 75 percent and then at lower levels. Do one last sprint, if you like, then wind down to 65 percent. Keep working out at low levels until your heart rate drops below 60 percent. Nice work. You're done.

That's our introduction to aerobic exercise. Do some kind of aerobic exercise four days a week forever. You'll get to love it, no kidding.

"Powder Rules Apply"

After soldiering through all this virtuous stuff, you may be thinking, "Is this struggle really worth it?" Well, yes, it really is. You'll feel better *all* the time, and once every so often you'll feel absolutely great. What follows is another payoff story. It should perhaps come after the strength chapters because it involves strength training, too, but you've been through a lot; let's go play in the snow for a few minutes.

One night, toward the end of the Aspen work/ski

vacation I mentioned, we have the dump of the year—almost three feet of new snow. In the morning, the ski patrol runs up the EPIC flag at Highlands, which doesn't happen often, and the powder hounds turn out in force. The powder hounds are the kids who can actually ski this stuff. They live in crummy places and tend the bars, make the beds, and give the massages, just so they can be here on days like this.

They're first in line, and when they get to the top, they head for the steepest places and go flying down. By long tradition, on days like this, they yodel and whoop as they turn, again and again, in the waist-high snow for the sheer joy of the thing. The tourists and the grown-ups, starting their breakfasts down in the town, hear them through the walls and feel a little uneasy. They're a little more petulant and demanding than usual with the young waiters. But the young waiters do not much care about the grown-ups this morning. They hear the whooping, too, and their hearts are in the hills.

My heart is in the hills, as well. Also my aging body. Because I heard about this on the radio when it was still dark out and went straight to the house of our pal Lois. (My wife, Hilary, doesn't ski this stuff.) I dragged Lois out of bed, over the modest objections of her husband and children. Because, on a day like this, it is recognized that ordinary commitments will not be met. The car or the dress will not be ready at four. Sally and Fred will not be at The Bistro at noon, after all. In fact, all bets are off, and Powder Rules Apply. That's the sign they put up in shop windows when they lock the door for the day and head for the mountain. And that's what I tell Lois and Tom when I get to their house, unannounced, at eight. It is not a concept that has to be explained to locals. Tom says that he will be the good guy this time because he really does have to work. Lois grabs a muffin, and we are gone. "Thanks, Tom. So long, Willy . . . Charley." Out of here!

Lois is forty-five, passionate (about everything), funny, and in super shape. She juggles a serious job writing funny stuff for *The New York Times* (that ain't easy), doing a lot of yoga, and taking care of the boys and the house. But not this morning. This morning, it is Tom's turn and, for us, Powder Rules Apply.

Everyone knows that powder skiing is supposed to be great fun, but frankly most people can't do it for squat. They fall all the time, and it takes forever to get up because there's no bottom to push off from. They get scared and sit back on their skis. Fall some more. Their thighs burn. They go home and don't come out again until the snow is packed down. Lois and I are not doing that. We are here. With the kids. And a few other grown-ups her age. And one old girl my age. I don't know her, but we nod to each other. There is an odd Freemasonry of old folks who do stuff, and we often nod to one another, as if we'd met before. This morning, the old girl and I nod and then she grins. Because the EPIC flag is flying and we are here. I grin back, introduce myself. We pat mittens and she says, "Go for it!" That's it.

Up top, it is blue and clear and the thick-laden trees are sparkling. One of those Rocky Mountain miracles you sometimes get. We should have warmed up on an easier trail, but that would have been a waste. The point of a dump is the steeps and deeps. We hustle over to Northstar . . . big, easy turns in deep powder on the upper part, big, steep turns down below. A couple of skiers have been here before us, but every turn is still in virgin snow. Everything is slow motion when you get this right. You're dancing. Very, very slowly, then very, very fast. You feel the swoosh, and the snow flies up over your head. A "face shot," they call it.

In the Bugaboos in the Canadian Rockies, they wear snorkels, sometimes, to breathe. Not here, but it's deep and the snow is incredibly light.

We are in the steeps now. There are always moguls on this pitch, but today they are deep under the snow, like bears asleep under the drifts. We point our skis straight down the steepest pitch, dance around the bears. The gravity pulls us down, the snow holds us up. And we dance in between, side by side. We grin, and we whoop, all the way down. Down the steep, open hill, down through the huge trees in The Glades. Up and across to the Ridge of Bell and into the steeps again.

We do every double black on the hill. Every place it's deep until it's all packed out. We race back up and swing back down. Half the time we are panting to get our breath at the end of a run. Some places, in the trees where the snow is really ridiculous, we struggle. By mid-morning, we are soaked in sweat and feel lovely. And we just keep going. Not in pain, I am thrilled to report. My old quads do not hurt, and they would have hurt like crazy ten years ago. Or twenty. I could not have done this then. Even Lois's quads hurt a little. Because she does not do enough weights. Yoga's great, but there's no substitute for the stinky weights if you're going to do this stuff.

Around two, we are cooked. We have been at it for almost five hours, with pit stops and a quick bite. We get beers and loll for a while at the bottom, with the other kids. Lois and I are exhausted but delighted with ourselves and with our day. We natter like children about this run and that. We boast and take turns praising each other. We think we are wonderful. We sure *feel* wonderful. Then Lois goes home to be there for the boys after school. I go home to bed. And sleep for three hours.

When I wake up, it is dark. I would not have needed that sleep forty years ago, and Lois doesn't need it today. But that's okay. This morning, when they flew the EPIC flag at Highlands, I was in my seventieth year. And I was a powder hound in the hills. And we danced and we whooped as we turned. For the sheer joy of our lives. And perhaps we were heard in the town . . . where the grown-ups were ordering breakfast.

CHAPTER NINE

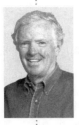

The Kedging Trick

et us have one of those candid moments we sometimes need in this relentlessly cheerful and optimistic book. Let us admit to each other that it is not easy to keep doing exercise six days a week, year in and year out, for the rest of our wretched lives. We may falter. We may slip off to the 7-Eleven . . . buy a pack of ciggies. Or start dunking the Oreos in the peanut butter. Take a jelly jar of bourbon . . . go watch TV. We may, in a word, say the hell with it and go sit down someplace. Scratch our butts. Never exercise again. Sometimes we need help. We *all* do. And, mercifully, Harry and I have just the thing. We are here to introduce you to the mystery of "kedging." Never heard of it? Fine. Nobody else has, either, but it's a terrific notion.

Sailing ships in ancient times—before the invention of the steam engine, the outboard motor and the mood-altering drug—often got becalmed and the crew had to just sit there in a funk. Which was all right some of the time, but not always. Sometimes there were enemy ships, drifting down with dark intent. Or a hostile shore getting closer. Or the sailors were bored stupid and couldn't take it anymore. It was in those circumstances, you will recall, that Agamemnon, desperate to get to Troy to wage war for ten years, sacrificed his daughter, Iphigenia, to whistle up a wind. How's that for an appealingly boyish scheme? Anyhow, it worked fine for a while but ended with appropriately horrid results for himself, his wife (who had to kill him, of course), his kids, and everyone in sight for a long, long time. But never mind that. Just accept that sometimes people get really, really stuck and desperate measures are needed. Kedging is one of the best. *So* much better than killing your husband.

It goes like this. The captain of a becalmed and threatened vessel has a light anchor (called a kedge) loaded into a longboat and rowed half a mile or so away. The longboat crew pops the anchor over the side, makes sure it's "set" on the bottom, and then everyone back on the big boat pulls like demons on the line, literally hauling the ship to the anchor. Then they do the whole business again, until they get where they want to go. Sounds like a lot of work, but maybe worth it if your ship is about to be overcome by Barbary pirates. Or if you, you precious thing, are about to be swept up on the rocks we chatted about, where the gulls and the crabs are waiting to eat your guts.

So . . . kedging: climbing out of the ordinary, setting a desperate goal and working like crazy to get there. To save yourself. Sounds nasty, but in fact all the kedges we have in mind are pretty pleasant. Demanding, but fun. Like signing up for a serious "adventure trip" of some kind, especially one on which men are not invited. Maybe a bike or ski trip (my favorites), or a yoga retreat (one of Hilary's favorites), or a hiking trip, or a week at a great spa. Training for an adventure trip and then doing it *hard* is one of the best kedges there is. The training and anticipation perk you up tremendously and give shape and purpose to your daily training. The trip itself is great fun and—if it's hard enough—gets you in better shape than routine training can ever do. Then the memory and the inspiration linger on for months. A triple-barreled motivator that's a joy to do.

Another, slightly indirect but still effective stunt is to spend too much money on a fancy piece of gear—the world's best bike, hot new skis, or whatnot—and see if that doesn't get you going again. If you're into biking and you buy yourself a snappy new bike, I *promise* you a new lease on life. *Promise it.* But whatever you do, figure out your own kedge. Then you may want to do it two or three times a year. I know this sounds dangerously like self-indulgence, but it's not. Life is going to be very long and you're going to need some tricks. You're going to need a damn good kedge.

Hilly and I just got back from a beauty—a deadly serious bike trip in Idaho with twenty-five close pals, age thirty (some people's children) to seventy (me). Most were in their fifties and sixties, most were couples and most of us had been biking together once a year or so, ever since a few friends casually started a "bike group" a dozen years ago. It began as weekend biking in Connecticut and morphed into serious trips all over the world. For a lot of us, it has turned into one of the nicest things we do. This last trip was a particularly good one.

It was in Idaho, which is about as pretty as it gets on this particular planet, and the company could not have been better. But the biking program was just a teeny bit brutal. Remember my friend Patricia, the Masters athlete? Well, she and her husband live out there, and she was asked to plan the trip. Which was a bold move. For example, the first day was fifty-six miles. *To lunch.* Then it got bad. Mercifully, there were sag wagons for the fallen. In fact, there were three sag wagons: two to pick up the injured and one for the dead. That Patricia, man . . . she thinks of everything. Actually, the beauty of a bike trip is that people can go at their own pace and adjust the length of the day to their own appetites. You want to be motivated, but you don't want to die. Patricia doesn't always remember that. Hilary and I did as much or as little as we wanted—sometimes with the A group, sometimes with B. And sometimes with Team Graceful, a group that I invented a few years ago that bikes harder than the Bs, a little easier than the As and has wine with lunch. Excellent.

But it was the nights that were magical. Especially for me, because I was deep into working on this book and spent most of my time talking to the women about it. There were a dozen women, all of them in semi-great to great shape . . . all of them bright, accomplished, and lovely company. They weighed in heavily on everything from menopause to sexism in the workplace, from empty nesting to "chick trips" to sex-in-your-fifties-and-sixties. There were varieties of experience, of course, but there was a surprising consistency . . . a center of gravity. They all agreed, for example, about the surge of power and confidence at fifty and sixty that I mentioned in the first chapter. Every one of them. And they all agreed about the wonder and importance of a women-only trip.

The Company of Women

have never been on a chick trip, obviously, but I've heard a lot about them and they sure sound like the ideal kedge for women. Happily, they are becoming very common.

The notion is that you and some of your pals make a long-range plan to go ski or hike or bike or do yoga or play serious tennis or some damn thing in some wonderful place and then do it.

The great trick is to put together a compatible group of women (easier than with men, but not a cinch), come up with a great scheme and go for it. The exercise component, I am told, is tremendously important, but it's only part of the magic. Listen to my pal Tina, a successful executive in her fifties: "I really believe in these trips. Women get a much-needed 'time out.' They can drop their roles—wife, mother, career person, errand runner, whatever—and just be a person who needs an opportunity to talk in the company of other women. There is an interesting dynamic when women get together out of their normal environment and are allowed to just be themselves for a while. They get personal, honest. They laugh at themselves and each other, and it's great." She went on to describe a recent adventure she and some friends had on the Salmon River, also out in Idaho. At one point the women all took their clothes off and sat around in a hot spring, laughing and talking. Then they hit the paddles again, hard, liking the realization that, Hey, girls, we can *do* this. For Tina, a chick trip "anywhere, for any length of time, is a real, healing luxury." Want to know something about Tina? She is way, way smart. Listen to her.

Hilary's yoga group goes to what looks to me like some godforsaken dust bowl in Mexico (I've only seen the pictures) and does serious yoga four or five hours a day. There are two leaders, including an excellent and stunning woman named Colleen. I have done a little yoga with Colleen, and I would go to Mexico to watch her play Parcheesi. Anyhow, they do some very serious and slightly competitive yoga—these ladies are in awfully good shape, a lot of them—and Hilary always comes home looking tan and fit. The food—heavy on veggies and beans—sounds nasty to me but is leavened with margaritas, which makes sense after a long day on the old yoga mat. But the conversation and communion, I gather, is the heart of the trip. I get this secondhand, obviously, but it's clear that the level of communication and intimacy goes well beyond anything I know about from coed trips, to say nothing of men's trips. It's interesting, isn't it, how few men's trips there are? And how many of them center around drinking and playing cards and killing stuff. What's that all about? We are a flawed sex . . . that's what. Women have an edge in this area, so take advantage of it. Go on a trip with your pals.

The Serotta Solution

Buying a serious new toy can also be a great kedge. Here's a nice example. When I turned fifty, a long time ago, some pals got together and bought me a sensational racing bike. I hadn't been biking or doing much of anything else for a while, and they thought that was too bad. They turned to a man named Ben Serotta for help. At the birthday party, a cheerful black-tie event, my son Tim rolled out this amazing blue-and-yellow creation to the oohs of the crowd. I still remember one line of his speech: "If Ben Serotta had gone into politics and become a governor, his would have been a happy and a prosperous people. Luckily, he decided to make bicycles instead . . ." And so on. Nice night. It was a serious racing bike and much too short-framed and tender for my modest skills. But it was so damn beautiful—there are few things better-looking on earth than a classic, steel bicycle—that I just couldn't stay off it. I got into biking, big-time, and have never looked back. It is at the heart of my exercise life. I've gotten other bikes since, but I still ride the Serotta now and then, and the rest of the time I keep it in my study in the Berkshires—it's behind me right now—because I'm so grateful to it for getting me back on my pins.

This spring, after a few weeks when I found myself thinking too frequently about Oreos, I went up to Saratoga Springs, New York, to finally meet Ben Serotta. He'd read our first book and said, come on up anytime. He's still an absolute maniac about bikes and a lovely guy. We went for a long ride, talked bikes for hours and hours, and then he set about building me a bright green Serotta "Ottrot," which has been recognized by leading biking magazines as simply the best custom-made bike in the world. What a joy. Once I got it, the vapors disappeared and I got passionately back on the program. Mostly on my new bike. Now Hilary's complaining that *she* has the vapors—which is a lie—because she wants one, too. Okay, in a complicated life, you sometimes need *two* anchors. Two bright green kedges to pull you along for the next twenty years.

Pulling to Paradise

Another toy story. Harry says no one rows anymore, except a handful of people who went to a handful of eastern colleges, so it's dumb or, worse, *elitist* to put pulling boats in the book. But I don't care. Rowing is not elitist. Decent people have been rowing for pleasure since the dawn of history. It is one of the blessings of humanity. What a genius that first person was who jumped on a log and paddled across a river while the enemies stood dumb-founded on the shore. And how about the one who figured out how to sit backwards and row? Or the excellent creature who invented the sliding seat and outriggers so we could row with our legs as well as our arms? Going about in pulling boats is deep in our blood, and the luckiest of us still do it. I do not say that the active woman who lives on the water and knows nothing but the inflatable and the Boston Whaler knows nothing of the sea. But she doesn't know much.

I have wanted a Whitehall skiff with a sliding seat and outriggers for as long as I can remember. Something to row in heavier weather and open water. When Harry and I sold our first book, I had already written the chapter on economy, so I did not squander my advance. But I did buy an overcoat of a curious design, which I had wanted since I was sixteen. And an incredibly beautiful blue pulling boat, made by the good people of Little River Marine, which I named *Yeats* after the poet. She has a lovely wineglass stern and hatchet-shaped oars that are nine feet long and lighter than ski poles. And she pulls like a train . . . one of the nicest motions in the water I have ever felt. There is no better exercise in the world than rowing a single scull or a Whitehall or any other good pulling boat. It's aerobic, of course, but it exercises your whole body while it immerses you in a rhythm and takes you to places that are good for your soul.

Consider Thanksgiving a while back. It was an unusually mild and sunny day for November, and I rowed all the way from Sag Harbor, Long Island, over to Shelter Island and back, a sweet, three-hour pull. There were no other boats. My pulse was a steady 60–65 percent most of the time, so I was adding thousands of those pesky mitochondria and miles of capillaries to my aerobic base, but I wasn't thinking about that. I was thinking about the swans beside me, at eye level, and the slap and whir of their huge wings as they rose off the water. About the seal who followed me for a little ways, curious as a dog. About the magic inlets in the tall marsh grass into which I pulled and sat, invisible, for a while. About the deep, steady rhythm of the rowing and the sweet glide of the boat through the water. And about the good, solid miracle of being younger this year, on Thanksgiving Day, on the water, in *Yeats*. For which I was duly grateful. A boat like this is the perfect kedge to pull yourself into . . . well, into eternity.

And by the way, some of the healthiest women in the entire world—regardless of age or whatever—are the women who row. It actually does something to women's bodies that nothing else can match. And it does it for a lifetime.

I remember a late summer afternoon recently, after a hundred-mile bike ride in the Rockies, with my pal Terry. We rode into the little mountain town of Frisco, where the ride ended, and there was a street fair going on in the middle of Main Street. And, weirdly, here in this remote mountain town, was this stunning woman trying to sell a modern, bright green single scull. What in the world was she doing here? It was as weird as a mermaid turning up on an Iowa farm, but there she was, with this stunning green boat, and we started to talk. She had been in a national championship eight-oared shell that spring. The three of us chatted for a minute, and then she gracefully swung this twenty-foot boat up over her head and easily walked down toward the mountain lake at the end of the road. Kedging at the high end.

The General Rule of Gear

There is one black-letter rule that you should know and act upon as you get older: *Get good gear.* This advice does not quite make it into the pantheon of Harry's Rules, but it makes fine sense. It is not so easy, after all, to bike a hundred miles a day when you're in your sixties, to windsurf in high winds in your fifties, to ski the deep powder in your seventies. Come to think of it, it's not *that* easy just to get out of bed in the morning and train, six days a week. So, if you're doing it, you deserve decent gear. Skimp on washing machines and junk like that. Buy good gear.

Bear in mind that gear has gotten so much better in most sports over the last twenty years. Parabolic skis have absolutely revolutionized skiing. Made it radically easier to be an intermediate skier and quite a lot easier to be an expert. Your 1975 Heads were hot when you bought them, but now they're dangerous relics. Same with bikes. I love my old Serotta, but it is not in the same league with the new one. And while there is still room in the decent heart for steel (especially if you can afford an elegant Richard Sachs), most steel bikes cannot compare with composites and titanium for a great ride. And peppy? These new bikes practically rear up and whinny when you put your foot down. Same with the equipment in a lot of sports. So buy new stuff.

I have had a hellish time with Harry on this subject, because he's so conservative. He was a serious biker as a kid and has a bike on which he literally biked across the country twenty-five years ago. Today, in my modest opinion, it is a lovable piece of junk. But will Harry pitch it and get something good? No! He has all those New England virtues, peculiarly including the one that makes spending money physically painful and the wearing of ancient clothes and fixing of equipment a spiritual lift. Harry owns one sweater. What a curse! Does he have any notion how long the sweater will last? Actually, I'm making some progress with him. He's seen the new Serotta, and he's beginning to yearn and plan. Get ready, Ben.

Buying is good. I am one of the handful of men who understand the urgency of buying good shoes, for example. I drag Hilary into shoe stores, not out. So I understand the shopping impulse. And the urgency of buying good gear rises above even the new-shoe imperative. Good gear is not a "toy," and it is most assuredly not an indulgence, as brain-dead husbands so often say of shoes. It is lifesaving machinery. No one can quarrel with this analysis. If your husband resists you on this, leave him.

A Bad Trip

All right, candor is the watchword for this chapter, so we're going to end on a candid note. These kedging trips can be luxurious (I'm thinking of my favorite Butterfield & Robinson bike tours). But not always. Sometimes they're not even safe. So I must urge you to be flexible in your expectations because, as I discovered last winter, it is possible to err. To get hurt. Humiliated. Ashamed. Here's a heartbreaking story. A while back, a pal named Cheeb, whom I've known since first grade, called to say he had an idea for the book: I should join him for his annual Masters ski racing clinic in Stowe, Vermont, in December. I could report on old folks at play, sharpen my skiing skills and have something to get in shape for. Fine. These things all sound fine, six months in advance.

I hadn't been to Stowe for thirty years, since I discovered

western skiing, and kind of wanted to go back now that I thought I was hot. Not Cheeb-level hot, but better than I'd been in 1970. I wanted to show off to the ghost of my old self. Besides, I had relatives up there. Sort of. A Quaker branch of Mother's family had farmed in Stowe for a hundred years before anyone thought about skiing. I had met the last of them, the three "Bigelow girls," when Mother drove us up there in September of 1941 in her green La Salle.

I loved that trip. Mother talking about Eliachim Bigelow (Uncle Like) mowing the fields with a yoke of oxen when she was a kid in the 1890s. Me getting a lesson in milking cows (I can still feel that cow's udder in my nervous hand, even though I haven't touched one in sixty-five years). And the Bigelow Girls, quilting, arguing, and "thee-ing and thou-ing" each other in Quaker-speak on the plain, covered porch. "Annie! Where is thy echustechon?" That's an ear trumpet. (Think of it: I saw a woman use an *ear trumpet*.) The girls would all be in the little cemetery now, behind the big white church in the middle of town, but that was okay. The farm would still be there. I could go see that. And I would stop by the cemetery and pay my respects.

I had only seen the farm a couple of times, but it was oddly important to me. Mother had gone there often when she was little, and she talked about it all the time. And the Bigelow Girls, who helped raise her, had lived there all their lives. That lovely old farmhouse, looking out over the Green Mountains, and a half-dozen other family farms in our past, in Danvers and Tiverton and Nantucket, which I had also heard about . . . they purred away in memory, just below the surface. Made me feel a little less scared in this hectic world as we go racketing along toward . . . some damn thing.

The cemetery was covered with snow. I never found the farm. And the ski part wasn't so great, either: it was scary and shaming. The hitch was Cheeb and his little pals. It was the Patricia syndrome. They were very serious ski racers. I do not mean "Last one to the bottom is a rotten egg!" I mean Masters racing. With gates. And strange costumes. And danger.

At some level, I had known this, and as the time came closer I tried to back out. I was not in good enough shape, I said. I'd been sick. I'd been traveling. The dog had eaten my homework. I told Hilary, and she said, good, she'd been afraid I'd get hurt.

"Oh," I said stupidly, "that's not it. It's the embarrassment. I'll look like an idiot."

Hilary paused for exactly one second. "You mean you're quitting because you're going to be embarrassed?"

I said petulantly that I wasn't "quitting"; I just wasn't starting. Because I had been sick. And maybe a little fat. Not in truly great shape.

"But this whole book," she said, "is you and Harry dragging these poor people out of their houses to gyms, where they're going to be embarrassed for months. And you're staying home because you might be embarrassed for five days? That's appalling!"

Yap, yap, yap. Then she called Harry and he piled right on. The toad. "If that's really it," he said when I took the phone, "I think that's a little raw. Besides, if you were humiliated some, it might be terrific for the book. Hilary's right that we may be a bit haughty here and there. This might be good for you."

"For *me*! What about you! There's no creature on earth haughtier than a nice warm doctor prescribing outdoor exercise for some fat, terrified old creature who wants nothing more than to sit and watch TV. If we need to be chastened, why don't *you* go to the stinking race camp?"

"Can't," Harry said serenely. "Too young. And I have a day job, as you know. Besides, it's not that you're *that* much haughtier than me . . ." He paused as he thought about that for a moment. "It's for the book in general. For both of us, really. And the reader. Very humanizing."

"I don't *need* humanizing, for God's sake. It's the one trait I have in abundance. *You* go." And so on. But of course he couldn't. Or wouldn't. He and Hilary were a wall against me. I sent in the check. And desperately tried to get in shape in three short weeks.

Let me say just a little bit about the training effort. It's pretty dull, but it does tell you a couple of things you should maybe know about cross-training, warming up, and virtuous stuff like that. To begin with, I started exactly the wrong way by trying to do too much. I wasn't in bad shape, obviously, but I was not quite ready for a Masters ski racing camp. Masters-level skiers are a different breed. So I leapt into a high-intensity conditioning class with lots and lots of quad-crushing crouches, leaps, and push-ups. When I joined the other boys and girls in class (none over thirty-five in this little cadre of killers), they'd been doing it for months. I thought, hell, I've been using my quads, hard, for years now. No problem.

Problem. It's the same muscles, but apparently you come at them a different way and they aren't ready. Biking and spinning are great, but they strengthen your legs in a narrow band. I was now outside that band. Way outside. It was kind of fun for a while. We'd leap over a nine-inch step and down into a deep crouch, our palms touching the floor, way off to one side. Then, quick, leap across the step into the same crouch, on the other side. Then do it again. About twenty times. Well . . . okay. I did that. But that took about two minutes and this was an hour-long class. It got much,

much worse. One little number I remember: jump up in the air ten times, then immediately throw yourself on the floor and do a matching set of ten push-ups. It just happens that, today, I can do ten pathetic push-ups . . . a miraculous improvement over five years ago when I couldn't do any. But that turned out to be an introductory bit of fun. Now do nine jumps. Now nine push-ups. And so on. And when you get to one, soaked in sweat and blood, do you quit? Not a bit of it. Go back to ten. Repeat entire progression five times.

I could not "repeat entire progression" once. So I stood there and watched, like a bull that has been cut a little too deep by the picadors. I had to quit long before they were done. It wasn't the aerobics, interestingly. It was the muscles. They were screaming.

I was crippled for days. Crippled so badly that it hurt to walk. Hell, it hurt to sleep. Okay, three lessons for all of us: One, if you're an old girl, don't go into a new sport or training activity at full bore. Let your muscles get used to it, even if you're in decent shape. Two, do some cross-training as a regular part of your routine, so you'll have some range and flexibility. Three, when you pop that kedging anchor into the ocean, let go before it hits the water or it will pull you to the bottom.

Going to Stowe: Real Women at Play

A Masters ski racing clinic is a coming together of fifty or sixty crazy people, in this case New Englanders aged forty-five to eighty-eight (sic), who are fond of ski racing. Terminally fond of ski racing. You are familiar, are you not, with the famous distinction between chalk and cheese? Well, the recreational skier (me) is as much like the racing skier (these birds) as chalk is like cheese. I had no more business in a Masters ski racing clinic than a golden retriever. For one thing, I am a rational man. Ski racers are crazy as loons, and the women are worse than the men.

Consider the scene on the third and worst day of camp. It's 7:45 in the warm-up hut near the gondola. This is *eastern* skiing. The warm-up hut is a huge, Spartan shed of the type used in Aspen to shelter large animals. There is a tiny commissary where nasty food is sold at low prices that would be astonishing if the food were edible, which it is not. That doesn't matter because the good folk who ski here are New Englanders, and they bring their own lunch in brown paper bags. Which they fold up and reuse, day after day. Their food is nasty, too, but at least they don't have to pay for it. They don't care about food anyway; they care about skiing. They care too much. It snowed a lot yesterday, but today rain is expected. Most of these folks have brought huge garbage bags in which to ski when rain really starts to come down. I do not have a garbage bag. I will not need it.

At one end of the shed, my new friends are putting on their things so they can be on the slopes by 8:00, when it may or may not be daylight up here. I have been skiing most of my life and am familiar with many of its little rituals, but there are some new things going on here. Not just the garbage bags. Worse.

A group of nice-looking women, in their mid to late sixties, are matter-of-factly strapping hard plastic protectors to their shins. Others are calmly strapping similar gear to their forearms. I am a bit of an equipment freak, and there is very little ski equipment of which I do not own several versions. I have never seen these things before. I have never *heard* of them. I learn that it's called "armor" and is favored by slalom racers all over the world. It's so basic, indeed, that one little old lady, who has left hers at home, is quietly cutting pieces off a big cardboard box with her own Leatherman knife and shaping them into homemade armor. She fits the cardboard to her shins and straps it on with duct tape. Which she happens to have with her. I feel ill.

An eighty-six-year-old man sits in a corner fooling with his helmet with *his* Leatherman. He is making sure that the face guard is securely screwed on. I have never seen a face guard on a ski helmet. Every person in the room but me has one. "What is this madness?" I ask Cheeb plaintively. "Why are we in this grim room, in the dark, with these elderly lunatics? And what are they doing?"

We are here, Cheeb explains cheerfully, and they are dressing up, because this is "slalom day." You, Chris, may be going a bit slower and will not have a problem, but these sexa-, septua- and octogenarians will be flying down the ice ruts and will want to protect themselves as they deliberately crash over the slalom poles that indicate where they are to turn. It develops that these poles, which obstruct the reasonable route down the hill, are on springs or gimbals and can be knocked down by the sturdier skier. Only the ski boots of these people will be on the "right" side of the poles. The rest of their screaming, wrinkled bodies will be canted dangerously over the poles, which must of course be gotten out of the way. So they'll smack them smartly with their arms, lower legs, jaws or what have you. It's what they like. They look forward to the day.

I do not. I wish to go to my home. I suggest to Cheeb that this might make sense. "No," says Cheeb, "you'll do fine. I've seen you ski for two days, and you'll be fine."

Well, that was a little lie. I did do it, but I was not fine. I went tearing down the dear old mountain at what seemed to me breakneck speed, screaming into and out of the icy ruts, smacking into the terrible poles (occasionally) and often shooting out of the course completely and heading for the woods. I was scared, clumsy, and embarrassed the whole day. Just as I'd known I would be. You cannot conceive how dangerous and unpleasant it is to ski a tight series of deep, ice-walled ruts, even at modest speeds, under the highly critical eye of people who have been doing it, on purpose, for fifty or sixty years. Never, never again.

But there were some wonderful things.

These people—many in their sixties but a good many in their seventies and eighties—were beautiful skiers. There was one elegant, sixty-five-year-old woman who had been first alternate for the 1960 Olympics and, believe me, she looked it. And the two men and one woman in their eighties . . . I could not believe how lithe they were. Not creaking along, not taking a last run for old times' sake. But skiing hard, with obvious pleasure. There was one woman—perhaps in her late fifties—who was one of the most beautiful skiers I've ever seen. A tall, handsome Scandinavian, she went sloping through those gates with incredible grace. Cheeb said she looks exactly the same at fifty miles an hour, which she hits routinely. I have never skied fifty miles an hour and don't intend to. But I might go back to see her do it.

Another reason I might *conceivably* go back, perhaps for a day or two, is that I have never learned so much, so fast. Terrific racing instructors helped a lot, but mostly it was my fellow skiers. They *all* felt free to give pointers to someone as clueless as me. The way grown-ups used to feel free to lecture everybody's children when I was little. One of the old ladies rounded on me sharply and said, "For God's sake, get your feet apart!" "I have got my feet apart!" I whined. "Oh, puh-leeze," she snorted. "Like this!" And off she sailed. Turns out that she was the near-Olympian. So I spread my legs a little.

One night, in a modest "chalet" with deep roots in the 1950s, there was a cocktail party—a Vermont cocktail party with five different kinds of potato chips and a dip made from dehydrated onion soup. It was fun. The group, a club of Masters racers who have been together for twenty years, knew and liked each other well. There was lots of ski talk, lots of race talk, and lots and lots of old-pal gossip. Good scene. We talk later in the book about the need to make new connections (and keep old ones) as you get older. These men and women had that project well in hand. That's a basic life tip, by the way: Make a sports or athletic group—like your bike or swim pals—into a "connect and commit" support group. Like a book group, only stronger. And weirder.

Talk about life-affirming! There was one handsome old gent whose brand-new wife had just joined the group. They were both serious skiers and absolutely blooming about their new life together. He was eighty-eight and she was eighty-five; they looked and sounded to be in their early sixties. Cheeb told John, the guy, that I had lived in Aspen for a while, and he was immediately curious. Turns out he had an interesting stake in the town. He was there the day it was invented. He had been in the fabled 10th Mountain Division at Camp Hale during World War II, one of the ski troopers who had fought ferociously in the Italian mountains and then become the founding fathers of skiing in America. This newlywed had led a group on overnight maneuvers from Camp Hale to what was then the dying mining town of Aspen. One of his troopers was the young (later legendary) Friedl Pfeiffer, who said, "This would be a great ski town. I'm coming back after the war." He did, and the rest is skiing history. And the new wife? She just glowed away as he told the story . . . reminded him of stuff he'd left out. A nice couple, and having a sensational time together. Starting at eighty-something. Happens a lot.

On the fourth day, I got a massive break. It snowed. A lot. Two feet, easy. A near record in this ice-hell. And it was powder, too, not the usual eastern muck. You cannot run races in that much snow, so school was out and we had a day of free play. Now, those old giants can ski anything, most assuredly including powder, but it was a bit of an equalizer. We skied until it was almost dark, men and women alike rejoicing in the powder like mad creatures. Including the eighty-year-olds, right down to the last run. I cannot tell you what a kick it was to go flying down those hills in deep powder, side by side with those people.

Okay, there are a couple of morals to be drawn. Doing stuff that scares the hell out of you—or embarrasses you or makes you feel like a dope—does have a place. In most cases it can't kill you, and the learning curve can be exhilaratingly steep. It opens your head up at an age when you're tempted to shut it down. Besides, scary is memorable. One of the curses of getting older is that time speeds up and the days seem much the same. Well, you want to slow time down? Remember some things? Go to race camp if you're not a racer. Go on a long bike ride if you're not a biker. I will remember that week in Stowe, clearly, until the day I die.

Last point: role models. I do not for a minute suggest that what real athletes like Cheeb and his pals do "informs" the lives of simple folk like you and me. But there *were* three octogenarians out there skiing. They did not all look great all the time, but they looked pretty damn good. My goal? I don't want to be a Masters skier, but I want to be out there. When I'm eighty-five. Or ninety. And I want you to be out there, too. Going for it.

Actually, "going for it" is what kedging is all about. There are as many kedging trips and kedging devices as there are good ideas, but the unifying theme is this: Make it serious. Make it fun. And go for it.

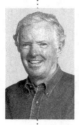

CHAPTER TEN

A World of Pain: Strength Training

How many times has someone slid up to you and said, "Hey, I've got a neat idea! Let's go down to the gym and lift incredibly heavy weights until it hurts like crazy and we have to stop!" Once a week? Once a year? Let me guess. Never? And why is that? Because lifting weights is stupid, embarrassing and painful, that's why.

I remember the first time I decided to venture into a weight room. It was when we lived in Aspen, where they tend to hide weight rooms in "spas," which look deceptively normal at street level. Lots of expensive shrubbery, lots of glass. A girl just inside the door takes your dough and signs you up for a year. It happens very fast. The pretty girl takes your credit card and says, "I'm Chanterelle, by the way. Let me show you the pool." Which she does. It's nice. Then the cheerful room full of aerobic dancers. The step machines and the stationary bicycles. Nice. It all looks nice.

Then it's time to get down to business: "So, look, do you, uh ∴ have a weight room?"

A cloud passes over Chanterelle's face. "Sure, sure. Let's go take a look." A hurried glance back at the counter and the mouthed words "Run his card!" Then down the rubber steps into an underground space that looks like a cross between the engine room of a World War I destroyer and a dominatrix's mudroom. Lots of tile and mirrors. Drains in the floor, so it can be hosed down when they're done with you. Huge steel machines with black pads all over. Lifting machines, twisting machines . . . machines to pull the teeth out of a Caterpillar tractor. And lots of sleek wires that seem to be used to tie women up and make them grunt. Men, too. Men with weird veins running all over their arms and necks. Like fat worms under the skin. Veins like macaroni on acid and biceps that look as if they've been blown out. This is a scary place.

"Listen, you probably have a lot to do. I'll just—"

"No, no," Chanterelle says quickly. "You've already paid. You're dressed. Let me just get Lance. Oh, Lance . . ."

Up hulks this guy with a deep tan and more teeth than you've ever seen in one mouth before. Sort of nice-looking, but something's terribly wrong. Like his body doesn't quite make sense. And the planes of his face . . . they're way too sharp. This guy is . . .

"Hi, let me show you around." It's Lance, and he begins this rap about the machines and his special training techniques. But you're not listening . . . you're just staring, nervously. At his body. Because it's becoming clear to you that he is almost certainly an android. And the manufacturer has scrimped on the little life-giving details that are so important. Maybe a foreign manufacturer, too, because he's dressed funny. His little red shorts look much too small on his huge thighs. And he's wearing a sleeveless T-shirt with enormous armholes through which it is impossible not to see his pecs, or whatever they're called. And his armpits. His armpits are the deepest and furriest you have ever seen. You could raise wolverines in there. You want to take a step back so he won't drip testosterone all over your new sneakers. You want to get the hell out of there . . .

Why, you ask yourself, why is this man telling me all this in a book promoting exercise? I am telling you this because I want to persuade you to find a strength trainer—maybe not as bad as Lance, but bad—and learn to do weights. And then do them two days a week for the rest of your life. And I want you to know that Harry and I realize this is not an intuitively appealing idea. Regular strength training for life sounds stupid, nasty, and scary. And we wouldn't even mention it if it were not one of the best pieces of advice in the whole damn book. Especially for women, who have to worry more about osteoporosis. Strength training will make you feel good and stay healthy for the rest of your life— once you get over the shame and terror and revulsion of going to the gym. In fact, it's so important that Harry has memorialized it in his Third Rule, which goes like this: *Do serious strength training, with weights, two days a week for the rest of your life.* Maybe three would be better; it's okay to do strength and aerobic stuff on the same day. You're allowed to do that.

The Payoff

You will perhaps remember how we talked about the tide that sets against you by the time you're fifty? The tide that threatens to wash you up on the beach where the gulls and the crabs are waiting to do unpleasant things? There are aspects of that tide to which women are peculiarly susceptible. Like crippling falls, disfiguring bone misalignments, and the like because of the wildly unfair business of losing bone mass at the rate of 2 percent a year that Harry will talk about in the next chapter. As he will say, lifting weights is the single most important thing you can do to resist that horror and keep your skeleton functional. Super important, obviously. You don't have to turn into a gym rat, but it sure does make a world of sense to do some weight lifting, starting right now and continuing for the rest of your life.

In addition to saving your bones, there's muscle mass. That goes, too. Out with the tide. Turning the sweet muscles of your youth into the dusty drapery of old age. Makes you too weak to do stuff. Like run across the street if you have to. Or get out of the tub. Or ski. No matter what, you're going to lose muscle cells as you age; that's one of the things you cannot change. But you can beef up the surviving cells—which have tremendous redundant capacity—to offset much of that loss.

Your joints—the meshing bones and the tendons and sinews and the goopy pads that make them work—are also important at your age because they go to hell first if you don't do something. The little grippers that attach tendon to bone get brittle and weak as you age. They atrophy. They let go without notice. And the goopy pads between the bones dry out and you make little crunching sounds when you move. And you hurt. The combination of all this stuff is aging joints, and it has more to do with your aging than almost anything else. When your joints go, you hurt all the time. You walk funny. You fall down. You get old.

Sounds bad, right? Well, here's the weird thing. Lifting big, heavy weights stops most of that. Lifting heavy weights every couple of days basically stops the bone loss . . . stops (or offsets) the muscle loss . . . stops the weakening of tendons, restores the goopy pads, and gets rid of the pain. Aerobic exercise does more to stop actual death—by heart attack and lots of cancers—but strength training can make your life worthwhile. It keeps your muscle mass from going to muck, your skeleton from turning to dust, your joints from hurting with every lousy step you take. This is key. We would not put you through the horror of weight training if it were not key. Here's another odd thing. After you've been doing it for a while, you kind of get into it. But we'll come back to that.

So what do you do? Hire a trainer, at least to get started. Trainers are expensive, Lord knows, but they're worth it, at least to begin with. Learning to do weights is a little harder than it looks, and a surprising number of people you see in the gym are doing it all wrong. Doing it wrong is both counterproductive and dangerous. Not "kill you" dangerous, but "hurt your joints and drive you away" dangerous. So hire a trainer for the first few workouts. And go back once in a while to keep yourself honest. Besides, for most of us, the world of weight lifting is such a strange land that it doesn't hurt to have a friendly guide to get you past the weirdness.

"Your Body Cannot Be a Walkin' Contradiction!"

Consider my favorite trainer, Audrey, a short, regular-looking Jamaican woman in her early fifties. She's no chiseled hardbody, but she knows exactly what she's doing, and how to get you to do what *you* should be doing. Interestingly, she is by far the most successful trainer in a fancy chain of gyms. She's tough, loves to laugh, and is remorseless. I told her about going on TV to promote these books, and she redoubled her exhortations. "Chrees!" she said to me in this lovely, lilting Jamaican accent. "This is see-ri-ous beesness! Your *bahdee, Chrees* . . . your bah-dee (pause for effect) cannot be (pause) . . . a walkin' contra*dic*-tion! Chrees . . . they will know you are livin' a *lie*!" And another twenty whatevers.

If money is an issue—money is *always* an issue—you can get started by reading a decent book on the subject. There are any number of books that offer good guidance and neat little drawings or photos of men and women doing stuff. But stay away from the books that promise to do it all for you in five minutes a week or some such nonsense. And avoid the temptation to buy one of those snappy gadgets on TV that promise to do all the work, without any unpleasant input from you. You're a grown-up, right? Then don't be a dope. The gadgets, or the weights, do not do the work. You do.

Okay, go to a decent gym and hire the nicest, smartest man or woman you can find. I was kidding about Lance and telling the truth about Audrey. There are some scary gym rats out there, but there are also plenty of informed people who are seriously interested in how bodies work and in making yours work better. It's a hot little field these days, and good people are going into it.

Do not make the mistake of hiring some person who just talks to you. Or listens. The gyms are full of women, in particular, who pay big bucks to have trainers chat with them and occasionally hand them a light weight. Chatting is good. We have almost a whole chapter on chatting and how it's the woman's great gift in the Next Third. But it ain't lifting weights. No. If you want to fool around under the guise of exercise, play golf. If you're going to do weights, do weights. It is not supposed to be restful.

Some Training Tips

H arry and I are not the ones to tell you what machines or free weights to use and how to do it; we leave that to your trainer and the books. But we do have a couple of points. First: You are forty, or fifty, or sixty . . . you are not twenty or thirty. Second: You are here to be younger *next year,* not next week. You don't want to make a mess of things in the first few days. So, much as it runs against my temperament to say it, take it easy. If you're one of the handful of women your age who's in great shape, take it *sort of* easy. If you're like the rest of us, take it *really* easy. In the next chapter, Harry will tell you that you can build muscle pretty quickly, even at your age, but joints take much, much longer. Strong muscles can pull weak joints apart. So, in the first few months, do less weight than you can handle and more reps—maybe twenty instead of the usual ten or twelve. Give your joints time to get in the game.

Women vary—surprise—but it is my observation that women, more than men, tend to dog it a little on weights. I see an awful lot of women in gyms with very light weights, going very slowly, with very long delays between sets. Lots of pausing to drink water, wipe the fevered brow, and all that. But sooner or later you gotta go for it or this stuff doesn't work. Go light, with high reps, in the beginning, when you're developing the all-important "muscle memory." Then go for it. Be strong, suck it up, do your job.

You may not think it, but using weights is a little like learning a new sport—not as complex as skiing or tennis, but a new sport just the same. And your muscles have to learn how. That's less true with the machines, which is why machines are more seductive and fun to use. And, tragically, why free weights are so much better for you. Free weights involve balancing and subtle corrections from side to side, all of which use and strengthen a whole bunch of other muscles and, more important, zillions of neuroconnectors, which are at the heart of your ability to function in the real world. It's not just the strength that matters, it's the *wiring,* too. The amazing message system that tells you where you are in the world and lets you function. By all means, use machines to get started and mix machines into your strength training indefinitely, but get into free weights, too.

This is just an aside at this point, but it goes to the free weight question. Riding a stationary bike in a spin class is analogous to using machines for weight training. It's wonderful, but not as wonderful as riding outside, the analogue to free weights. When I ride a real bike, outside, my heart rate routinely goes 15 percent higher than it usually goes in spin class. Not because I'm trying harder, but because real biking is a little harder—and thus a little better for you. There's more going on. There's all that balancing all the time . . . all that looking around at the real world to see where you are and what's coming up. And there are those millions of tiny adjustments every minute to take account of the real world and balance and Lord knows what else. That stuff takes energy. And it's super for you. It brings all those pesky neurotransmitters back to life and makes them strong. The stationary bike cannot do that. Moral: *Free weights are much more complex and much better for you.* So get into them eventually. But let's be fair: doing any weights is a torment and doing machines is just fine if that's all you can stand. Most days, it's all I can stand. I hate free weights. And fear them. Seems reasonable.

Eventually you have to get to heavy weights and low reps. You have to do weights "to failure" some of the time. That means a touch of pain. That means lifting weight that

The "Bulk Up" Fantasy

Whenever I talk about this stuff, the one thing I always hear from women is that they're afraid doing weights will make them "bulk up." This is absolute lunacy. First, it doesn't happen. Second, so what if it did? And third, this is the silliest excuse for idleness you'll find in an area where silliness is the rule.

The fear, I guess, is that muscles on a woman will make her look too masculine and drive the poor boys away. Or, much worse, she'll get big meaty thighs. But working out does not make thighs meatier. It makes them *work better*. It makes them *stronger*. It makes them more shapely. Besides which, women who happen to be blessed with strong legs and thighs to begin with are the truly lucky ones. We are mammals, after all. And the fun of being a mammal . . . the essence of being a mammal . . . is moving around. On our legs, for God's sake. If you want to have scrawny little pins and sit around like a fern, okay . . . but that's not what we're for. We are designed to *move*. That's what makes us feel right. And having a good set of wheels, having strong calves and thighs, is one of the high blessings for our breed.

Finally, the notion of what looks good in women's bodies is, blessedly, changing. Title IX has swept through, and athletics are now part of women's lives. Women are no longer supposed to lounge on divans and be helpless, like Daisy in *The Great Gatsby*. Women do stuff today. And they look it. And those who are not idiots like what they see.

you can lift, say, only ten times before you literally cannot do it anymore. Sounds nasty, doesn't it? Sounds like a guy thing. But it's not. That's how this process works. Men's and women's bodies do not vary one bit in this important respect.

You build muscle by tearing it down. It's all part of the growth and decay business that Harry is teaching us about. But this goes beyond inflammation. What you actually do—and this is Harry's language—is "microscopically damage" your muscles by lifting heavy weights. When they grow back, they're bigger and stronger. Your bone mass increases at the same time. And you gain tendon strength. And neuroconnector strength, which may be the most important of all.

To make real progress on the strength front, you may have to go to three days a week. (My trainer says two days is for maintenance; three days is for getting stronger.) If you do go to three days, rotate the areas covered. Your muscles need a day, or even two days, to recover from a serious weight session. If you don't rest between sessions, it's all teardown and no buildup. Not good. And don't forget aerobics. No matter what, you have to have at least four days of aerobics each week.

Women Especially Should Default to Quads

f you run out of time (or passion) for doing weights, do whatever you can for your legs, especially your quads. This means squats, or one of those big machines where you sit down and push a weighted sled up a ramp with your legs. Or any of several other machines and exercises aimed primarily at your quads. Do your hamstrings, too, maybe using the machine that makes you pull back with your heels.

A lot of people seem to think strength training means barbells and biceps, and they forget their legs. Not smart. When your legs give out, you're cooked. That means the cane, the walker, and the chair. *Especially for women.* If you don't keep up your bone density, the great threat over time is that you will fall and break your hip. Remember, weights build bones. Weights build hips. Busted hips mean infirmity and death. Nothing is more important than heading that off. And nothing helps more than doing serious weights with your quads and hamstrings.

Strengthening your quads is also the best thing you can do to prevent bad knees. Strengthening your quads, the shock absorbers of your body, means you're much less likely to fall and get injured. And strengthening your quads, the biggest muscles in your body, means they will burn more calories, even on "idle." So, when in doubt, default to quads.

The Nursing Home Miracle and Other Payoff Stories

t's never too late to start a serious program of strength training. Quite the contrary. The later in life, the more important it is. There was a study done a while ago in a nursing home. They got all the residents, including the ones who were on walkers or bedridden, to do weights. It worked miracles, even though some of these people were in their nineties. Almost all the bedridden got up on walkers. The ones on walkers went to canes, and so on. *Moral: Weight training is serious therapy to halt or reverse the ravages of aging.* Do it early and you can skip a lot of aging altogether. Do it late and you can reverse a lot of it. I have felt those results myself, big time.

Here's another little payoff story from a while back. It

was 15 degrees, early in the morning in New York, and I was down by the East River, walking Aengus, the selfish dog. Bright sun, wind on the river. And all of a sudden I felt like running. Not for exercise or to show off (no one was around) . . . just for the hell of it. And I did. Cutting this way and that like a hundred-year-old football player. Astonishing the dog, who joined right in. Strange. Nice. I remembered, later, another time when Aengus was running around on the lawn like that. Like a lunatic. I said to Hilary then, "Gee, I wish I felt like doing that." And here I was, running around like a lunatic, out of sheer exuberance. Because I felt like it. Strength training does that for you. It makes you look a lot better, too. No matter how old you are. Makes it more fun to take your duds off and climb into bed at night with Old Fred or whomever, too. It's worth the pain, ladies, worth the pain.

The real reward for lifting is feeling great the rest of the time, when you're just walking around. Especially in your joints. That reward isn't instantaneous—it can take months—but it's a big deal. In my case, when I took this up seriously, I had a lot of sore joints: hips, shoulders, elbows, wrists, Achilles tendon . . . the works. I was starting to totter around like a little old guy, even though I did a fair amount of aerobic activity. It was creepy. I was going to an odd, sidearm tennis serve, which was useless and made me look a hundred. Sometimes just reaching for something on a shelf gave me a little twinge. Aging. I was aging. And you will, too. Unless . . .

When I started weights, *all that went away*! Not my arthritic hands, but the rest of it. I am not exaggerating. I remember how I used to creak and wobble and hurt a little, first trip down the stairs in the morning. Gone! My hips do not hurt anymore. Or my feet. Not even my shoulders, which were the worst and took the longest. My serve still stinks, but it's no longer sidearm. Even my Achilles tendon, which I suffered with for decades, has responded. All because of weights. Harry warns that some of my aches will come back as I get older, but not for quite a while and not as bad. I'll take that.

Part of what I was curing was mild arthritis, which is nothing more than inflammation, often brought on by idleness. Women often tell me that, gee, they can't do weights because they have arthritis and it hurts. I tell them they probably hurt and have arthritis because they *don't* do weights. Think about this: For most forms of arthritis, the prescription is a six-week course of physical therapy. But physical therapy is mostly just six weeks of supervised weight training. Six weeks because your insurance coverage runs out after that. But you shouldn't be doing it for six weeks, you should be doing it for life, two times a week (maybe three). *That's* how to prevent most forms of arthritis if you don't already have it. And to make it better if you do.

Here's another huge change in my life, once I started doing weights: I quit falling down. One of the truly alarming things that happened in my early sixties was that I began falling for no reason at all. Two or three times, I was crossing the street or just walking on a city sidewalk and stumbled over a little uneven place or a rise in the pavement. I'd catch the bottom of my sneaker and go flying, as if I'd forgotten how to walk. And I wasn't even old. I was in decent shape and pretty damn active, but I was falling down. Talk about hearing the waterfall. I thought I was going over.

Once I was carrying a lot of stuff and had Aengus on a lead, running across Park Avenue as the light was about to change. I caught the bottom of my foot on the pavement, and down I went. The light changed, and I was in the middle of the cars. Aengus was loose and terrified. I was dazed and surrounded by broken packages. Horns were honking, and a woman in the median actually screamed because she thought I was going to be killed. I thought so, too.

Something similar happened on a mountain hike out west, about ten years ago. The steep part, the challenging part, was over, and that had gone fine. Now we were on the flat, half a mile from the parking lot, and for no reason I tripped and tumbled off the trail. Landed on top of my own leg and broke it. Was put into a cast and couldn't exercise all summer. I thought, so this is aging. Great!

The happy fact is that it did not have to be that way, and it isn't anymore. The reason I was falling, Harry tells me, is that the neurotransmitters that coordinate balance deteriorate with age. Which is to say, your balance goes and you walk into stuff as if you were an idiot. Harry says that, for all of us, simple walking is really a series of near falls followed by a million tiny adjustments and recovery. When you age, the wiring that manages that stunt falls apart, and so do you. You no longer catch yourself. And here, of course, is the pleasing news. Lifting weights fixes up the wiring and cures the problem. Not a hundred percent, Harry says, but damn near. In my experience, anyway. I have not fallen in years. Don't even stumble much, or come close. Presumably because I do the stinking weights. I tell you, I swear by 'em. And you should, too. This is so important for women, because of the bone loss problem. It is super important for women not to fall down. Doing weights keeps you from falling. Doing weights builds up your bone mass so that, if you do fall, it is not catastrophic. So, do the weights.

Luckily, you don't have to take all this on faith or in reliance on one old boy's experience. Harry is going to explain the science, and All Will Be Made Clear, in the next chapter. To me, it's holy writ. I didn't much like all that falling down.

CHAPTER ELEVEN

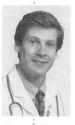

The Biology of Strength Training

Aerobic exercise is primarily about your muscles' ability to endure. Strength training is primarily about your muscles' ability to deliver power, which, surprisingly, has as much to do with a special form of neural coordination as actual strength. That's a critical point. Strength training causes muscle growth, and that's important, but it's the hidden increase in coordination that changes your physical life. This is not eye-hand coordination; it's the coordination of fine muscle detail through the elaborate networks of nerves that link your brain and body.

Generally, we aren't aware of nerve decay as we get older, but it's the main reason our joints wear out, our muscles get sloppy, and our ability to be physically alert and powerful begins to fade. And it is reversible with strength training.

It's easier to illustrate how this works by example, so let's look at what happens when you take a single step up a single stair. That might sound too simple, but in my first year of medical school I sat through a two-hour lecture on the neural coordination required to swallow a single bite of food.

A Single Step

Think about how much play your knee tolerates in simple walking: the moderate amount of bending and jarring you subject it to during each step. Now imagine standing at the foot of a flight of stairs. Climb the stairs in slow motion, two at a time. Notice that your thigh and calf contract, hard, at the very beginning of each step, and the first thing this does is pull the knee joint instantly into a very tight alignment *before you actually move.*

You might think this is just the result of tightening all the muscles simultaneously, and you are partly right, but it is also critically important that each muscle tighten to just the right degree to put your joints in perfect alignment to do the mechanical work you're asking of it. A mechanic tightens the fan belt on your car to a specific tolerance and then bolts it in place. Your body is far more sophisticated, and adjusts the fan belt for maximum efficiency and safety with each step. Each joint is automatically pre-tensioned to just the right position for each step.

Now hold this book out in front of you with both hands and stand up slowly. Focus on the precise delivery of power from your muscles throughout the motion. It involves all the major muscle groups in your lower back, buttocks, thighs, calves, and feet, as well as a host of minor, stabilizing muscle groups in your spine, torso, shoulders, abdomen, and pelvis. Seriously, stand up from your chair in slow motion, noting the muscles involved from your head to your toes.

You go through these coordinated cycles tens of thousands of times in the average day. Each step, each coordinated movement, involves thousands of nerve fibers, which together form a neural network. You have millions of potential neural networks in your body, and you shift between them with each step. Your body grows and your brain learns the tiniest amount from each one. They have to, because C-6 is in the background, helping them to forget all this, just a little bit, every day.

The trouble comes when your muscles, brain connections, and the controlling spinal reflex arcs get sloppy and weak from years of a relatively sedentary existence. The casual motion of daily life is not enough to turn on the C-10 of growth. Pushing your chair back from the desk, or driving to the mall, are insultingly trivial tasks for your physical brain, and over the decades large parts of it have deliberately gone to sleep in protest. Remember the threshold for C-10? It takes a critical amount of effort to cross that threshold and secrete enough C-6 to trigger the production of C-10. Below that threshold, all you have is the C-6 of chronic decay. You need to do strength training to cross that threshold for power and coordination; to get C-10 into your neural networks, into the meat of your muscles, into your joints, and into your tendons.

Aerobic exercise takes you across the threshold for endurance, circulation, and longevity, but you need strength training for power and neural coordination. A single step on level ground doesn't turn on C-10. Nor does climbing a few stairs. But climbing stairs until you feel your legs burn will turn on C-10. Lifting weights until you can't lift them anymore . . . that *really* turns on C-10.

The Brain-Body Connection

Strength training creates an intimate connection between your body and your brain. It's easiest to look at this from the top down, starting with your brain and nervous system. Your physical brain—the remarkably complex, physical brain—integrates the millions of messages coming up from your body and coordinates them with all the impulses it's sending down to move your muscles against resistance. The neural impulses to create coordination and power blaze a trail through your neural circuits. Each time you use them, you directly strengthen the balance, power, and muscular coordination centers of the physical brain. And the trail gets broader, smoother and faster.

Athletes have come to realize the benefits of strength training over the last thirty years. But the interesting thing is that the greatest advances have come not in the strength sports, like the shot put and weight lifting, but in the coordination sports—the ones that require grace, skill, and coordination, like figure skating and skiing. Those improvements are due largely to increased coordination and muscular integration, as well as the increased muscle power available for jumping and landing, developed through strength training. The same can be true for you. You still have the circuitry to do a triple jump on skates or, more realistically, to run across the court and hit a powerful backhand, but it's a shadow of what it could be. Indeed, the last time most of us used these neural connections to their full extent was during fourth-grade recess.

Consistent strength training can change all that by bringing your neural connections out of hibernation. For example, even though it *feels* as if you're contracting 100 percent of each muscle involved in level walking, only

10 percent of the cells in those muscles are actually in use. These cells are distributed evenly throughout each muscle, so every part of it moves, but 90 percent of the cells are resting . . . going along for the ride. With harder exercise, you recruit an increasing number of cells. Walking up a real hill or a long flight of stairs, you might use 30 percent of the muscle cells during a given step. Lifting the heaviest weight you can handle, you might even use half the muscle cells at once, but that's about it.

The ability to choose which muscle cells get activated— and the degree of contraction—gives us an amazing physical potential. Running across a tennis court to hit a forehand requires subtle shades of coordination for the direction, arc, spin, and force of the shot—which means that each of the muscles in your legs and arm has to play its own part in a simultaneous symphony. Hundreds of thousands of nerve cells, controlling hundreds of millions of muscle cells. A massive harmony that lasts a split second, just to hit a ball across a net. That's the neural information superhighway we talked about earlier—the billions of nerve signals flying around your body every minute of the day.

Slow-Twitch, Fast-Twitch

The nerves that control your muscles contain thousands of individual cells, each of which splits further into hundreds and hundreds of tiny branches. And each branch goes to one—and only one—muscle cell. There are over a million muscle cells in the large muscles of your thighs, and perhaps ten thousand nerve cells, bundled into a couple of main nerves, controlling them all.

This gets detailed, but stick with it. You have two types

of muscle cells, built for strength or for endurance, and they are different. This is a critical point, so I'm going to repeat it. Your muscles have strength cells and endurance cells, and they are different.

Muscle endurance cells are known as slow-twitch. They have more mitochondria, more endurance, and less power. Muscle strength cells are known as fast-twitch: fewer mitochondria, less endurance, and much more power. Each individual nerve cell sends all of its tentacles to either strength or endurance cells, but never both. This means that each individual nerve cell ends up signaling for either strength or endurance. Remember that, in your thigh, for instance, each of these nerve cells has thousands of tiny branches, going to thousands of muscle cells, all either strength or endurance. Your quadriceps muscle, the big one in the front of your thigh, has over a million muscle cells. The big nerve that controls it has around ten thousand nerve cells. Each one of those nerve cells controls a few thousand muscle cells, called a motor unit, in a specific pattern.

Now we can look at how you actually move. Your brain can activate any combination of those motor units to perform specific movements. The choices your physical brain makes, instantly, between the thousands of motor units in each muscle are what give you the ability to dance, spin, jump, or just wiggle your toes. You activate only a fraction of the nerve cells with each step, but it's a very carefully chosen fraction for each individual muscle. It's a little daunting to think of the complexity of all this, of the millions of split-second decisions your physical brain makes just to keep you on your feet, let alone dancing. Luckily, you don't have to think about it; you can take it for granted. It is vitally important that you understand that it's there, but you can go years without worrying about it if you take care of it.

Chris talks about skiing as a strength sport, which is true enough, but the equally important point is that it's a *coordinated* strength sport. Strength training makes both the power and the coordination possible and delivers them in the integrated package that lets you ski well at seventy, or eighty, and will let you live well at any age.

With this as background, let's look at strength training vs. endurance exercise. When you walk, your body predominantly recruits endurance units and rotates through them so each one gets a rest period between steps, which means that each unit gets only a fraction of the exercise you think you're giving it. Certainly not enough stress to generate the powerful regeneration of C-10.

As you start to run, your body uses more endurance units with each step. Each unit may be used every third step now, and that's enough stress to trigger high levels of C-6 and then C-10. If you're running up a hill, hard enough to go beyond the capacity of your endurance units, your body adds in strength units. The longer you run, the less rest time the endurance units get. The more strength you demand, the less rest the strength units get. At some point, you will push them beyond their recovery cycles. They will fatigue, and the fatigue will damage them. Taking them to fatigue is what turns on the surge of C-6—the good stress of exercise that turns on C-10.

By the way, this is why you have to sweat when you do aerobic exercise; at low levels of demand, your endurance cells alternate too much to get fatigued. This is also why you have to push to the point of muscle fatigue with weights— to that burning feeling in your muscles that most of us hate and would skip if it were up to us.

Peak Fitness: Who Needs It?

You do not build new muscle cells with strength training; in fact, you continue to slowly lose them as you age, regardless. What you do instead is build new muscle mass inside each remaining cell: the protein, the substance—in short, the red meat. And the potential growth in those remaining cells is extraordinary: certainly enough to keep you strong and fit for the rest of your long life.

Put another way, you can lose half your muscle cells over the course of your life, lose half your peak fitness, and still end up stronger at eighty than you were at twenty. Besides, when were you ever at your peak fitness? No one but Olympic athletes and professional tennis players ever get there.

Weight lifting remains a relatively minor sport among men and women, but it's the place to look for peak strength. The strongest American woman in the 165-pound class is able to stand up with 407 pounds on her shoulders. She is in her twenties, and that's how strong her legs are. She can stand up with the equivalent of two firemen on her back. The American record for women over sixty is 231 pounds. The woman who can lift 400-odd pounds in her twenties will be down to 230 pounds by the time she reaches her sixties. She will lose 40 percent of her peak strength. But so what? She will still be able to pick up one fairly overweight fireman.

When you hire that personal trainer, he or she will eventually make sure you lift enough weight to cycle all the way through the reserve capacity of your strength cells. To use them ten or twelve times in a row, and then do it again.

Done right, you will drain them of all their energy and *then* force them to contract a few more times. That's the critical part; that's how you intentionally damage your muscle cells. Not your muscles, just the muscle cells. And you damage them quite a lot. On purpose. Electron microscope pictures of muscle show extensive damage at the cellular level after a weight workout. That's fine and what your body needs. Lots of C-6, lots of inflammation, and then lots of repair and growth. Your muscles will quiver and burn, which is not fun, but inside you will be forcing your brain to activate *all* your strength units. Do this for three sets, and you will have forced your body to *damage* all those strength units, which then forces it to *repair* all those strength units. Growth, strength—youth.

This is why you shouldn't do strength training six days a week. If you've done it right, you've done some real damage. Unlike endurance units, which recover from aerobic exercise overnight, your strength units need to enter a forty-eight-hour repair cycle. Two days a week of strength training is enough. Three days is the maximum.

Doing It Right

B y the way, you want to be very, very careful not to confuse damaging your muscle cells by *exhausting* them with damaging your muscles or joints by *overloading* them. It's tempting to use heavy weights so you can exhaust the muscle cells with fewer repetitions, because, frankly, the repetitions hurt. They feel lousy, and eight is a lot easier to tolerate than twelve or fifteen. But you are not young. You will be *younger* next year, but you will not be *young* next year. Your trainer will almost certainly be younger than you are and may not understand this in his or her bones, so you are in charge of not getting hurt. Also, as you get into better shape and get stronger, your brain will secrete more adrenaline when you exercise. You will start to enjoy the weights and look forward to going to the gym. The downside is that the adrenaline of strength training will activate your primitive impulse to compete, to push yourself to your peak performance, where injuries happen. Don't go there.

The Balancing Act

Now it's time to think about your brain and a concept called proprioception—the deceptively simple notion that you have to know where the different parts of your body are at all times. It's how we stand up and how we move. We stand on two feet like a ladder standing straight up into the sky, not leaning against anything. That's an amazing feat on our part. Try balancing a ladder straight up. You have to make constant adjustments to keep it from falling over. Our bodies are just the same. And that's the simple stuff. Try running around the yard holding a ladder straight up. Try to spin around and throw to first base holding the ladder straight up. Try to do any of the amazing things we do all the time standing on two feet. And then try it standing on one foot!

Your body is aware of exactly where each limb is in space every second, because each muscle, tendon, ligament, and joint sends thousands of nerve fibers back to the brain through the spinal cord. Those fibers signal every nuanced gradation of contraction, strength, muscular tone, orientation, position, and movement at every moment of the day. Close your eyes and concentrate on your index finger. You know exactly where it is to within a couple of millimeters, automatically; same thing with your big toe or left elbow. Keep your eyes closed and do a quick survey of where each part of your body is right now. Your brain keeps careful track of the location of every muscle and joint in your body every second, all day, every day, waiting for you to need the information. And it sends millions of signals throughout the day just to keep you upright and aware of where you're standing.

Strength training works on these signals. Pushing a muscle hard sends a blaring signal back up to the brain. Remember adjusting the fan belt, the instant tightening of your joints on the staircase? This is important stuff for your body. If your brain slacks off for an instant, and you don't make the split-second adjustments, you might get hurt. You will pull a muscle, sprain an ankle, or break a leg. In nature, you can die from a minor injury. The endurance predator, or a forager laid up for two weeks with a sprained ankle, might never come back. So the signals to your brain from strength training are loud and important: priority news. And they create growth—first in the signaling pathways themselves, blazing that direct trail through the forest of neural networks, and second in the muscles, tendons, ligaments and joints directly. With this growth comes a new integration between your brain and body. They have always been fused; we just forgot it. This is how you reconnect them. It's a literal, physical reconnection: nerve fibers you can see under the microscope, brain chemistry you can see on MRI scans, reaction time you can measure in the lab. It's skiing better, feeling stronger, feeling better.

It's also *not* falling down. As Chris mentioned, you're much more likely to fall as you get older unless you stay in great shape. This is a major public health issue, because you also fall harder and do more harm to yourself. C-6—*hiss* and, literally, *bump* in the night. Falls have been carefully studied, and it turns out you do not stumble any more often as you age; in other words, you catch your toe just as often as you did at twenty. But instead of easily recovering your balance, you're more likely to hit the pavement. There are two reasons for this. To begin with, you have let your proprioception slow down a critical bit. It takes a split second longer before your brain realizes you're falling, and in that split second momentum and gravity turn against you. The other point is that it takes strength to recover from a stumble. Your toe stops on the pavement, but your body keeps going, building up speed and momentum in a Newtonian drive toward earth. By the time you move your leg, your entire body mass is moving forward and down with increasing speed. It's like jumping off a low wall. Your legs have to be strong enough to stop your momentum, or down you go. And if you've happened to let your bones decay, to get osteoporosis, down you stay.

Osteoporosis: Shattered Bones, Shattered Lives

As we go through the basics of osteoporosis, keep the following mantra running in the background: *"Osteoporosis is optional, osteoporosis is optional, osteoporosis is optional."* You need to do that because learning about osteoporosis will scare you, as it should. Let's start with the numbers:

• Twenty million American women have osteoporosis, a *preventable* disease.

• There are one and a half million fractures each year from osteoporosis, and the large majority of them occur in women.

- You—yes, you—have a 50 percent lifetime risk of breaking a bone from osteoporosis, and the vast majority of those fractures are caused by falls that you would have bounced right up from in younger years.

- Americans—mostly women—suffer 300,000 hip fractures *every single year.*

- Hip fractures kill more women than breast cancer.

- Twenty percent of women who fall down and break a hip die within a year.

- And of those who survive, *half* will never live independently again.

- Twenty-five percent of women who break a hip will end up in a nursing home.

- Twenty-five percent will be at home, but dependent on a wheelchair or walker to get around the house, and dependent on someone else to get through each day.

- There are a million spine fractures each year in the United States and about a quarter million wrist fractures, most from osteoporosis.

- Only half of spine or wrist fractures heal back to full function; the rest become lifetime disabilities.

Take a hard look at the grim reality of those numbers, what they mean for older women and what they would mean for you. Now let's look at the stunning news that the vast majority of those fractures *never need to happen.* You, and almost all women, can skip osteoporosis, broken bones, and nursing homes altogether.

All you have to do to avoid this epidemic of broken bones and broken lives is 1) keep your bones strong, and 2) don't fall down.

1) Keep your bones strong. You reach your peak bone mass by age thirty, and then, in an instant, the tide turns and you lose bone for the rest of your life. The average

American woman loses up to one percent of her bone mass *every year*—from thirty to the onset of menopause. The pace picks up after menopause; the tide rushes out faster, so you lose around 2 percent each year in the first decade after menopause. By age sixty, before you know it, you've lost up to 30 percent of all the bone you ever had to see you through to the end of your long, long life. It's like having a third of your retirement money vanish without a trace. And you have no idea this is happening to you, because osteoporosis is a completely silent disease. *Osteoporosis does NOT hurt—ever.* Broken bones hurt, quite a lot, but none of your aches and pains have anything to do with osteoporosis. Your bones silently melt for decades, but you feel fine. The first time you hurt is when the first bone breaks.

But you don't have to lose bone, or at least not much, if you're willing to commit to two, and only two, lifestyle interventions: adequate calcium intake and the right kind of exercise.

Only 10 percent of American women get all the calcium they need from diet alone. If you have to ask which foods contain enough calcium, you are in the other 90 percent. We recommend some excellent nutrition books in the Appendix, but start taking calcium supplements . . . and take them for the rest of your life. Calcium supplementation is only mildly effective, but it's safe, and you need all the help you can get because your bones have to last. As of this writing, premenopausal women should take 1,200 milligrams of calcium a day (usually a 600 mg pill when you brush your teeth in the morning, and again at night); after menopause, take 1,500 milligrams a day. You also need vitamin D to absorb the calcium, so take a supplement that contains this as well (800 IU is the recommended daily dose). Calcium citrate may be better absorbed (Citracal is a popular brand). You will read a lot about other minerals your bones *might* need, like magnesium, phosphorus, selenium, and so on. The truth is that no one yet knows enough to make a sensible recommendation; stick with the calcium and vitamin D for now, and check in with your doctor yearly as recommendations may change over time.

That's the calcium story—modest benefit, but well worth doing. The real key to *preventing osteoporosis altogether* is exercise. Actually bending your bones a tiny bit, over and over again, by jumping up and down on them or by picking up heavy weights, is what you need to do. High-impact, weight-bearing aerobic exercise builds bone, but you're going to have to wade through a lot of misinformation about weight-bearing exercise if you want to avoid osteoporosis. Walking is great low-intensity aerobic exercise, but it does not prevent osteoporosis. It slows down bone loss, which is a big help, but it's still not enough for most women. *High-impact* exercises like aerobics, with lots of running or jumping and landing, actually build bone but are awfully hard on your joints and very few people tolerate truly high-impact exercise past the age of forty. Walking is a *medium-impact* exercise and has only a modest benefit for your bones. Walking a couple of miles, which is a half-hour to forty-five minutes, just does not put enough stress on your bones to stimulate them to grow. Perhaps walking four to six miles does, but the studies have shown that moderate walking is a modest help, not a true treatment.

What does work is strength training. Pure and simple, brute-strength training. Women who strength-train *gain* a little bone mass every year, as opposed to those doing aerobics alone, who are just slowing down the pace of loss. Real strength training has stopped bone loss cold in multiple studies. Fit women live long; strong women live well. And don't skimp on weights for fear of bulking up. Women who strength-train usually put on muscle mass in their chests and shoulders, but not in their hips and buttocks, where strength

A Word About Arthritis

People with arthritis often see it as a barrier to strength training. But arthritis is rarely a contraindication. Quite the contrary. The combination of strong muscles and improved proprioception protects the joints from further damage and lets them heal. Most arthritis patients report about a 50 percent reduction in pain and limitation with several months of strength training; minor arthritis usually disappears entirely. All those aches and pains do make it trickier to get started, however, particularly if you have significant arthritis. If that describes you, talk to your doctor about having a physical therapist guide you in the initial stages of your weight-training program. If the arthritis is in your hands, talk to a physical therapist about strength exercises for your hands. But, unless your doctor tells you to stop, never let arthritis keep you from exercising. (Your doctor letting you off the hook because you ask does not count; she has to actually forbid the exercise.) There are a few types of arthritis that exercise exacerbates, and a small number of patients may have so much pain from severely eroded joints that such exercise is impossible. But those two groups make up a tiny minority of arthritis patients, and doctors can guide patients there. For everyone else, remember that arthritis is an *inflammatory* condition. It's a disease of C-6, so treat it with C-10.

training is actually trimming unless you get to bodybuilding levels.

Medications come in if your bones have thinned past a critical point. Most women who start this early enough, and stick with it, will never need medication and will never break a bone.

2) Don't fall down. The other part of the equation is this simple admonition. You can live the rest of your life with thin bones, and never break one, *if you don't fall down.* Strength training gives you the power to fight gravity and stay on your feet. Even if you do take a fall, having strong reflexes and powerful muscles changes it from a head-on collision to a softer impact. Like the crumple zones in your car, your coordinated muscle action softens the blow. You will fall less if you're strong, and you will fall better, dramatically lowering your odds of serious injury.

Falls aside, strength training lowers your chance of injury with all forms of exercise—in large part by speeding up your proprioceptive reflexes, but also by strengthening your tendons, ligaments, and joints. Tendons and ligaments are living tissue, but they grow more slowly as you get older. Pulling hard on a tendon strengthens the nerve connections and makes the tendon grow a bit farther into the bone, strengthening the attachment and rendering it more resistant to injury.

Find a Strength Sport

Weights are satisfying, perhaps even mildly addictive, but they're not fun for most people—which is why you need to see the payoff. Our advice? Find a strength sport that you like, or learn to like one.

Bicycling, skiing, tennis, squash, kayaking, and canoeing are great ways to feel the measurable benefit of your time in the gym. Golf does *not* count as a strength sport, but most women find that strength training also markedly improves their golf game.

Once you're fit and pretty strong, you might try yoga. Whereas weights build specific muscle groups in isolation, yoga integrates strength and balance training. The rich sensory stimulation of using muscle groups in different combinations, and linking this with breathing, mind exercises and stretching, creates a more profound neurosensory and proprioceptive integration than Western exercise. *But beware*: The injury potential from yoga in our culture is quite high. You have to be reasonably fit to start yoga; after all, it was created by people who were already living a very physical life. Moreover, we have an aerobics class mentality that asks us to do more and better each day. If you do try yoga, think about starting with individual instruction for five sessions. It's expensive but well worth it, and if the instructor doesn't teach you how to listen to your body, find someone else. Group yoga classes, once you understand the basics, are among the best deals around, going for ten or fifteen bucks in most places.

Whatever you decide to do, *do it.* Strength training is critical to the rest of your life, and you can start at any age. Women can double their leg strength with a few months of training. At any age. In one study, women in their nineties showed marked gains in strength with training. Think about these benefits, and stack them up against the fact that only 10 percent of Americans over sixty-five even *claim* to be doing any form of regular strength training.

That's appalling. It should be clear by now that everyone—certainly all women over fifty—should be doing

And a Word About Kegels

You may wonder why the subject of incontinence is covered in a chapter on strength training. Certainly, treating incontinence may not be the first benefit you think of from strength training, but this is not some editorial error. Most women who have given birth, and many who have not, develop incontinence as they get older. This is largely because the "kegel" muscle that controls urination has been stretched beyond its natural design. (Other factors can contribute to incontinence, so check with your doctor, but weakness of the kegel muscle is a major factor in most women.)

There's nothing special about the kegel muscle itself. It's tiny, but it's the same tissue as any other muscle in your body. And that means it gets stronger with exercise and atrophies without it. So you need to exercise it every day. Here's how: The next time you urinate, stop right in the middle *without clenching your buttock muscles*. That's the key. Keep the large muscles of your butt relaxed and stop peeing. You'll feel yourself using an internal muscle that runs front to back along the floor of your pelvis. That's your kegel muscle. Clench it as hard as you can, and hold that contraction for the slow count of ten. Then relax and do it again. Do this three times in a row, three times a day (more often if you feel like it). Most women will notice an improvement in incontinence within a few weeks, but this only works as long as you keep exercising that muscle. So if kegels work for you, do them for the rest of your life.

real strength training two or three days a week. You can do a quick routine in half an hour, or spend an hour or more if you get into it, but don't skip it.

The Frail Elderly

That's the horrible, but descriptive new terminology for weak, old people. It's where you do NOT want to end up. The Frail Elderly are defined by their loss of lean-muscle mass. They are simply weak, they are infirm, they are . . . frail. And it's hard to be strong in spirit and mood when you're frail. There are some wonderful people who manage it . . . whose spark is strong enough that it rises above the flesh. But most of us depend on the direct connection between our physical and mental health. Take a moment to fast-forward ten, twenty, or forty years, and visualize yourself as old and fit. Hiking with your grandchildren or your friends, active and appealing. Now visualize yourself as old and *frail*. Bent over a walker. Tentative, passive . . . dependent. That's the huge difference we are pounding away at in this book. That's why we are so insistent about daily exercise and building connections.

You really are likely to live long enough for one of those two scenarios to come true. Active or dependent. You pick. Remember, aerobic exercise saves your life; strength training makes it worth living.

CHAPTER TWELVE

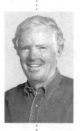

Chasing the Iron Bunny

H ere's a dreary chapter about personal economy that you may be tempted to skip, but I am *begging* you to read it. Because the topic is *so* important to women. Let's start with a nasty little statistic that should catch your attention . . . or make you slap the book shut and go to the fridge. Listen to this:

Half the women in America approach the end of their lives *at or near the poverty level.* As if women were expendable, you know, and no one cared what happens to them after Old Fred dies or runs off with someone. Sound okay to you? I thought not. It's awful. And you don't want to go there. And you certainly don't want to let some mutt send you there, just because he wasn't paying attention or didn't care enough to make a plan when there was time to do something about it. Like cutting back a little on your life-style today—making it a hair less fun for now—so it won't be just god-awful for you when he's gone. Take a peek at this chapter to make yourself at least start thinking about it.

It is so important that we've given it its own rule, and there are only seven rules. And it is so hard and complicated and vicious and hateful that the rule itself has three parts.

It goes like this: *Spend less than you've got.* What that means is a) take a look at your dough; b) make a plan; c) get real. Translation? Take a look at all the stuff you own today. Houses, securities, insurance, social security . . . whatever you've got. Especially, especially, *especially* if what you come up with is "not much." (Hint: Count social security as "not much.") Then take a look at what you and your partner are going to make between now and the time everyone retires (if you are going to be able to retire). Now take a wild stab at how long you and he are each going to live (assume, just for fun, that you'll live to be ninety and that you will outlive him by six years if you are the same age) and see if there's going to be enough dough to live on for the rest of *your* life. And if there's not—and *no one* is going to have enough, believe me—then make a plan. Spend less today. Buy some insurance. Sell the big house. Get a financial adviser, if you can afford it. Read stuff. But do some damn thing. *Think, plan, get in a crouch.* Get ready.

And get real. This means starting right now to implement that plan, no matter how half-baked and pathetic it may be. Because acting on any plan in this critical part of your life is much better than just averting your eyes and going off a cliff. Or into the dumpster. You're worried about your looks in old age? Dumpster diving is an extremely bad look. So get real about the rest of your financial life, even if it hurts, which it will for a while. You are far better advised to take a little pain today—when it will do some good—than to take a gang of pain tomorrow. When it won't do any good at all.

Look, this is hard. Because most people will quickly

realize that they should spend a good deal less today so things will be okay tomorrow. And that kind of long-range behavior is not an American virtue. Good old American optimism teaches us that everything will be okay. Well, everything will *not* be okay, and you will bear the brunt of it. So take a deep breath and face the facts. Actually, making a change in this area is easier than you think and much easier than lying to yourself, which is probably what you are doing now.

At some level, you know right now almost everything you are going to learn when you Take a Look and all that. And it is making you deeply, if silently, anxious. Talk about *hiss, bump* in the night! There's almost nothing worse for you than constant, unfaced financial anxiety. It's awful for your sex life, awful for marriages, awful for kids, awful for older women. Especially awful for older women during those eight or ten years or more they live alone. Getting real may hurt, but at least the silent, gnawing pain—which is worse—will go away.

Think of getting real about your financial life as a magic pill to prevent half the anxiety and pain of retirement. Remember that wonderful slogan from the sixties, "Be here now"? Great stuff . . . lots of fun. But that was then and this is now, and it doesn't make one whit of sense anymore. *Think ahead* should be your mantra now. Figure out what's going to be left when you're old and *be there now*. And if it's awful, fix it. Fix it today because you can't fix it tomorrow. Get Old Fred involved and committed, but know that, in the end, it's up to you to take care of you. Of course, you can just start being a little nicer to the kids . . . assume they'll take you in when you're old. There's a plan. Sort of.

You—and Fred, too—may have trouble even *hearing* this. People go into a fugue state on this stuff. They go off to a land of dreamy dreams and assume it will somehow take care of itself. Well, it won't take care of itself. It will take care of you. And Fred. And your little dog, Toto. You will all be way out of luck unless you force yourself to look this one in the eye and plan a little. If you don't, when the fog lifts, you may be on the rocks. You do not want to be swimming away from the wreckage alone at seventy.

Harry and I are not financial advisers, for sure, but we ask you to sit down right now and make a realistic estimate of how much income per year you're going to have in retirement. Figure it out for the two of you and for you alone, after your pal's gone. Next, unless your income is inflation-protected, adjust it downward. Then assume things will be a bit worse and cut it 5 percent more. You may also want to take a hard look at some of your prospective sources of income, calculate coldly just how reliable they are and make appropriate adjustments. Okay, that's your annual income. Teeny, isn't it? Now come up with a lifestyle and a plan—a more modest house in a less expensive town, etc. etc.—that will let you live on less than that. And that will leave enough for you to live on during the six or eight or ten years when you're likely to be alone. Do that and you will be safe and happy. No matter how small the house or how tight the lifestyle, it will be joyous when contrasted with the lives of those who don't do it.

Living within your real income—and expectations—is one of the great secrets in life. As for getting there, there is, as always, good news and bad news. The good news first: Above the poverty level, there is no correlation between money and happiness. Elaborate surveys say this is so. Think about it. You've been struggling for more dough all your life, and there is no correlation between money and happiness. How can that be? I don't know, but apparently it's true.

So what's the bad news? Deciding to live on less is way, way hard. We think we are what we own. Or drive. Or eat. Or wear. We are material and status junkies. And like all junkies, we are absolutely convinced that we gotta have it. Gotta have money/status/power. We've been trained to chase the iron bunny like the greyhounds at the racetrack, and we cannot get over it. We have so much invested in what we make . . . how many empty rooms we have in the house . . . how big the gas piggy is. The whole economy and the wonderfully powerful media/advertising complex focused all our attention on these things. And like dopes, we bought it. As workers and as consumers, chasing the iron bunny. And we barked and wagged our tails and ran like lunatics. Not for the nourishment, God knows, but because that was the game. And now we have to quit.

It's not hard to quit *eating* iron rabbits. But it's very hard to quit *wanting to eat* iron rabbits. You have to persuade yourself that that game is over. Never mind whether or not it was a good game or how terrific you were at it . . . it's over. Time to quit playing and come inside. Come inside your family's income. Try to do it early. As with smoking, you can recover. It takes time and earlier is better, but do it. Get over the game or it will kill you.

It's entirely possible that you and Fred are going to have to work for much of the rest of your lives. That probably wasn't the plan, but it may be the reality. If it is, the earlier you know it and act on it, the better. You'll want to figure out what you can and want to do. Maybe some retraining makes sense, some schooling. Whatever. But think about it. And start now, before you have to. And save like a lunatic. Every dime you save today is fifteen cents (or whatever, depending on interest rates) you don't have to earn tomorrow.

The difficulties of turning your back on old spending habits run deep in our being. What we're really talking about here is stepping out of the endless struggle for status in the pack that ran our lives for the last forty years (and ran the pack's lives for a few million years before that). That's the subject of some serious talk in the final chapters of the book, and it involves some very serious and difficult issues. Briefly, it goes like this. From the time you were a teenager, you were obsessed—and encouraged to be obsessed— with your status in a particular pack. Your clique in high school . . . your colleagues at work . . . the other families on your block or at the club. It's hard, but you have to try to get over it. Live within your means and forget how it looks to the rest of the pack. They're over at the dump now, anyway, sniffing for fresh garbage. Look after yourself. As you know now, there's lots of Darwinian stuff programmed deep in our bones that is *not* in our personal best interest. Caring about pack status when you're in your fifties and sixties is one of them.

A little example, close to home. Hilary and I had a nice weekend house. Good for us. But we were also a teeny bit in debt. More than a teeny bit, actually. So, taking our own, excellent advice, we put that house on the market and found another that suited us better in a slightly less fashionable place for about half the price. The idea was that we could pay off our debt, have a place that would be easier to maintain, and, in candor, be more appropriate to our slightly unfashionable selves. We were getting real, just as we say in this book. But we took a "bridge loan" to buy the new place before we sold the old. A great idea, but, wow, did we pay along the way. The sale of the first place took forever. With lots of near-deals and heartbreak. All to a drumbeat of articles about how the "real estate bubble" was about to burst. Thinking about that risk made us almost physically sick with constant, deep anxiety. As a trial lawyer, I thought I was more or less immune to stress. Wrong. Financial stress is different. This was not just *hiss-bump,* this was terror. Lots of lost sleep, lots of feeling half sick without knowing why, lots of depression. Our little saga turned out okay, but the point is this: Financial stress is just plain awful. It can make you sick. It can ruin your life. "Deprivation"—denial of your God-given right to drive a Lexus or whatever—is a tiny price to pay for avoiding financial stress.

This is a very short, almost flippant chapter on a very serious subject, and we were tempted to skip it altogether. But Harry rightly felt that we had to say something. That it would be irresponsible to write a book about the Next Third and skip this one. Failure to make a financial plan is like bone loss. You may not see it; there may not be any symptoms. But it can ruin your life. In fact, it can kill you dead.

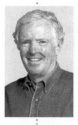

CHAPTER THIRTEEN

Don't You Lose a Goddamn Pound!

H arry and I are serenely aware that an $88 billion check is waiting out there for the person who comes up with the next blockbuster diet book that says his or her gimmick really does work and will make you lose fifty pounds in two weeks and keep it off for the rest of your life. Because there are a hundred million chubby Americans who are panting to believe it. Well, tough. It's not true. And we're not going to take your money.

The dreary, persistent fact is that diets don't work: 95 percent of them fail, which is why setting weight loss as a goal is generally a bum idea. The almost certain failure can infect your whole attitude toward fitness, while the yo-yoing up and down actually makes you gain weight. So don't diet. That's the headline. Our advice is, basically, forget about it. But exercise six days a week and follow Harry's Fifth Rule. Which is: *Quit eating crap!*

Now the small print. Will there come a time, way down the road, when you lose a pound or two on this regimen?

Just for fun? Not dieting? Why yes, that could happen. You might lose forty, as a matter of fact, the way I did. There's a pretty good chance of it, to tell you the truth. If you do, just send us the $88 billion when you have a moment. But not now, please. We won't take it. The thing to do now is *get in shape*. Go back and read the first few chapters and start to exercise! Because exercise does work, whether or not you're fat as a walrus. It is always the first step, the bit of magic that changes everything. So focus on that, quit eating crap, and forget about weight loss over the next two weeks or twenty-one days or whatever. If you have a year and are game for a little effort, we can talk.

"Quit eating crap" may seem a little vague, but you'd be surprised how much you know right now. I urge you to sit down and make a list of the mountains of garbage you're eating that you *know* you should quit eating altogether. I bet you get it 85 percent right before you read another word. (Hint: French fries. Almost all fast food. Processed snacks and breakfast foods with names that end in "O." And all sugar-swamped soft drinks, like full-strength Coke and Pepsi.)

Exercising and not eating crap is not a diet, and you won't fail at it. If you don't lose weight, you will still be radically better off and functionally younger. If you lose weight, it's a bonus.

The God That Lied

Dieting is the False God of the last thirty years. And women, since they care a little more about how they look, have wasted more time and dough at its temple than men have. But the differences are minor; the whole country has been on an extraordinarily expensive and feckless binge of diets and misery for a long, long time. We have spent billions on them, too, and what did we get for our money? We gained forty pounds apiece. A handful of guys got rich and the rest of us got fat. Not a good use of our dough. Or our time. Or our hope. In fact, it was a ridiculous, shaming, and debilitating waste. So maybe we should cut it out.

As you might expect of a False God, the various bibles of dieting are not very reliable or consistent. The rich protagonists who preach the True Faith cannot begin to agree on the sacred texts. I am not just talking about fad diets like the "hot dogs and ice cream" diet that ripped through parts of Colorado a few years ago. The big guns in the field are just as wild. Consider the head-on conflict between Pritikin-Ornish (low fat, low fun) and Atkins (high fat, high fun . . . until poor Dr. Atkins died and his successors-in-interest backed off a bit from the eat-steak-till-you-drop claims). These are two of the biggest in the field and one of them has to be crazy. Or at least wrong.

And now take a peek at the convolutions our own government has gone through in the last dozen years. In 1992, back in the days of carbo-loading and the war on fat (by everyone but Atkins), the USDA came out with a new, much-ballyhooed "food pyramid" that looked like the one at the top of the next page. Take a minute to check it out. . . .

Looks familiar, doesn't it? It should. For years, it was on every box of Wheat Thins and Triscuits in the country, and not a few boxes of breakfast cereal. Yum! Cracker makers and bakers and purveyors of French fries loved it.

Trouble is, it was almost totally wrong, as almost everyone now agrees. On the latest government pyramid, white bread, pasta, white rice, and potatoes went from the top of the list to the very bottom. Vegetable oils went from worst to just fine. And so on. The fact that the nation's own experts can go

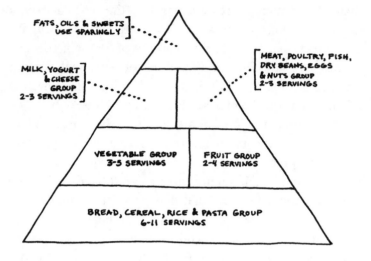

through such wild swings in a dozen years does not inspire much confidence, does it? Actually, Harry and I think the government is getting warmer this time. Much warmer. And honoring the new pyramid would not be a bad idea, especially, of course, the USDA's startling, new recommendation of serious daily exercise. But still, the nagging question persists: Does anyone out there know what they're talking about?

The answer, I'm afraid, is "yes" and "no." On the "no" side, most diets are utterly unproven scientifically or medically. Not because their proponents are all dopes or charlatans, although there are certainly some of those. Or because there's some massive conspiracy of corporate farmers, fast-food restaurants, lobbyists, and rotten politicians that's responsible, although they play a very robust part. Rather, as Harry points out, there simply is not a lot of good science on specific foods available. The real difficulty is that every bite of food you take is a hugely complex blend of thousands and thousands of chemicals that interact in millions of important ways with different parts of your body. No one has taken the deep dive into the biology and chemistry to see what happens. Indeed, no one knows if it's possible to do so. So it's no surprise that no one has begun to devise tests to evaluate individual foods.

Harry puts the problem in an interesting light. He talks about President Kennedy's decision in 1961 to spend a fortune and put a man on the moon within the decade. Which we did. But, Harry says, if Abraham Lincoln had said that and spent the same amount of money, nothing would have happened. Same thing for Teddy Roosevelt. Or FDR. You cannot go to the moon with steam engines; the fundamental science has to be in place. That would be the problem today if a theoretical president decided to "solve" the national obesity problem with a breakthrough pill or diet or whatever it took. You could spend the dough, but you wouldn't get there, because the core science does not exist.

Which is not to say that we have to sit here and eat pizza and French fries for two hundred years while the scientists beaver away. There are, for example, broad population studies suggesting that the Okinawans live so long because their diet is so rich in vegetables, fish, and soy. Personally, I take greater comfort in the fact that the Mediterranean diet also gets high marks. I find it a little more accessible. Lots of yummy vegetables, olive oil, some meat, and a sufficiency of red wine . . . I'm there. It may occur to you that these are mighty broad-brush evaluations, deciding that a whole country or all of southern Europe is eating "good" food. Sounds a little rough, doesn't it? In fairness to the nutrition community, narrower, more scientific population studies are very hard to conduct. Ideally, they would involve large numbers of normal people and last for, oh, ten years, testing this and that food. Broccoli, say. Well, who in the world is going to eat broccoli for ten years and keep a record of it? And who is going to volunteer to be in the control group that has to eat rat poison with their broccoli? So it is slow work. But we know enough to set out a few rules.

Yes, Virginia, Calories Do Count

Once-popular books to the contrary notwithstanding, calories do count. They are, ultimately, the only things that count. So one can say, with utter confidence, that the secret behind getting fat is eating more calories than you burn. Surprise. As far as getting fat is concerned—as opposed to getting heart attacks and cancer and whatnot—it doesn't much matter what kind of calories they are. For obesity, 100 calories of spinach is no better and no worse than 100 calories of French fries. It's the old gag about which is heavier, a ton of feathers or a ton of lead? Same deal here: Calories are calories.

Well, not exactly the same deal. Some foods take a certain amount of energy just to digest. Those yummy fibers, for example. All that bran. (They taste it, too, don't they?) If you can hack it, it makes sense to eat more of those, because they fill you up and keep you filled while they work their way endlessly through your digestive system. They contain some good health stuff, too.

Start to get an idea of what an ideal level of calorie consumption should be for you. That depends on your age, the shape you're in, and the general level of your activity. It's a sad fact that your base metabolism (the rate at which you burn calories automatically, without doing a damn thing, which is the vast majority of all the calories you burn in a day) goes down as you age. Once again, the free ride of youth is over and you have to go to work to have a good life. The falling base metabolism rate—and the sedentary habits of older people in our society—is where that gut comes from after forty. Or fifty. A normal American woman in her fifties or sixties has to get her caloric intake down to roughly 1,400 calories to lose weight. Up to, say, 2,000 a day is maintenance. Unless she gets some serious exercise. Or has a huge aerobic engine.

Want to hear something smug and annoying about me? I had my resting metabolic rate tested this spring. The way the test goes is, you lie down in a darkened room and breathe into a mask for fifteen minutes. And this clever gadget tells you your base metabolism: how many calories you burn a day *before* any normal activity (we all burn some 800 calories a day just walking around, putting our shoes on, gardening, and so on) and before any exercise (which in my slightly peppy case would burn up another 400 or so calories a day). They wired me up, but, alas, it didn't work. The results were goofy. The machine was busted, the guy said, so I was told to come back two days later, to try taking the test again.

Here's the annoying part. The machine was not busted … it was just that my results were off the charts. Because I am an insufferable workout nut with a wonderful aerobic base. It turns out that, before I take a step, I burn twice as many calories a day as projected for my age. And the reason, Harry tells me, is twofold. First, I have added more lean muscle mass by doing weight training. And second, I have that nice aerobic base, which I put together, one day at a time, over the last five years. You know, the millions of new mitochondria and miles of new capillaries and stuff that make it possible to run and jump and play when you're an old person like me. That base is a hound for calories, whether you're using it or not, even when you're sleeping. It's like the "feed me!" plant in *The Little Shop of Horrors* ... gotta eat, all day long. What a break.

Until you become such a hell-for-leather biker or whatever that you don't need to worry, it makes sense to learn to count calories. Sounds dull and it is, but not as dull—or as hard—as you think. You don't have to be perfect at it, after all. You just want a rough idea of how much you're eating every day and where the excess, if any, is coming from. That's not hard. First step is probably to get one of those little calorie counters and look up a few of the things that you eat most often. That won't take long, because most of us eat in a surprisingly narrow band ... same stuff, week in and week out. And you don't have to worry much about the fruits and vegetables and fish, because they are so low-calorie that they're almost free (if you don't slather them with butter or sauces). So it's mostly a matter of keeping track of the carbs, the meat, and the sugars. And the booze, if you're still drinking. As I say, you don't have to be perfect. Just get good enough so that you have a realistic sense of how much you're eating and so you can't lie to yourself. If you want to stay where you are, try to get along on roughly 2,000 calories a day. If you want to lose a little, eat less. Easy? Try it.

Lying-to-yourself reaches epidemic proportions among the so-called experts. In one lovely example, a bunch of nutritionists (the very people we pay to yell at us about our disgusting habits) kept careful track of what *they* ate over a period of time. And *they lied to themselves* to the tune of some 20 percent of the total. Here is a handy, two-step process to help you get over your own damn lying. Step one: Try hard, every meal, not to lie. Step two: Add 20 percent to your total regardless.

A brief word about portion control. We are nuts in this country when it comes to portion size. Partly, as you must have read by now, it is the fault of the greedy, manipulative fast-food industry. They are able to offer "supersize" portions of fries and colas for a pittance, with little cost to themselves. Sounds like a deal, so we waddle in and gobble 'em up. Big mistake, as the movie *Supersize Me!* graphically illustrated. The same attitude spills over into restaurant portions in general, and finally at home. Our very *plates* have gotten bigger. Harry, who is such a Puritan that his advice in this area is deeply suspect, suggests that we all buy a set of salad plates for our main meals and allow ourselves only one plateful. That may not be as odd an idea as it sounds to me. Take a look at the frozen Lean Cuisine meals, which I sometimes rely on. One big secret to their low calorie count is that the portions are very small indeed. Adequate but small. Maybe we should all go there. Okay, so maybe the rule should have had two parts: Don't eat crap. And don't eat so much of it. And stop with the business about cleaning your plate out of respect for the starving Armenians. Do not eat like a little piggy and call it virtue.

Short-Cycle Hunger Spikes

Another important point, as Harry is about to tell you, is that some foods—especially carbs and sugars—spike short, intense cycles of renewed hunger. You feel hungrier, sooner, after a plate of French fries than after a bowl of spinach. Because almost no one can resist those hunger spikes, it makes plenty of sense to limit—not eliminate—carbs and simple sugars. Personally, when it comes to carbs, I don't have to wait for the hunger spike. I can eat them until I drop. Eat the whole loaf of French bread and butter, before the menus are passed out. Eat the entire bucket of popcorn at the movies. The whole bowl of pasta. I am never tempted to eat spinach or codfish like that. Sadly.

But even if you have more willpower than I do, you should sharply limit your consumption of white bread, white rice, pasta, potatoes, and sweets. They are at the tippety-top of the new pyramid, and they belong there. Incidentally, French fries, which I adore with all my heart, deserve their own circle in hell. They should be the flagpole on the top of the pyramid. They start as potatoes, so they're carbs at the core. Then they're routinely cooked in saturated fats, which makes them much, much worse. If there is evil in the universe, it is made manifest in the design of the French fry, which tastes so heavenly and is in fact the devil's own food. The devil's own drink, of course, is full-sugar cola.

Which brings me to those things that are so awful for you that they should be banned altogether—a list that is going to vary from person to person. My personal diet guru, the wise Stephen Gullo, has great advice about how to deal with food we know is rotten for us but love: Drop it altogether. His favorite quote to me was "For those who are given to excess, abstinence is easier than moderation."—John Drybred. Best nutrition advice I ever got. For me, as you may have guessed, that means no French fries. Maybe for you, too. And having no bread is way easier than a little bit. I have lapses, but not so many. And I know enough to feel guilty!

Quit Eating Fast Food

The science of nutrition is imperfect, and our understanding is weak—but not so weak that we do not know that the brightly lit fast-food signs are guiding us to a dark place. I don't want to spend the rest of my life in court, so why don't you take a look at the new food pyramid, then at the McDonald's menu, and let some things speak for themselves. (Burger King or a host of other joints would do as well.) Remember, before we begin: Calories count. Red meat, white bread, potatoes, sugar, and saturated fat are bad. Okay, McDonald's . . . what have we got under the golden glow?

I just drove over to the nearest McDonald's, up here in the Berkshires, to see what's cooking. Happily enough, things are better than they were a year ago, the last time I looked. There are big ads in the windows for various salads, and the pleasant guy behind the counter—at six-thirty in the morning he's got time to talk—says that some people actually order them. Not many, but a few. But, he says, the big sellers by far are still the basics: the Big Mac, the Quarter Pounder with Cheese (and not infrequently the Double Quarter Pounder with Cheese), the large fries, and the large Cokes. Which makes all the sense in the world; that's what these places have been about since the early days, and that's what we all come for. Change may be coming to Fast Food Nation, but it's coming slowly and the old ways are dying hard.

The fast food people know how to make food that tastes good, and they can make healthy food that tastes good if they put their minds to it. The McDonald's Caesar Salad with Grilled Chicken, for instance, is terrific. It's only 220 calories, too, a real bargain all around. Fruit and walnut salad, which is heavily promoted, is also pretty tasty and it's only 310 calories (although why they candy those nuts is beyond me). Still, give the devil his due.

But let's not kid ourselves. Most of us are not here to buy salad. We buy the Big Mac and the Quarter Pounder and the large fries and large Coke, which were promoted so hard for decades, and for that we pay a terrible, terrible price. Not in dough; this stuff would be a great buy if it weren't for the fact that it's killing us. The price is calories and fat and sugar, and none of us can afford it.

Take the Big Mac meal. The sandwich is 560 calories, with an appalling 30 grams of fat (half of them saturated). The fries are 520 calories, with 25 grams of fat, and the Coke is 310 calories, all of it from added sugar or corn syrup. That's 1,390 calories—enough to see you through the entire day—and almost all of it rotten for you. Sugar, some starch, and a lot of fat, much of it saturated. Not good. And if you're a little hungry and decide to add a 32-ounce "triple thick shake" for dessert (they only come in triple thick), you can add another 1,160 calories, almost all of it sugar. Yum. Now you're up to 2,550 calories, almost every one of them rotten for you. And all you've had is *lunch*. Keep this up—as so many Americans do—and guess what? You're gonna get fat. Maybe a bit sick.

So what do you say about these places? They have quit pushing "supersize" portions. (So they do have *some* shame, after all.) But the "large" portions are not a hell of a lot smaller (the large fries are a whopping 10 percent smaller than the old super size. Thanks a lot.) And they have created some salads. Great. But you don't go to McDonald's for salad. Most of us don't, anyhow. You can *get* conversation in a whorehouse, but that's not why you're there. If you want to stop eating crap, stay out of fast-food places. Period. Recovering alcoholics should stay out of bars, even though they sell ginger ale as well as whiskey. Those who want to change their ways should stay out of fast-food places, even though they sell salad as well as Big Macs. Isn't that obvious? C'mon!

One Very Small Raspberry for "Food Liberty"

By the way, it is my position that grown-ups should have the legal right to eat themselves into wheelchairs if they like. But I do think that fast-food joints—which are, after all, getting rich on making you fat, miserable, and sick—should have to give effective *notice* of what they're doing. By putting the calorie count up there as prominently as the low, low price. But after that, it's up to you. And your kids. It's a free country, after all.

That last point was put forward, as if it were serious, in a wonderful message this past Fourth of July from the Center for Consumer Freedom. "Consumer freedom," ladies . . . gotta have it. Oh, and look! The patriots behind the message turn out to be . . . why, bless my soul! . . . among others, the great Americans at Wendy's, Coca-Cola, Tyson Foods, and other stalwarts of the fast-food industry. And do they *care*. Listen to this, which I've cribbed from a Paul Krugman op-ed piece in *The New York Times,* July 4, 2005: "'Too few Americans,' says the CCF, 'remember that the Founding Fathers, authors of modern liberty, greatly enjoyed their food and drink.' . . . Now it seems that food liberty—just one of the many areas of personal choice fought for by the original American patriots—is constantly under attack."

Don't you just love it? The Founding Fathers fought for "food liberty," God bless 'em. I am a slightly serious student of the American Revolution, but I don't remember that aspect of the conflict. I do know that one of my heroes, the Boston bookseller and artillery general Henry Knox, was awfully fat. And that he died from getting a chicken bone stuck in his throat after the war. But I don't remember much talk of fighting the British—or even the evil Hessians—for the right to pig out. Maybe I missed something.

No, I didn't. The fact is that there is simply nothing these folks won't say or do to make a buck. I don't mean to be a fussbudget, but promoting "food liberty" as part of the nasty fight to keep fast food in the nation's schools strikes me as disgusting. Incidentally, Coke has lately wrapped itself in the cloak of decency with a tiny ad campaign to promote exercise. And they scrupulously do not mention Coke in their ads for exercise, because they don't want to taint that noble effort with commercialism. Right.

Look at the Label

Okay, back to the main business at hand. You get several shots at not eating crap: in the food market, when you buy things; in your home, when you decide what to cook; and at the table, when you decide what and how much to put in your greedy mowzer. At each of those stages, try to think just a little bit about what's good for you and what's rotten. And try to act like a grown-up.

You also get three choices with restaurants. One, you do not have to go to places that specialize in food that's horrible for you. Two, in the restaurant, you can order things that are good for you (and ask the waiter to take the bread away, immediately). Three, once the damn stuff is on your plate, you don't actually have to eat it all. Three strikes, ladies. Think about each one.

In addition, you should take grateful advantage of food labeling. Lord knows how it happened, in this militantly capitalistic/laissez-faire nation, but labeling is required by law, and it's pretty good. The type is small, but the information is huge. Learn to look at the label. Learn not to eat much with saturated fat in it. And try to stay away completely from the real killers, the trans fats. (The reference is to "partially hydrogenated oils" of one kind or another on the label.) And stay away from foods with lots of calories. Or lots of carbs. Easy-peasy. Eventually, looking at labels becomes kind of fun. You are often surprised to find really tasty stuff that is superlight on calories. You are even more often stunned to see how many calories and carbs some of your oldest and best-loved friends have been packing all these years. I pick up a box of pasta from time to time to see if it's still true that this pleasant little package contains, say, a thousand calories. I used to empty those packages into my tummy and thought I was doing myself a favor. Not so. Read the label!

Anyhow, cruise the shelves and look for food that tastes good, that's made of good stuff, and that doesn't have a million calories. It's a scavenger hunt. Be super careful to check the portion size that goes with the calorie number on the label. They are little cheats. On a can of soup, for instance, you'll find that a "portion" contains only 110 calories. But then you discover that the little can allegedly holds seventeen servings. It's not lying, exactly. It's just deeply misleading.

It Is Possible to Eat Fish

We are deeply wired to eat; you're not going to change that. But we can substitute good stuff for crummy stuff . . . fill our tummies with things that taste okay and don't make us fat or sick. We have all reached a certain age, and change does not get easier. But it isn't impossible, either. When I got on this kick, I'd been eating crap, happily, eagerly, compulsively, for sixty years. Most of my life, I had gotten away with it. Starting at about fifty, my luck ran out, and I went from 155 pounds to 207. Not nice. Then I met Harry, got into the Sacred Rules, and over time my weight drifted down to about 170, which was a joy. I'm about 180 now, which I can live with.

Along the way, I learned some interesting things from Harry and on my own. The most striking example: I have always hated fish. *Hated* it. Ate it, under protest, twice a year. I kept being told, however, how great it was for you and what a key it was to weight loss and weight control. With reluctance bordering on horror, I tried it again. Never mind the details, but I now eat fish five nights a week. And I do it for pleasure. And those rye crisp crackers that are made out of cardboard and twigs and taste horrible? I now eat them like peanuts. *Love 'em.* And I never eat the popular crackers that were the beloved staples of my youth and middle age. You can retrain your palate. Takes time, but it can be done.

Lose Twenty Pounds

Okay, time for a little shift in emphasis. Maybe it wouldn't be such a bad idea, after all, if you lost twenty pounds or whatever it would take to get back to your true weight. No rush. And no diet. It will just take care of itself, because once you start exercising seriously, you'll see yourself differently and you'll start to feel a little odd being overweight. You probably feel a little odd now, but that's not what I mean. Once you get in shape and get into the business of working out, it will start to seem, oh, inappropriate to be overweight. I don't know quite how, but it just happens. Then, whether gradually or in a plunge, your weight starts to drop. You really could lose twenty pounds. Without going nuts and without going on a diet.

A good trick is to have the right picture of yourself in your head. Exercise makes that much easier. Working out, you automatically have the picture of your young self in your head. It feels natural to get rid of the excess that just doesn't *belong* there . . . like putting down a package you've been carrying for too long. Like putting down that enticing box of white rice.

Incidentally, whole societies, whole countries, find obesity so profoundly at odds with the picture they have of themselves that it just doesn't happen. Not because of different genes or even different food, but because it's just out of the question. Think of how many fat Japanese people you know. Or those Frenchwomen we've been hearing so much about, come to that. In their countries, it isn't done. Make obesity *your* taboo. Draw a picture in your head—of you on that bike or in the hills or on the boat—so strong and sharp and clear that being heavier than you want is just out of the question. Sound a little mystical? Far-fetched? Try it. Once you've become younger, sometime next year, you'll want to look it, too. And you may.

Exercise and Weight

Few of us are going to lose weight directly by exercising, because it takes far too much exercise to burn off significant fat. Olympic endurance athletes burn 4,000 to 6,000 calories a day, but they're working out like maniacs four, five, and six hours a day, every day. You're not going to do that. You'll actively burn off a lot more calories than a sedentary woman, but not enough for major weight loss. But, as you will remember from the tiresome story of my wonderful metabolism, you get an amazing lift from having stronger muscles and a bigger aerobic base, even when you're not working out. Build the sucker and it does become a "FEED ME" monster. Once you get in shape, you're constantly burning much more energy. And remember, some 60 percent of all the calories you burn are those "maintenance" calories. Harry says—and it is certainly my experience—that you can increase your basal metabolism by 50 percent with rigorous exercise. That is huge.

The other way exercise works, of course, is that it really helps your self-image. Take a look around the gym. You'll see a few fat people, and it's entirely possible to pursue a heavy exercise regimen when you're very heavy yourself. I've done it. But it's not common. Look around a yoga class, and you'll see what I mean. Maybe they're all self-selected, and they looked like that the day they walked in, but I doubt it. I think that, like me, like a lot of people I talk to in gyms around the country, they just lost the weight somehow once they got in shape . . . once they got that new picture in their heads. I remember sitting on my bike in spin class those first months. The rooms are always mirrored, as you know, and I could not take my eyes off myself. I found myself staring, hypnotically, obsessively, at the folds around my gut. I didn't want to lug the flab around, now that I was doing all this vigorous stuff.

But again, we're talking about being younger—and thinner—next year. And the year after that. We're talking about a fundamentally different lifestyle, and it will take a while to kick in. That's all right; you're going to live a long time. So exercise hard and get interested in life. Thin will take care of itself. And, did I mention . . . Don't Eat Crap!

CHAPTER FOURTEEN

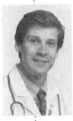

The Biology of Nutrition: Thinner Next Year

The message from thousands of studies, over decades of medical research, is clear: *Never go on a diet again.* The only way to lose weight is to embark on a program of steady, vigorous exercise, avoiding the worst foods being thrust upon you in our national diet, and eating less of everything. I wish that were not true, but it is. This is not a diet chapter; it's a nutrition chapter. So, as Chris already told you, quit eating crap. Here's why.

As you might expect, we'll be going back to nature and how your Darwinian body reacts to various foods. This way, you'll understand what we mean when we urge you not to go into "famine mode," which will make you fat. And you'll understand why we urge you to avoid the junk foods that make you ravenous and are inflammatory for your cells.

The first and most basic point is that your Darwinian body does not know what to make of excess. It does not know what to do in the face of steady doses of too much food. It was not designed for *over*abundance or idleness, and it reacts in crazy ways. It reacts as if they were signals of famine.

Back in nature, every calorie was precious, so our early ancestors developed very specific—and very successful—ways to handle predictable swings in the food supply. There are seasonal variations in the fat content of our bodies that are as old as time. Winter, the dry season, migration: We have faced episodic famine since the beginnings of life. Our bodies respond by storing up fat and cutting down radically on the use of energy. This biology is locked deep in our bodies—and in the bodies of every other animal on the planet.

You might think—from our own reaction to plenty—that all animals would pack away as much fat as possible whenever there was extra food at hand, but that's not true. Animals put on or drop fat in response to more subtly perceived need. Fawns, for example, stop growing in October and start storing the calories they eat as fat to survive the winter, regardless of how big they are or how much food there is. In the spring, they start to use the calories to grow again, to build bone and muscle, and *they don't get fat* no matter how much food there is. They grow bigger if there's more food, but they don't store fat. Humpback whales store massive amounts of fat as they feed in their summer grounds in the North Atlantic and then, using their blubber as fuel, migrate thousands of miles to their calving grounds near the equator. They do not eat at all for six months, surviving by using every calorie of stored fat to its maximum potential. Migrating birds, feeding on shrimp in Chesapeake Bay in the fall, double their fat reserves in less than a week and then fly nonstop to Africa, but in the spring, when there is even more food, they grow muscle and bone, and the females lay eggs. They don't get fat.

The fundamental reaction to *springtime* for most animals is to invest extra calories in lean muscle and growth. To grow stronger and bigger, not fatter, even when there is plenty of food around. For males, it's the time to grow new tissue, like muscles, bones, and sinew: partly to hunt, but also to compete for mates. For females, it's all of this, but it's also time to invest every extra scrap of energy in pregnancy. Women do store some fat to prepare for pregnancy, but not a lot, and it's not the same thing as obesity. There is a natural time to become fat, but it's heading into winter, not springtime. Fit-and-lean is the natural reaction to springtime. Game abounds, you are a healthy predator, and you surely do not want to burden yourself with an extra thirty pounds of fat.

But in times of incipient famine, that is exactly what you would want to do—like a bear going into hibernation or a deer on the edge of winter. So what are the signs of famine for humans? For us, the primary signal of famine was sedentary life. In the absence of food to hunt, we just sat around, conserving energy in that slow race with death. It's the sitting around that your body hears. Lock that image in your head. Your body reads idleness as a sign that you are starving to death, *no matter how much you eat.*

Exercise Against Decay

The signals of approaching famine may differ between humans and other animals, but the biology of our reactions is essentially identical. It is the biology of decay. As you know by now, this whole book has one core message—either you grow or you decay. And sure enough, that's the essence of the biology of nutrition as well. Put simply, the chemistry behind obesity involves decay. Shutting down every system you possibly can so that you can survive winter, drought, or famine. The fact that there *is* enough to eat today, or even vast excess, doesn't change this. If you are sedentary, your body reads the bacon cheese-burger as the carcass of the animal that starved to death just before you—your last-gasp chance to gorge. And here's an interesting thing. This biological response is turned on by our old friend C-6 and turned off by the C-10 of exercise. Scientists have known this for only a few years, but it makes perfect sense. C-6 and C-10 are, after all, the fundamental messengers of growth and decay.

That is why the single best thing you can do to stay or reverse obesity is to be physically active—to exercise con-sistently enough to send those springtime signals every day. The point of exercise is *not* to "burn off" calories, but rather to tell every part of your body to grow, to invest in building new tissue, and to run at a higher metabolic rate all day and all night long. Burning those extra calories is what does the job, even while you sleep. Losing weight will take some time, but it will occur. Ultimately, you will have to eat less, because you can overwhelm the most active metabolism with sheer caloric volume, but this becomes easier as you get in shape. Your body doesn't want the excess fuel, and your self-image changes, automatically and unconsciously, over a few months or a year.

So keep portion control in the back of your mind. Let it percolate through your sense of self, and someday you'll find yourself feeling full after the appetizer and enjoying a salad for lunch. Until then, just focus on cutting out the stuff that's killing you.

Quit Eating Starch: The White Foods

One of the foods that are killing you is starch (refined carbohydrates), which means the current buzz about bad carbohydrates is basically correct. (How refreshing to have a major food fad turn out to make some sense.) Bad carbs are the white foods—potatoes, white rice, and pretty much everything made with refined flour. The good carbohydrates are the ones found in nature—in fruits, vegetables, and whole grains, which have relatively few calories per pound. Starch is bad because it continually signals you to take another bite. Fat and protein signal your body to stop eating after a certain point, but carbohydrates, whether good or bad, don't. In nature, you had to eat prodigious amounts of them to get enough calories to stay alive, so a full stomach was the only shutoff signal you needed.

Even though the starch we eat today comes packed with calories, there's still no "turnoff" signal when you've eaten enough. Worse than that, it sparks a short-term surge of renewed hunger shortly after you eat. Starch is addictively appealing, packed with calories, has virtually no real nutritional value, and makes you ravenous again thirty minutes after you eat.

Starch is so bad for you because it's basically sugar, and sugar plays a key role in how your body "reads" its own food supply. Briefly, the accumulation of sugar tells your body how much you just ate. That sounds odd, but it's true, and here's why it's important. The chemicals you use to digest food are powerful and dangerous. They are designed to destroy and absorb the things you eat, like meat. That means they can destroy parts of you, too. Gastric acid, for instance, can burn right through your stomach wall, and too much insulin—a critical agent of digestion—can kill you in no time. So you need to secrete just the right amount of acid and insulin to digest the food you ate. No less, because you need to absorb all the energy you can, but certainly no more, because you don't want to start digesting yourself. And you need some reliable signal from the food you ate to regulate the flow of those digestive elements.

Sugar is that signal. In nature, sugar content was closely proportional to the available fat and protein in each meal, and the ratio was surprisingly steady across most plant and animal species. The rise in free sugar in the bloodstream after a meal was a remarkably accurate indicator of how many calories were just consumed. That's why it became the most important control signal for your digestion. Not the only one, but the most important one. The amount of free sugar in food is known as the glycemic index, and it's a critical marker of nutrition. It's not listed on packages, but diabetics who take their disease seriously know glycemic numbers cold.

Since there isn't much free sugar in nature, a small rise in sugar signals the end of a pretty big meal. And remember, the whole digestive cascade—insulin and all—keys off these changes in blood sugar.

But this carefully balanced response, developed over hundreds of millions of years by fish, birds, and dinosaurs, goes haywire in a fast-food world. Think back to when we were hunter-gatherers. Before we invented agriculture, we ate over two hundred different plants, fruits, and nuts and as many as a hundred different game animals, snakes, worms, and insects. There was precious little starch or sugar in any of them. Grains like wheat and root vegetables like potatoes, which are phenomenally high in starch, are the creations of agriculture, introduced only 10,000 years ago. That feels like a long time to us, but it's a nonevent in the evolution of our digestive tracts.

For a long time, we could barely harvest enough of the stuff to survive. But now we have a vast excess. And, in combination with sedentary living and saturated fat, it is killing us.

Here's something to think about at dinner tonight. There's more free sugar (the stuff that flows right into your bloodstream to trigger your digestive response) in mashed potatoes than in table sugar. And here's something else. There's as much free sugar in a single can of cola as in five pounds of venison. And what about this? There's more free sugar—to say nothing of saturated fat—in a supersize side of fries than in five pounds of elk. How does your body respond? With confusion. Because the signal you send with a 1,000-calorie meal of soda, fries, and a burger is that you have just eaten 10,000 calories of "natural food." And your body goes nuts, rushing out insulin and other digestive chemicals in response.

That's the real problem with starch. You have called for ten times the amount of digestive power you actually need. Ten times the insulin, gastric acid and a few dozen other dangerous chemicals. And things start to happen. First you hyperabsorb every last calorie from the food you ate. Second, because you obviously just killed a huge animal, your body tries to store every excess scrap of energy as fat. Third, because you now have enough insulin to digest a large animal but have killed only a soda and some fries, your blood sugar plummets and you're hungry again. Very, very hungry, and so you eat, usually quite a lot. What your poor Darwinian body reads is that you've gone from gluttony to starvation and back to gluttony in a couple of hours—*and it has no possible explanation for this!* This ultra-rapid cycling between gluttony and starvation has no parallel in nature. We talk about the signals you send with exercise, or by being sedentary, but our modern diet is so far outside your original design parameters that you are not sending *any* coherent signal. The whole system breaks down in a welter of hyperabsorption and decay. It's like rock stars smashing their guitars onstage. Noise comes out, but no more music. Adult diabetes is one of the results of this breakdown. Obesity, arthritis, heart disease, cancer, and stroke are some of the others.

So back to the simple message. *Do not go on a diet, but quit eating crap.* No matter what else you do, cut out the junk. Cut out the starch and the sugar, and replace them with fruits, vegetables, and whole grains—primitive, unrefined grains like pumpernickel and seven-grain bread. Quit eating more than you want. Say no to supersize portions, whether it's fries at the fast-food place or popcorn at the movies. Seriously consider ordering an appetizer and a salad as your full meal. Even that is usually more calories than you need, but it's a start.

Fat for Fuel

Now that you know how the insulin surge from eating starch drives your body to absorb every last calorie and store it as fat, it's only appropriate to start thinking about fat. And fat is going to surprise you. It has three roles in your body, and spilling over your belt is the least of them. You think of fat as storage, as that lump around your middle that grows steadily, year after year. But in nature fat is supposed to be active, dynamic tissue. The only time it turns into that inert lump is when winter comes. Active fat is healthy, essential, wonderful stuff. It's the inert fat of winter that does us in.

First, let's look at *active* fat, which we absorb and burn up every day, fat that we might store for a few hours, or a couple of days, but that moves in and out of our bodies as easily as it does in migrating birds flying to Africa. It's the healthy, "unsaturated" fat you've been hearing about. This fat, which is supposed to be the majority of the fat you consume, is the basic fuel for your metabolism and a key building block for your body.

Your body depends on the steady energy that fat supplies night and day throughout your life, and that's how you start to lose weight with exercise. Think of the hundredfold surge in C-6 that comes with running a marathon, and then the flooding river of C-10 that comes after it—the wave of inflammation that rips out all the tired, damaged muscle. The ensuing wave of growth that sweeps through your body, rebuilding your muscles and carrying the signals to grow into every corner of your body. That's all fueled by fat.

The wave of repair and regeneration goes on for hours after exercise, and your body runs in high gear the whole time, burning extra fat to replenish the energy in your muscles, to rebuild the glucose stores and the tissue so you can hunt again tomorrow. You burn far more fat recovering from exercise than you ever will on the treadmill. It's the great hidden trick to weight loss—stepping out of the gym, but still running your metabolism hard for the rest of the day. And even after the regeneration is complete and the muscles are rebuilt and recharged, your metabolism keeps ticking over at a higher rate than it does for the sedentary guys—even while you're sleeping. Your muscles are meat, not metal. You can't park them in the garage overnight; you have to feed them twenty-four hours a day. Sedentary women gain weight eating 1,800 calories a day. Serious women athletes, in peak condition, can lose weight eating

4,000 calories a day. You're not going to get there, but you can probably increase your resting metabolic demand by 50 percent with good, stiff, daily exercise. That means you burn 50 percent more calories each day just sitting around, *in addition* to whatever you burn at the gym, and that is key. Those extra calories you burn sitting around are how you lose weight.

Fat for Growth

Not only do you burn unsaturated fat, but you build with it. Your cell walls, for instance, all forty billion of them, are largely fat, as are all the connections between our brain cells, our sex hormones, and many of our chemical messenger molecules. You couldn't live a moment without the scaffolding of healthy fat that supports each living cell in your body. Indeed, you can't make a new cell without fat, and you make new cells all the time—more than twenty billion a year—especially when you're getting younger.

Your body is a massive, ongoing construction project, and unsaturated fat is one of the key building materials.

Fat for Storage

The fat that dominates our diet today is saturated fat—the form of fat we use to store energy for hard times. In nature, it's great stuff—an incredibly light and compact way to store energy. That might seem a little counterintuitive looking down at your belly, but it's true. Fat stores about twice as much energy per pound as sugar does. Another surprise, again counterintuitive in a Dunkin'

Donuts world, is the fact that, in nature, even this fat comes off you with comparative ease. In modern life, however, in the perpetual winter we have created through sloth and gluttony, your body uses every possible trick to lay down extra calories as saturated fat and to hold on to them like grim death.

Saturated fat has the longest shelf life, both in your body and in the Oreos on the supermarket shelf; it's warehouse fat. That's why the food industry loves it. Those people don't hate you, or want you to die young; they just love that saturated fat is chemically stable, has a long shelf life and carries flavor well. Too bad your body likes the shelf life, too.

And now for some more bad news. Saturated fat is not a passive player; it's an inflammatory messenger in its own right, an automatic signal that it's time to decay. Add it into the diet of lab animals, and they immediately start to produce C-6. Obese people are five times more likely to have inflammatory proteins in their blood than lean people, and the most sedentary people, even controlling for body weight, are four times more likely to have inflammatory proteins in their blood than the most fit. Inflammatory proteins, remember, are the ones that can kill you with heart attacks, strokes, and cancer. Which is why rates of colon, breast, and ovarian cancers in populations around the world are directly proportional to dietary levels of saturated fat.

It's because winter never lasted for decades before, and C-6 never lasted for decades before either. Blood markers of inflammation, such as C-reactive protein (not coincidentally, a marker of heart attack risk), rise progressively with obesity, which makes sense: being sedentary triggers C-6, which tells your body to start laying down fat. The fat in turn triggers more C-6, leading to more decay and more fat deposits, which triggers more C-6 . . . and so on. In

The Good Fat

The dominant fat found in nature is unsaturated fat. It moves in and out of our bodies easily, burns cleanly as fuel and builds strong, resilient cells and tissues. Unsaturated fat, a mainstay of the natural diet we no longer eat, is found in wild-game meat, most vegetable oils (especially olive and canola oils), nuts, fruits, vegetables, and especially in fatty fish like mackerel, salmon and sardines. In our primitive diet, 30 percent of our calories came from fat, but it was mostly good, healthy, unsaturated fat. Ironically, our modern diet also gets about 30 percent of its calories from fat, but it's mostly the bad, unhealthy, saturated fat.

We have less unsaturated fat in our diet for two reasons. The first is economic. Free-range animals have only about 10 percent body fat, and it's mostly unsaturated. Once you ship them to the feedlot, keep them from moving and fatten them up, their percentage of body fat goes up to 30, and most of that is saturated. Profits zoom (there's a lot more money in a fat cow than a skinny one), but so do your weight and cholesterol. So cut way, way down on your consumption of red meat. Limit yourself to lean cuts and smaller sizes . . . and don't eat too much of them, either.

The other problem with unsaturated fat is that it goes rancid faster than saturated fat. It's not storage fat; it's active fat, ready to use throughout your body, but harder to store and ship. So the food industry—rationally enough from their point of view—has taken it out of our diets as much as possible. Unsaturated fat has become a trickle in our diets, accounting for a tiny percent of what it did when we lived in nature.

response, white blood cells invade your fat tissue, creating a pool of decay, and then the white blood cells themselves secrete their own C-6, creating a vicious and deadly cycle of fat-inflammation-fat-inflammation. Even worse, your fat tissue secretes C-6 faster the fatter you get.

C-6 also makes it harder for your body to listen to the changes you do make in your diet. Researchers have found that mice, and patients, with high levels of systemic inflammation, those headed fastest toward their heart attacks, are the most resistant to cholesterol reductions with diet. Up to 40 percent of the cells in fat tissue in an obese person are not fat cells at all, but rather inflammatory cells—the same white blood cells we talked about in the walls of your arteries. And they release a steady trickle of C-6 day and night, but never enough to trigger C-10. You might hear the C-6 if you listen carefully when you open the refrigerator door in the middle of the night: *hiss-bump, hiss-bump.*

Is all this sounding familiar? It should, from reading about heart attacks in Chapter Five. Disturbingly familiar. The same white blood cells that invade your arterial walls to form plaque invade your fat tissue to cause the inflammation of chronic obesity. Even the minimum maintenance repair cycles begin to break down. Without enough unsaturated fat to build with, an obese person's body substitutes saturated fat. It builds the stuff right into your cell walls. But it's a slightly different shape than unsaturated fat and it doesn't quite fit. Imagine building a wall where some of the bricks are just a little off: that would be your cell walls. And so they don't work quite right. The other problem is that the saturated fat is still inflammatory, triggering local inflammation, which produces tiny drops of C-6 that collect throughout the cell walls of your most important tissues. Let me say it again: *Heart disease, stroke, cancer, and even*

Alzheimer's disease are all strongly linked to the inflammation caused by the saturated fat in our diet.

Saturated fats (and cholesterol) are found in full-fat dairy (butter, cheese, milk, and cream), but skim milk, nonfat yogurt, and nonfat cheese are pretty good for you. Eggs are probably fine in moderation, though no one knows for sure, and meat is generally bad. Chickens store fat under their skin, so chicken cooked without the skin is fine— unless you decide to fry it in a vat of oil! Very lean cuts of beef and pork are okay but hard to come by, and bacon and sausage, which I love, are terrible. You also have to steer clear of trans fat, a hidden, artificial fat the food industry came up with. Functionally, it's just the same as saturated fat. It's in almost every fried food, every doughnut, every cookie, pie, pastry, and almost every cracker you can buy in America. Pick up a bag of potato chips and add up all the fats listed on the label. Then look at the total fat number. They won't match. The "missing" fat is the trans fat. And it's very, very bad for you.

That's enough on the dark side for this short primer on nutrition, but I hope the core message is clear. Stop eating crap. Eat less. And exercise *hard* six days a week.

What *Can* You Eat?

Get ready for a quick canter through a list of the good stuff. Go as heavy as you can on fruits, vegetables, and whole grains. That's important for two reasons: fiber and micronutrients. Fiber is simple. It's roughage— indigestible roughage. It slows down the absorption of fat and keeps your colon working, clean and free of cancer. It's also the bulk you need to fill you up so you feel like you had a square meal. We had a ton of it in our original diets but have almost none now. Fiber content is listed on packages, so read those labels. High-fiber cereals and breads have about three grams per serving. Since your goal should be about forty grams a day, you can see how far we have to go.

Micronutrients, mainly trace minerals and vitamins, are also important . . . and just a little odd. There are hundreds of them, and no one knows for sure how much of each we need. We know they are critical to thousands of chemical reactions in our bodies and in short supply in our modern diets. We know they include chemicals that are essential to our immune systems, muscle and brain function, heart health, bone health, and blood formation, as well as the antioxidants that protect us against cancer. We know they abound in fruits and vegetables, and that you can't get them from supplements. In addition, we know that individual needs differ. Your body needs a slightly different mix of micronutrients than your neighbor's body. But there is no way to figure out which ones you need, or in what concentrations (though you can spend thousands of dollars getting your hair, fingernails, urine, and blood analyzed by people who will tell you differently). So take that multivitamin, but don't fool yourself into thinking that a breakfast of vitamin pills substitutes in any way for a healthy diet. Instead, eat a wide variety of good stuff, and your body will pick and choose what it needs with unerring accuracy.

The latest official recommendation is to eat nine servings a day of fruits and vegetables. Yes, it's a huge amount of leafy stuff, but work at it. Your colon may even start acting normally again! It makes very little difference which ones you eat, but try to eat at least four different colors of fruits and vegetables each day (shades of green count). And don't listen to people who malign fruit on account of its sugar content. That's nonsense. Fruit is loaded with nutrients, and in the context of the sugar load of our modern diets, worrying about the downside of fruit is silly.

Whole grains and legumes (beans) are the other major healthy food category. Before grains are processed, they contain a broad range of nutrients and not much free sugar. (Refining flour breaks down the cell walls of the grains and releases the sugar, which is why it makes food taste so good. But it also strips out most of the micronutrients and fiber.) Most "whole wheat" and multigrain bread in the supermarket doesn't count as truly whole-grain, which you'll understand if you read the labels. The first ingredient in the supermarket "health" breads is unbleached but *refined* flour. (Bleaching it makes it into white bread, but it's the refining part that turns it into starch.) The only good stuff is the heavy bread that comes from the health food store — seven-grain, twelve-grain, pumpernickel, and so forth. Whole grains (whole wheat, whole rye, etc.) have to be the *first* thing on the ingredients list, not the last, or someone is misleading you. Whole-grain breads have richer flavors than refined-flour breads, so it doesn't take long to get used to them and come to like them. (Refined flour does not taste any better; it's just that you're used to the sugar, and sugar is an acquired taste.) Luckily, as you get older, your taste buds don't like sugar as much and you can appreciate other flavors. You can get used to coffee with no sugar (or at least coffee with fewer than ten sugars); it takes only a month or so. Breakfast cereals are an easy place to win with this. Cheerios have whole wheat as the first ingredient, followed by things you don't need, but are still respectable. Shredded wheat has only one ingredient: whole wheat! Add some skim milk and a banana, or frozen blueberries, and you're a third of the way toward a healthy day.

Protein will not be a problem if you come even vaguely near a healthy diet . . . especially if you force yourself to like skim milk and other nonfat dairy. (Again, give it a month.) Eat lots of fish, the oilier the better. Eat white meat chicken, too: not as great as fish, but much better than red meat. Obviously, you're going to eat some red meat—this is America, after all, and it does taste wonderful—but take it easy. Eat much, much less, and get it as lean as you can, especially for burgers. In fact, start thinking of meat as a flavoring rather than a staple; a little bit goes a long way.

Salt is also pretty easy to discuss: We eat too much of it. We're supposed to get two grams a day, but most of us get eight to ten without even lifting a salt shaker. Since food manufacturers add salt and sugar to everything they make, just stay as close to fresh foods as you can and never add salt again.

One more tip: Remember that whole grains, vegetables, and fruits now take up much of the new food pyramid. Food purveyors like to say there's no such thing as bad food, there's just sometimes too much. Well, that's not quite right. Some things are so much worse for you that it makes sense to see them as just plain bad.

And another thing: If you buy it, you will eventually eat it. Good nutrition happens in the supermarket, not in the kitchen. Eat a good meal before you shop and make a list of all the healthy stuff you want to buy before you head out the door. Guess what? You will be thinner next year.

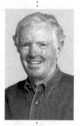

CHAPTER FIFTEEN

"The Drink"

n Ireland, the people have a special relationship with whiskey and other strong waters. They call it "The Drink," with capital letters in their voices. As one might say: "Then it was The Drink, I suppose, that took him away, the dear creature." As if to explain that the departed had been in the grip of forces larger than himself and was not entirely to blame. Being a quarter Irish myself, I have a wary respect for The Drink. And a deep and abiding affection for it, too. As for a wonderfully amusing old uncle, or perhaps a charming niece, who once in a great, great while ... murders someone. Once a month, say, but nothing you can't forgive in someone who is so much fun the rest of the time.

The Drink is such a joker in the deck of our lives that it is hard to know what, if anything, to say about it. Harry thinks it's so scary that we shouldn't talk about it at all, because, if you're going to talk about it, you have to mention the good side and that can be dangerously misleading for some people. He worries that you will just hear what you want to hear and tumble into addiction. Harry says, if alcohol were a medicine and had the side effects that it does—i.e., maybe 20 percent of users become *abusers* at some point in their lives—it would never get FDA approval. My reaction is respectful, as always of Harry's views, but a little different.

First, wine and liquor already have the equivalent of FDA approval and have had it for about ten thousand years. They tried to change that during Prohibition, and it didn't work so well. It's here; it's already in most of our lives; and it's not going away. So it makes sense to talk about it. Second, there is the troubling but stubborn fact that, for some of us, wine and liquor are among the great joys of life. Third, there are some remarkable population studies that indicate that drinking *in moderation* (you'll want to remember that part) is terrific for you. So, it is a tricky story, with the good news and bad news we've become so familiar with.

On the Bright Side

The good news is astonishing. I've been drinking for a while, but I was stunned, on New Year's Eve 2002, to read in *The New York Times,* and later in *Scientific American,* that steady drinking in moderation (which means two drinks or less a day for men; one for women) is not just fun . . . it is powerful medicine. (Before you get too excited, a "drink" is one and a half ounces of booze, or five ounces of wine.) Booze, used regularly and in moderation, is terrific for just about everything that ails you. Not, let me quickly say, if you become an alcoholic. Then it kills you. And lots and lots of perfectly nice women do become low-level (and high-level) alcoholics in their sixties and seventies; that's what scares Harry. Indeed, there have been recent studies that show that women over sixty are peculiarly and perilously subject to alcoholism . . . something we do need to talk about. And we will. But, in moderation, alcohol can be good for you. There are so many of these studies, and the results are so clear, that it is hard to argue with them, unless you want to step onto some kind of religious or moral ground. Here's some of what I read that day in the *Times*:

"Alcohol has become the sharpest double-edged sword in medicine. Thirty years of research has convinced many experts of the health benefits of moderate drinking for some people. A drink or two a day of wine, beer or liquor is, experts say, often the single best nonprescription way to prevent heart attacks—better than a low-fat diet or weight loss, better even than vigorous exercise. Moderate drinking can help prevent strokes, amputated limbs and dementia." (Amputated limbs? Yup, amputated limbs. Worth thinking about, for you clumsy do-it-your-selfer moms.)

The reporter, Abigail Zuger, went on: "'The science supporting the protective role of alcohol is indisputable; no one questions it anymore,' said Dr. Curtis Ellison, a professor of medicine and public health at the Boston University School of Medicine. 'There have been hundreds of studies, all consistent.'"

"In a study of more than 80,000 American women, those who drank moderately had only half the heart attack risk of those who did not drink at all, even if they were slim, did not smoke and exercised daily."

"Among more than 100,000 California adults, moderate drinking after age 40 was associated with reduced death rates during every subsequent decade of life—in some people by as much as 30 percent."

The *Times* piece pointed out that the studies at last

explained the endlessly pleasing "French paradox," which arises from the fact that the French eat more cheese, butter, and other fats than you can shake a stick at and still "their hearts are relatively free of fatty blockage." This also explains the Italian or Mediterranean paradox, to say nothing of the Chris Crowley paradox. It is good to have these things cleared up. Harry takes a wary, if not actually hostile, view of all these paradoxes. He suspects bad science in there somewhere. I, on the other hand, suspect his Puritan roots.

It doesn't matter what you drink. There is still some lingering thought that red wine is a damn fine antidote to cancer, but in general it doesn't matter. As long as you're steady about it. Drink a little every day, they all say. No bunching up . . . no bingeing. Every day. I can just see your partner sticking his head into your room: "Honey, have you had your martini yet?" Or, *Drink your wine, damn you! Do you want to die?*"

So, there you are . . . what we should have known all along. Wine and beer and booze are marvelous for us. At last, the scientific community is talking some sense.

The Dark Side

Okay, those same *New York Times* and *Scientific American* articles do make oblique reference to teeny problems associated with too much alcohol. In fact, they say the risk of too much alcohol takes almost all the fun out of the good news. And the notion of what is too much cuts in pretty early.

From that same *Times* piece: "Heavy drinking raises the risk of high blood pressure, heart failure and half a dozen forms of cancer; it may cause diabetes, pancreatic failure, liver failure and severe dementia. Heavy drinkers have mortality rates far higher than moderate drinkers, statistics which do not even include the effects of car accidents and alcohol-fueled violence that destroy not only the drinker but others as well."

Then they go on to make the dreary point that "The net health effects of alcohol are heavily influenced by its dangers. The World Health Organization estimates that, over all, alcohol causes as much illness and death as measles and malaria, and more years of life lost to death and disability than tobacco or illegal drugs." Not so great.

And for women over fifty-nine, the news may be quite a bit worse, as a 1998 study by the National Center on Addiction and Substance Abuse indicates. It reports that some 1.8 million older women are addicted to alcohol. That is a huge number, and the consequences are grizzly, partly because doctors (and women) fail to take due account of the fact that women's tolerance for liquor is lower than men's and that their tolerance goes down as they age. You should also bear in mind that the consequences of problem drinking can be radically compounded for those who also abuse prescription drugs (especially psychoactive drugs taken for anxiety or depression), which is also common among older women. Finally, the study says, if you happen to be nuts enough to still smoke at your age, the cocktail is truly toxic. When you hear "substance abuse," you don't automatically think "old girls," but you should. Happens a lot, and with appalling consequences (lots of sickness, suicide, and God-knows-what-all). So watch it.

For instance, pay attention to the fact that it takes less booze to make you stupid now. The CASA study says one drink a day is the max for mature women and problem drinking cuts in at two and a half drinks a day. And you may be better placed, psychologically, to start drinking more in your sixties, maybe because you're alone ... maybe because you're in the hole financially ... maybe you've got less structure in your life and more stress. In other words, you get a new shot, in your sixties, at becoming a drunk. A frighteningly good shot, according to the CASA study and Harry's experience. And it doesn't just happen to dopes and losers, Harry says. Successful, solid women with stable families and all that suddenly take a funny turn. So do not assume you can handle The Drink just because you've been doing so for the last forty years or because you're a great woman. It may not be true.

More grim news. Addiction or alcoholism is not the only downside to drinking. The ever-thoughtful Harry sent me a story on a study of heavy but functioning non-alcoholic drinkers. Men who drank a little more than three glasses of wine a night were shown in MRI tests to have measurable brain damage. "Our heavy drinkers sample was significantly impaired in measures of working memory, processing speed, attention, executive function, and balance," according to researcher Dieter Meyerhoff in the May 2004 *Journal of Alcoholism*. "Heavy drinking damages your brain ever so slightly, reducing your cognitive functioning in ways that may not be readily noticeable. To be safe, don't overdo it." The study didn't say what the cutoff level was for women, but obviously it's less than three drinks a day. In other words, while a little booze is good for a girl, more than a little is bad. And the sweet spot is awful damn small.

My trainer once made a terrifying point about drinking. I was feeling puny, I told him, because I'd had most of a bottle of wine the night before. I couldn't lift as much or do as many reps as usual. "That figures," he said. "Drinking too much ages you." *What?* Here I am, working like a crazy man to be younger, and my beloved Drink is making me old? Yep, it's true.

Okay, here is my serious, bottom-line advice, which is similar to what the experts say. If you don't drink, don't start. Too risky. That's mainstream advice. If you do drink, don't stop—*if you're able to do it in moderation.* Which is not so easy. If you *are* able to drink in moderation, you're golden. But remember, the cutoff point is one drink a night. When was the last time you stopped at one drink? I don't see it much, I must confess. And remember, as few as three-plus glasses of wine a night for men (less for women), over time, is bad.

Here is the golden mean that I suggest: Have a glass of wine a night as a magical garnish with your meal. A gentle push into a pleasant evening. Perhaps one night a week, feel free to have two. And quit. If you notice the "gentle push" getting a teeny bit urgent—like an old pet that is suddenly starting to growl and act funny—stop. 'Cause that sucker can bite you in a heartbeat, and the wound can fester for the rest of your life. At our age, things can get a lot worse a lot faster than we imagine.

But at our age, we also need as much joy as we can get our mitts on. For me, that most assuredly includes a glass or two of wine most nights, until death. Occasionally the exquisite, the life-enhancing martini. But watch it.

CHAPTER SIXTEEN

Menopause: The Natural Transition

Until a few years ago it looked like the "solution" to menopause, and the health problems of the years beyond, was to put almost all women on hormone therapy. Hormones not only relieved the symptoms of menopause, but also appeared to prevent heart disease, stroke, Alzheimer's, and a host of other terrible illnesses. If you look back at books on menopause from just a few years ago, it seemed like malpractice to deny women the benefits of estrogen replacement therapy. Then, in 2002, the Woman's Health Initiative study showed that hormones not only had *no* net health benefit, but actually *increased* the risk of serious illness by a small amount.

That single study brought the era of putting every menopausal woman on estrogen to a sudden halt. Perhaps more significantly, it changed the scientific model of menopause from a disease requiring treatment to a natural transition managed only as needed for symptom relief. According to a recent National Institutes of Health consensus panel, most women move through menopause without major problems; there are effective treatment options for symptoms, but they carry risk; and, most noteworthy, *menopause is a phase of life, not a disease.*

Hormones, acupuncture, and some alternative supplements work well as short-term solutions for specific symptoms when needed. But lifestyle—the platform of serious exercise, good nutrition, and emotional integration—is the most important therapeutic option for moving through menopause. Above all, lifestyle choices are the foundation for embracing the thirty years that most American women will have *after* menopause.

Think about that for a moment. Most American women will live for thirty years after menopause. That means that menopause is nowhere near the finish line; it's more like a *starting* line for a whole new phase of life ... one that will last for three decades. And every morning of those thirty years, you will wake to that fundamental biological choice: Do you want to decay or grow? That's the good news. The bad news is that the question takes on more urgency now, because the tide sets against you with menopause. The stakes are higher. The pace of decay picks up speed. Your rate of bone loss doubles. Your risk of heart disease—a small fraction of men's before menopause—catches up within a decade and then pulls ahead. You can still swim against the tide without too much trouble, but you can't afford to drift anymore.

Back on the savannah, your hormonal cycles, from puberty until somewhere in your forties, were precisely controlled to maximize your chances of successful pregnancy. Stress, sedentary living, and poor diets affect women's menstrual cycles to different degrees, because in nature those were all signals of peril . . . of dangerous times to carry a child. So menstrual cycles may not always look like they're precisely planned in modern times, but your body has a remarkably clear sense of what it's doing . . . up until around age fifty-one, when menopause starts for most women.

And it has an equally clear sense of what it's doing *after* menopause, usually by age fifty-five or so. Your body has moved into a new phase, no longer influenced by your estrogen cycles, but regulated by the daily balance between growth and decay that is built into all of us (women, men, antelope, dolphins, penguins, squid . . .).

Menopause is the hormonally tumultuous transition between these two highly ordered states, unpredictable, and different for each woman. It's a period of temporary chaos. Somewhat like the turbulence of the Middle Ages between the long stability of the Roman Empire and the creative explosion of the Renaissance. The important point is that medicine and alternative treatments can only alleviate the *symptoms* of menopause, and they all carry small risks. To affect the underlying biology, it's up to you to give your body guidance by managing your exercise, diet, and emotions as you head into your own renaissance years.

A Short Detour for the Healthy Skeptic

t would be natural for you to ask how much is really known for sure about menopause, and what you should believe. After all, a few years ago the notion that most women should take estrogen after menopause, probably for life, approached religious dogma. How did the medical profession swing from that certainty to a diametrically opposed certainty so quickly? And where did the information come from, anyway?

These are important questions to ask, because you are going to be a critical consumer of medical information for the rest of your life, and the media will bombard you with new recommendations and studies on a daily basis. Most of those stories will be inaccurate, and most of the recommendations will be wrong or, at best, partly right. The story of hormone replacement in menopause is a perfect illustration.

Let's start with what it means biologically to say that we "know" something. In everyday life, we think of knowledge in terms of yes/no answers. We know or we don't know. It's like a light switch that's on or off, making the room either light or dark. But in medical research, it is *never* that simple. We can't put people in test tubes. We have to study them in real life, where there are hundreds of different influences on health, *in addition to* the drug we are giving them. Most of the time the drug effect is just a faint biological whisper that we try to hear above the roar of growth and decay. We *try* to factor out some of the major lifestyle issues, like the influence of smoking, cholesterol, and so forth. And we *try* to include enough people that all the other influences average out, but it's an impossible task. We do our best, but the reality is that we *never* know for sure. Biology is like a huge jigsaw puzzle, and we only have bits and pieces. Sometimes we can connect enough of them to make a really great educated guess, and many times we have enough pieces to make a decent guess. But other times we know only enough to make dangerously bad guesses, cloaked in the guise of authority.

And while good researchers spend their lives thinking hard about these issues, the media, the pharmaceutical industry, and many doctors simply ignore them. A study of twenty people means almost nothing scientifically, but the reporter on the ten o'clock news may think it's just as newsworthy as a study of ten thousand people. And then there's the issue of bias. Ninety percent of the studies published by drug manufacturers show that their drugs work as hoped, but independent studies show that only about half of them do. Are the industry's studies outright lies? Generally not, but they are deceptive, because they present uncertainty as statistical probability, and then the willing media and many doctors present it as fact.

We should just say "we don't know" when the studies and statistics are marginal, and many doctors do. But others don't, because humans don't like uncertainty. This goes back to our basic neural biology. No human likes uncertainty. We are wired to make rapid decisions, and we get very anxious if we can't. When there is no hard information, we choose the fastest route to a decision — any decision — to end the panic of uncertainty. You can measure this in the lab, and experimental psychologists have shown over and over again that humans will *reliably* make blatantly bad decisions to end the feeling of uncertainty. So doctors, who after all are human, talk themselves out of uncertainty. And medical reporters, newspaper and magazine editors, and patients all do, too.

This was the case with menopause and hormone therapy. The science was equivocal, and no one really knew for sure what hormones did to women's bodies. In that context, doctors, as a profession, forgot the critical distinction between the proven and the promising. Seduced by the possibility of offering women important health benefits, and with a strong push from an aggressive pharmaceutical industry, rafts of studies that provided partial answers were pulled together to provide what we assumed was the truth.

A host of "observational" studies over the years had looked at women *who had already chosen,* before the studies began, whether or not to take hormones. In those studies, the women who chose to take estrogen did better than those who didn't—50 percent fewer heart attacks, fewer strokes, fewer cases of Alzheimer's, less osteoporosis, albeit with a slight increase in the risk of breast cancer.

It seemed apparent that hormones were the answer. Luckily, just before the "answer" became completely locked in as established medical fact, the National Institutes of Health, under the leadership of its first woman head, Bernadine Healy, MD, was charged with addressing (and redressing) decades of gender bias in medical research. And so began one of the largest, most ambitious, and most successful public health studies in history: the Woman's Health Initiative.

The WHI is a massive national research study looking at heart disease, breast cancer, colon cancer, hormone replacement therapy, and osteoporosis in women from age fifty to seventy-nine. The hormone part of the study is over, but the rest of the study is continuing and will provide critical information on women's health for decades to come. With an initial budget of 625 *million* dollars, the WHI is studying more than 160,000 women at forty research centers across the nation. The hormone part of the WHI involved thousands of women who—and this is critical—didn't choose whether or not to take estrogen. They agreed to be randomized, to have the researchers flip a coin to assign them estrogen or placebo. The WHI is so accurate and powerful because all those women bravely agreed to leave their treatment up to a coin toss at a time when the benefits of estrogen seemed so clearly established that some thought putting women in the placebo group was unethical.

The WHI illustrates how ferociously difficult and expensive it is to do good science and how *dangerous* it is to confuse the proven with the promising. In the case of hormone therapy, the theory made all sorts of sense biologically. Women are far healthier than men until menopause, but then they catch up—especially in terms of heart disease. And all those observational trials showing that the women who took hormones did better were real studies. You can go back and read them today and think they are very convincing, until you realize that they are wrong.

What happened was that the researchers did not appreciate how central lifestyle is to our long-term health. The women who *chose* hormone therapy were not identical to the women who did not. They were, on average, more health-conscious. They exercised more. They ate better. And despite the fact that they lived in the same neighborhoods, went to the same doctors, and quit smoking at the same rate, they got sick less often and lived longer. It was the lifestyle differences—not the estrogen—that accounted for the 50 percent reduction in heart attacks and the reductions in strokes and Alzheimer's. The estrogen was just a marker for healthier lifestyles.

That marker effect is, by the way, why I have reservations about studies touting the health benefits of moderate, daily alcohol. Moderate drinking may be just a marker for a more connected lifestyle, which is the actual benefit. Sitting down to dinner *en famille* is at least as likely an explanation of the French paradox as the bottle of Bordeaux on the table.

Most studies try to "control" for lifestyle, but whether you're researching alcohol, estrogen, vitamins, antidepressants, or cholesterol medications, lifestyle is too huge and varied an engine for health or sickness to ever truly control for it in an observational study. If you're lucky, an observational study will generate the most important questions.

Then you have to do a real study to answer them. The problem is that real studies are hugely expensive, like $625 million expensive, so we can answer only a small handful of the most important questions with certainty. Those are the studies that are supposed to generate headlines, congressional hearings, and fundamental changes in the way we practice medicine. The rest of the studies—99 percent of the research published—are not supposed to be news. They are just scientists talking to one another and should never see the evening news. So why do the media make it sound as if immortality lies just around the corner and every study is a major advance or retreat? Because they need headlines more than they need news, and no one would buy a newspaper with the headline TINY ADVANCE IN MEDICAL SCIENCE POSSIBLE. CONFIRMATION IN A DECADE. Luckily the NIH asked some important questions about women's health and menopause ten years ago and dedicated $625 million to answer them. As a result, women today have more accurate information about menopause than we have arguably ever had about any major health issue.

So, What *Do* We Know?

With that as background, let's look at what the hundreds of thousands of women who participated in the WHI and other studies have to say about menopause.

Natural menopause can start anywhere from your early forties to late fifties, but *on average* menopause in American women starts at age fifty-one and lasts about four years. The caveat is that no woman has an average menopause. Each experience is different, and the variations are enormous.

Half of all women report only minimal symptoms, while others have significant symptoms throughout menopause and a few have problems for more than a decade on either side.

The studies showed that menopause itself has only a few true symptoms. More than 50 percent of women will have hot flashes, night sweats, and mood swings, and about a third will have significant vaginal dryness. There is a small increase in urinary problems, and a small number of women have sleeping problems beyond those caused by the night sweats. Sexual satisfaction dips during menopause for some women and increases for others.

Hot flashes are caused by sudden dilation of the blood vessels in the skin, which brings warm blood from the core of your body to the surface. This is the normal mechanism your body uses to cool off in hot weather, but the control mechanism is somehow short-circuited by the changing estrogen levels of menopause. The temperature of your skin can rise as much as eight degrees in a matter of seconds during a hot flash. Each generally lasts around five minutes, though on occasion they can last as long as thirty minutes. The cooling mechanism is so effective that a long episode can leave you chilled and shivering.

Night sweats are hot flashes that happen at night. Your temperature drops a little when you sleep, so the proportional rise in temperature is greater; besides, you tend to be under the covers, so the heating leads to more sweating than during the day. Also, because your temperature regulation system works more slowly when you're sleeping, the episodes tend to last longer, meaning they can significantly disrupt sleep. Apart from the sleep deficits caused by night sweats, the overall rate of insomnia in surveys remains about the same before, during and after menopause. That doesn't mean some women don't have worsening insomnia during menopause. Some do, while some sleep better, but the average stays the same. Most of the sleep trouble that women notice from age fifty onward is related to lack of exercise, stress, artificial light and noise, late-night TV, and the natural shortening of the sleep cycle that comes with aging.

Symptomatic vaginal dryness affects about a third of women and makes sex less comfortable for about half of women. In the absence of estrogen, the lining tissue of the vagina atrophies, which can make urination painful and can limit the amount of lubricating fluid your vagina can secrete during sex. Surveys of sexual satisfaction in women without symptomatic dryness give mixed results, with some women reporting increased sexual desire and satisfaction, and slightly more reporting less desire and satisfaction; overall, women report about the same level of sexual satisfaction and frequency after menopause as they did before.

Mood swings are often the most disruptive symptom of menopause, and like the mood swings of adolescence — to which they are chemically related — they are unpredictable and different for everyone. They often begin years before menopause itself and can surge through the limbic and primal brains as great and powerful waves. Emotion is stronger than thought, preceding it both in evolution and in the wiring of our brain, so an emotion — frustration, rage, sadness, sexual desire, fatigue — can take on a reality independent of external circumstance. Because these mood swings can begin years before menopause, many women don't see them as chemical events until long after they start. They seem to come out of the blue, which is generally the hardest part. Most women find that understanding the mood swings as the perimenopausal symptoms they are — as actual, physical surges of chemicals flooding through the brain in response to fluctuating estrogen levels — makes a big difference. It does not change the intensity of the emotion, but it does help keep it in perspective as a temporary, physical state and not a symptom of mental illness.

That's a key point, and the research is crystal clear on this: *Mood swings are not a mental problem,* and they don't trigger mental illness. For years, the link between menopause and a wide variety of mental illnesses was simply assumed. Well, it's simply not true. Menopause has *no* association with depression, anxiety, or any other psychological disorder. Women go through depressions and other problems during their menopausal years, but at the exact same rate as before and after menopause. As intense as the mood swings can be, they have no impact on your fundamental emotional health.

According to hundreds of thousands of women who have participated in careful research studies, those four symptoms — hot flashes, night sweats, vaginal dryness, and mood swings — are the only major symptoms of menopause. So why is menopause linked with so many other problems? Because menopause happens during the years when the tide begins to set against you. Depression, weight gain, mental slowing, sleep troubles, joint problems, fatigue, and anxiety affect women and men alike as our forties turn into our fifties. These problems are not caused by menopause; they are caused by C-6. They are caused by decay ... which is good news, because your options for dealing with menopause are limited, but your options for dealing with decay are not. So here's what we know:

There is no increase in the rate of depression or other mental illness during menopause. The mood swings of menopause, however bad they get, bear no relationship to mental illness. They do not trigger depression, and they are not permanent. Women (and men) get depressed in their forties and fifties at the same rate as before and after menopause.

There is no weight gain associated with menopause. Women (and men) gain weight steadily in this country, but there is no statistical spike upward during menopause. Just that slow, steady march toward obesity caused by being sedentary and eating too much. Of course, the tide changes more rapidly in some people than others, and there are plenty of women and men who gain fifteen pounds in a single year somewhere in their forties or fifties. No matter what the timing looks like, the studies show that it's not menopause. Male and female alike, some people just hit a sudden riptide of decay in those years. Their metabolic rates plummet and the pounds pile on. It's demoralizing, but avoidable. . . if you run to the gym and cut your portions down. If you need encouragement, consider this: studies show that there is *no difference* in body fat percentage between serious, postmenopausal women athletes and those in college. A few more wrinkles perhaps, but no difference in body fat, from twenty to old age, as long as you stay fit.

There is no decline in mental functioning associated with menopause. The benign trend toward forgetting where you put the car keys continues apace in both sexes, but there is no decline in cognitive abilities during menopause.

Women can experience waves of fatigue or aching as part of their mood swings, but there is no link between arthritis or chronic fatigue states and menopause. These symptoms are real, but they are symptoms of decay, not the absence of estrogen.

The Lifestyle Treatment

Exercise remains the foundation for reduced menopausal symptoms. The studies on this are largely observational, but both aerobic exercise and strength training reduce mood swings, hot flashes, and night sweats. Morning exercise seems to be a little more effective than exercising later in the day, but both work well. The increase in lean muscle mass and baseline metabolic rate that come with serious exercise are your best weapons for fighting steady weight gain; in addition, exercise is by far the most effective preventive strategy for osteoporosis. (That doesn't mean you can forget your calcium: 1,500 milligrams a day, with 400 IU of vitamin D. Take 500 milligrams when you brush your teeth in the morning and at night, and another 500 milligrams on your way to exercise every day.)

Diets high in soy may help with all the symptoms of menopause (including vaginal dryness), probably because soy is a distant chemical cousin of estrogen. Japanese women, whose diet is naturally high in soy, almost never have hot flashes; in fact, there is no word for them in Japanese. But if you're not into soy, try a lighter diet high in fruits, vegetables, whole grains, and unsaturated fats. Sugar, caffeine, alcohol, chocolate, hot or spicy foods, overeating, stress, and sedentary living all trigger hot flashes and night sweats. Since the triggers are so individual for each woman, there may be other triggers for you. It often helps to keep a detailed diary of symptoms, diet, and exercise for a month to see what the correlations are for you.

Attitude counts! Studies show that a positive attitude reduces the frequency of symptoms. Women who report positive attitudes going into these years do best in terms of reported scores of life satisfaction and seem to have an easier time managing symptoms. Formally structured behavioral techniques like meditation and relaxation exercises have also been effective in a number of studies, and some women find it helpful to have the support of meditation classes and other groups.

Vaginal dryness does not respond to most lifestyle changes (other than possibly soy). It helps to start using a lubricant immediately if you notice discomfort during sex. This works well for most women, though for some it's not enough. In that case, talk to your doctor about whether hormone replacement is right for you. It's important to address this early on, because the less often you have sex, the more fragile the lining of your vagina can become, and this can set up a cycle of painful sex, less sex, and even more painful sex.

Pills, Supplements, and Other Treatments

f lifestyle alone is not enough for you, the medical treatment options are simple and effective. Acupuncture helps a number of women, and the risks are minimal, or you can replace the estrogen your body used to make with either hormones prescribed by your doctor or herbal supplements. It's important to understand that herbal supplements are still hormone treatments. They seem to work because they have plant-derived estrogens rather than the animal-derived estrogens of the pharmaceuticals. Which is safer is anyone's guess, since no good studies have been done. The likelihood is that it makes little difference where the estrogen comes from; however you look at it, you're accepting risk in exchange for relief.

The risk you accept with hormone treatment, according to WHI data, is a small increase in the possibility of invasive breast cancer, heart attack, stroke, and blood clots in the lung. Putting them all together, there is a 0.3 percent increase in the risk of serious illness for each year you take hormone therapy. Balancing it out, your risks of hip fracture and colon cancer go down by about 0.1 percent with hormone therapy. Assuming that each of these events, good or bad, is equally important, then on balance there is a 0.2 percent net increase in the risk of serious illness for each additional year you take hormones. Another way of saying this is that for every thousand women taking hormones, two will face serious illness each year as a result and 998 women will be fine.

The WHI also found that low-dose hormone therapy is very effective for the *symptoms* of menopause. For women with severe hot flashes, vaginal dryness, mood swings, and night sweats, the benefits may be worth the small risk. For most women, they are not. The WHI study was stopped early because the risks became apparent, and all the women who were on hormone therapy stopped it at that point. Most of them (75 percent) stayed off hormones. But 25 percent resumed hormones because, for them, the symptom relief was worth the risk. Most women use hormones for a relatively short time, stopping within five years, and move into the postmenopausal biology without further trouble, but there are a small number of women who find that estrogen improves their long-term quality of life enough that they choose to use it indefinitely.

The Decision Is Yours

t would be nice if our news was that the right exercise, nutrition, and attitude revolutionize menopause, and that you will skate right through with no symptoms if you adopt the healthy lifestyle, but it's not. Women report over and over again that being strong and fit, eating right, and taking charge emotionally make a major difference to their menopausal experience. It helps *every* woman; for some, it makes all the difference in the world. That should be reason enough to give it a whirl. But the *real* reason to change your lifestyle is that menopause kicks off the tide of decay like a hurricane. For whatever biological reason, decay is slower in women than in men up until menopause. After that, the increase in bone loss and the dramatic acceleration in heart disease, cancer, arthritis, fatigue, obesity, and depression is like being on a bobsled run. But it's all just decay, and decay is optional.

The bottom line is that whether your menopause is easy or hard, it's only a stage of life. Like adolescence, graduate school, or raising toddlers, it has its own finite time frame. No matter what you do, it will last a number of years, and then it will end. The thirty years of the renaissance that then lie ahead of you are the real reason to exercise, to eat right, and to connect . . . because the end of your menopause is the starting line for the rest of your life.

PART TWO

Take Charge of Your Life

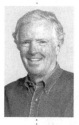

CHAPTER SEVENTEEN

"Teddy Doesn't Care!"

When I was sent off to first grade in the fall of 1940—to the very same school Harry was sent to a hundred years later—my father and his brother Ben (two people of tremendous energy and charm) had me pumped. They cared like crazy, and they passed it on. I was urged to grab a seat in the first row on the first day, which I did. I was told to listen hard and to get my hand up fast, and I did that, too. I duked it out with Deedee Bethell for the monthly spelling prize, which went mostly to her but sometimes to me. That delighted Pa and Uncle Ben.

One kid named Teddy took a different line. He sat in the back and was not much interested in what was going on. When pressed by the teacher one day, he astonished me by saying, with perfect serenity, "I don't care." That was it. The teacher let it go. I went home that afternoon, absolutely flabbergasted. I told Pa and Uncle Ben and the others, "Teddy doesn't care!" Again and again, that day and later, "Teddy does *not* care!" I couldn't get over it. The phrase became a joke in my family. My beloved sister Petie still says it sometimes, when I press her to do this or that and she doesn't want to. "Teddy doesn't care," she says and ruefully shakes her head. Won't budge after that. It still stumps me.

At this stage, you may think that I must have been a *nightmare* as a child. And as an old man. True. But think about this: *Caring* . . . being interested enough to get up every day and give it a shot . . . to do new stuff, do old stuff . . . to keep on going when you wouldn't mind sitting down for a while . . . that is a gift of God. Or Darwin. Or The Shore Country Day School. It is *the* great theme of this entire book, and a true blessing. At some juncture, some dark and stormy night when you can't sleep, some dreary Monday morning when you've lost interest in yourself and others, there is an almost irresistible temptation to say, "Who am I kidding? Who cares if I get up and do my exercises today? Or eat a vast tub of popcorn at the movies? Or work on that project I've been so excited about? Really, who cares?"

I respectfully submit that the answer better be "I do." Or you're cooked. That is the message of the last few chapters of the book in particular, which is why it rises to the level of being Harry's Sixth Rule. Harry's Sixth Rule reads, in its entirety: *Care.*

Care is a triple-barreled message, a Gatling gun of advice. First, we urge you to care enough about exercise and nutrition so that you have a decent body and a good attitude going into the Next Third. Lord knows, that's important. But the book veers off into new territory at this point and we mean something a little different. Up until now, it has almost all been about your body and being *physically* younger next year. Critical stuff, obviously, and the foundation for the rest of your life. But that's only part of it, and not necessarily the most important part. With exercise, you have given yourself a great set of wheels. But that doesn't amount to much unless you go out on the road. The rest of the book is about life on the road. Once you've taken charge of your body, you have to think about taking charge of your life.

Isak Dinesen Cared

Many women, by no means all, have a much greater flair for connecting and committing to other people than men do. But it's not at all clear that women have a concomitant flair for just plain *caring*, which is a little different. Those are the women who use menopause or retirement (theirs or their husband's) as an excuse for giving up generally and saying the hell with it. You know . . . the children are gone, so they might just as well go sit on the goofy bench and knit granny squares . . . wait for the end.

Remember that Isak Dinesen quote from Chapter One? Look at it again, if you wish. "Women," she wrote, "when they are old enough to have done with the business of being women, and can let loose their strength, may be the most powerful creatures in the world." To get a little idea where Ms. Dinesen was coming from, consider that she held on to that notion with ferocity until the very end of a life much tormented by terrible illness (syphilis visited upon her by her husband) and pain. She wrote right up to the end and stayed involved and passionately interested always. Listen to this, from a letter to a young man she befriended and traveled with as a frail, old woman:

"I shall not forget you, and I beg you, too, to remember that altogether we have salted away sweet hours, made the years rewind, eaten all the ripened heart of life, and made a luscious pickle of the rind."

"Made a luscious pickle of the rind," by heaven! That's what we want in life, my beloveds! That's caring! That's the Next Third!

Most of us have no legitimate business dreaming of greatness, I suppose, but we don't have to be mutts, either. And it is the serious business of all of us to come as close to greatness—or some personal version of it—as our gifts and characters will allow. It is the first thing to care about. And caring is the great gift in life. The engine that pulls the train, the magic that fills the sails.

Well, that got a little highfalutin there for a minute, didn't it? Actually, much of caring is a matter not of aspiring to greatness but of caring about and for others, connecting and committing to other people. As a matter of fact, that's Harry's Seventh Rule: *Connect and commit.* It means rededicating yourself to family, friends, companions. Get involved in groups and do communal things, whether work or play. That, as we will be saying, is peculiarly the woman's gift. But there is a strong temptation, for women as well as men, to do less on this front as we age, and that is a huge mistake. Because, it turns out, we were literally built to be involved with and to care for one another, and that does not change one bit as we age.

That's what being a mammal is all about. That's Harry's next chapter, and it is powerful stuff. If we don't exercise our social skills—if we let ourselves become cut off and increasingly solitary as we age—we will become ill and die. Hundreds of fascinating studies have demonstrated the point. So "caring" also means caring about other people and being involved with them . . . acting like the pack animals we are, right to the end. But it also goes beyond that.

It means getting involved in a kind of caring that satisfies what may be a core element of our rational brain as well as our essential human character. We believe that we were built to aspire to things beyond the interests of ourselves or our immediate pack . . . to "care" in that exalted sense about larger than human goals. There is at least a possibility that this "higher caring" is what being a human is all about.

Harry and I don't want to say much about this higher caring because it's so very personal. For many people, choosing how to work for the greater good is influenced by their notions of spirituality, a topic we simply can't deal with seriously within the compass of this book. But we can say that finding the selflessness within you—getting that one right for you—may trump everything else. Caring at every level is one of the most important things you can do in the Next Third of your life.

Keep a Log or Lose Your Command

Back to earth and some very mundane advice about the mechanics of caring. One of the great keys to caring about your own life is to *watch it*. And to keep track as if it mattered a lot. Which it does. If you're going to have a good life, a full life, a life that you and others care about, it must be the *examined life*. And that means writing stuff down. It sounds banal, but it works. It's so easy to look out at the rain and give it the Full Teddy—"I don't care"— and go back to sleep. If you know you're going to have to admit it, in writing, you're more likely to get up and go.

So keep a simple diary or log in which you write down, every day, these three things: 1) what I ate, 2) what I did for exercise (or didn't), and 3) what I did with my life—sexually, socially, morally . . . whatever you care about. It is a tremendous help to know, as you decide from minute to minute what to do, that "All Will Be Written" and "All Will Be Known." It is a talismanic business, a sign that *someone cares*. Even if it's just you.

Keeping the log—and keeping it accurately—has been the sacred duty of captains and commanders from the earliest times. Those who tampered with or kept a false log faced grave penalties, certainly including loss of command. That's a good phrase, actually. If you do not keep an accurate log, you will lose command. Of yourself.

I first learned this log stunt from my passionate one-on-one diet adviser, Stephen Gullo. He had a sensible regimen and a hundred clever tricks. But his first trick was that he cared. His real trick was that he taught me to care. And his most important device was the keeping of a log.

Every day I had to fill in a sheet, listing every damn thing I ate or drank, and then fax it to him. Once a week, I had to go sit in his office while he lectured and cheered me on. After he and I were done, I kept up my log and became my own cheering section. I already knew what not to eat; everyone does. The big thing was teaching myself to care. The price of fitness is eternal vigilance, and the greatest spur to diligence is the daily log. Works equally well with your efforts to connect and commit. Write stuff down and you become a serious person, in the sense of someone who cares. A daily log is a crutch to lean on when you're weak. A shield to ward off boredom when you're tired. A sword to symbolize resolve when you falter. It is a practical tool and a magical device that stands between you and the relentless thought "You know what? I just don't care." A couple of times I lost my log and, *without fail,* went straight to hell. In my experience, there is a perfect correlation between dropping the log and going to hell. So now I carry it everywhere. And I keep it religiously.

But whether you try the log or not, remember: The great trick in life is to care. On the surface and at the deep heart's core. Teddy died young, by the way. Teddy didn't care.

CHAPTER EIGHTEEN

The Limbic Brain and the Biology of Emotion

U p to this point, the book has been about our bodies and how to grow physically younger for years to come. Now we want to talk about the emotional and mental sides of our lives, because the choices we make there have just as much biological impact as the choices we make for our physical bodies. Staying emotionally connected, in particular, turns out to be a biological imperative, a critical part of the good life—and a real challenge as we age in our society.

Through some mix of nature and nurture, many women are better at creating and maintaining emotional connections than men, but it takes a major, sustained effort to stay fully connected as you age no matter your gender. The stakes are enormous. And it all comes back to biology, the biology of connection and love.

We evolved as highly social animals, like chimps, wolves, and dolphins. It's not a choice; our survival depends on being part of a group. No one has ever gone into the Amazon jungle and found an isolated person; it's always a tribe. There is no such thing as a solitary human in nature, because isolation is fatal. We were designed to be emotional creatures, which is to say that we are mammals.

"So what?" you ask. "Why is being a mammal so special?" After all, a hundred million years ago we were furry, insignificant little rodents, trying not to get stepped on by dinosaurs, barely holding on to our evolutionary niche. We are special, and we triumphed, because we invented a second brain.

Remember the primitive, reptilian brain? The extraordinary, runs-your-body-perfectly, does-exactly-what-you-tell-it-to brain? Well, mammals built a whole new brain that sits on top of the reptilian one. You can think of it as the emotional brain, but its real name is the limbic brain. Roll that word around on your tongue: *limbic*. You're going to find it coming up over and over again in your conversations after you finish this book. Chris now uses the word incessantly and enjoys it immensely. It's an actual, physical chunk of brain that runs our emotions, and in many ways it's the most important brain you have. You can scoop this brain up and hold it in your hand. You can see it work with functional MRI scanning. You can trace its development back a hundred million years. Complex emotions, from the limbic brain, are the reason mammals succeeded—the reason we survived when the dinosaurs did not. We are social and emotional creatures from start to finish.

Fear and Anger, Love and Play

Reptiles developed our primal negative emotions. So it's your physical, reptilian brain that has the control centers for fear and aggression—our deepest and most primitive emotions. Killing prey, territorial defense, fight or flight, sexual predation, and ruthless self-interest are the legacy of our earliest ancestors. Surges of adrenaline, morphine, serotonin, and scores of other chemicals flood the crocodile's brain when the prey dives into the river. We have that brain, and those chemicals, today. They are our automatic, chemical responses to the environment, to threat or prey, and they work!

The brilliance, the absolute triumph of mammals, is that we took the same chemistry, the same neurological pathways, the same wiring and turned it around to create positive emotions. Reptiles run purely on negative reinforcement. Mammals invented love, joy, pleasure, and play, all of which are enshrined in our DNA, in the chemical and neurological pathways in our limbic brains.

But the reptiles were doing pretty well with anger, fear and aggression. Why go further? What's the biological point of love or friendship, of being happy, sad, optimistic, or enthusiastic? Why invest extra energy in building a whole new level of brain structures? The answer is to raise our young and to work together for the survival of the pack.

Nature hardwired our reptilian ancestors for their own *individual* survival. Apart from a drive to have sex, reptiles have no real social or parental instinct. Most of them cheerfully eat their young, which is why they're programmed to lay eggs and get out of town before they hatch. Remember, those reptilian instincts are still a deeply powerful part of us. Our primitive brain still runs our most basic functions, giving us a fierce, primal drive for our personal survival. What it doesn't give us is a concern for the survival of our children or the ability to sense the emotions of others.

Our limbic brain gives us these two critical advantages over the reptiles. It lets us love our young and work in groups. Its first and most powerful creation is the emotional cascade triggered by the sight and sounds of our own off-spring. The overwhelming biology of parental love swamps our more basic, selfish instincts — don't eat the baby! As time went by, the limbic tool kit allowed us to build the second great advantage — working in groups — through a complex neurological array of positive reinforcement for the sharing of food, warmth, shelter, information, and parenting.

Parenting and Living in Packs

Mammals succeeded because we learned how to invest much more in our young than lizards do. "Don't get between a mother bear and her cubs" is wisdom known to all of us. But the words "Don't get between a turtle and her eggs" have never appeared in print before.

Live young take much more energy before birth than eggs do, and actually sticking around to raise the young takes even more investment in each offspring. "Prey mammals," like mice, have a relatively modest commitment to their young. They have large, frequent litters and expect to lose quite a few from each. Genetically, they are protected by their numbers more than by their parents. Predator mammals, like bears and humans, on the other hand, have few offspring, take a long time to raise them to independence and safety, and are profoundly connected to them. The loss of a predator child is a major genetic blow to the parent, and we have a much greater emotional attachment to our young as a result. That attachment is choreographed by the limbic brain, your mammalian brain, which controls your reptilian brain, turning its selfish instincts into love, attachment, and social connections.

Here's a critical point. Your limbic brain is physically in control of your primitive brain and deeply wired into it, but it's only in *partial* control. It has a series of small control centers that sit on top of and around the physical brain. Each center is primarily responsible for different moods, but they are cross-wired so they talk to one another all the time. In a very real sense, your emotions and moods control your body's basic, physical chemistry.

Think of the physical reaction you have to anxiety. That's the limbic brain kicking your reptilian adrenaline into action, like a rider on a big, powerful horse with a mean streak. If the rider is good, she has a lot of control, but the horse will always be a bigger, stronger animal. If the rider isn't so good, or if the horse spooks, she can get thrown and the horse will take off without her. The same

Some Practical Advice on Sleep

As you get older, you need about an hour less sleep a night, but that sleep is more important. The biological catch-22 is that you don't sleep as well as the years go on, which means you have to work harder at it. My advice is embarrassingly simple, but here it is: Go to bed an hour earlier than you usually do, in a room that's truly dark. Try it for a month and see how much your quality of life changes. The best way to ensure that you wake up halfway through the night and get poor-quality sleep is to drink alcohol in the evening, with caffeine after lunch a close second, so watch what you're drinking. Finally, if you don't get a good night's sleep, try to sneak in a nap after lunch.

holds true for your primal instincts. If you work at it, your limbic brain can become a good, even great rider, but the horse will always outweigh you by a thousand pounds; you will never be as firmly in control as you would like to think. In practical terms, that means you will pay a steep physical price if you don't get the emotional structure of your life into fairly good shape.

Luckily for us, although the limbic brain responds to both positive and negative reinforcement, it responds best to the chemistry of pleasure: We feel good about our offspring and about being part of a working group. Back in nature, packs let us forage with a collective eye out for predators, hunt more effectively, and share child-raising. Packs also let us sleep: a surprisingly important activity, which we spend a third of our lives at. Mammals can sleep at night and doze during the day because their limbic systems synchronize throughout the pack. At least one animal is always in light sleep and will wake the others if there is a threat. Reptiles can't synchronize their rhythms and therefore can't rely on a pack to let them sleep. They can never relax . . . never rely on the group to watch their back when their eyes are closed.

Sleep is still largely mysterious, but one of its major functions is to give our metabolisms downtime for routine maintenance, which is especially important because we are warm-blooded. Being warm-blooded lets us run at full speed whenever we want. We can hunt at night, or in the predawn chill, because we keep our muscles at 98.6 degrees, ready to go, all the time, but running at high speed all the time takes its toll. NASCAR drivers wear out a $75,000 engine with each race, and then it's back to the shop for a new one. We are not far off. When we're on high alert and stressed, we secrete a steady river of adrenaline and cortisol: our stress hormones. They keep us in high gear for the demands of kill-or-be-killed but, like the race car, at a cost. Our bodies need a constant repair effort, and it can only happen when we're not racing. In effect, adrenaline and cortisol prevent us from diverting energy to repair when we might need it to survive. When the environment is not threatening, when it's time to relax, another set of chemicals are released, like serotonin and relatives of morphine and Valium. These are the signals that it's safe to wind down and go into the shop to replace the engine, rebuild the transmission, and get ready for tomorrow's race. This balance between high alert and repair mode fluctuates throughout the day, but the major repair period is when we sleep.

The downside of being warm-blooded is that we have to maintain a constant body temperature, which is not a trivial issue when the weather turns nasty. Snuggling is about as cheap (and beneficial) a way of heating yourself as possible. Mammals, it turns out, are actually drawn to one another—to physical, social contact. Touch produces serotonin, which feels good. We want more of it, and we seek out contact. The snuggling, the warm safety of the pack, releases more serotonin in our brains, and the serotonin blocks the release of adrenaline and cortisol. It's the physical signal that the hunt is over, that it's time to wind down. Time to let our body repair itself after a day of hunting, gathering, and not being eaten. In the bad old days of evolution, being eaten or starving to death were not abstractions—they were daily realities. Striking the right balance between fear, high-alert mode and calm, relaxed, repair-and-feeding mode was critical. Emotions let us do this collectively rather than individually, which puts us a half-step ahead of the competition.

But the reptilian brain was always there, lurking below the surface of group living. You—the individual—still have to survive in order to reproduce. So our limbic and reptilian brains learned to work together, balancing the individual with the pack. Balancing the primal emotions of fear and aggression with the new emotions of love, joy, pleasure, and play. Being part of a pack takes constant positive reinforcement; if we don't experience it, if we isolate ourselves, the negative chemistry of our reptilian brain takes over. That's why play turns out to be such a surprisingly important mammalian achievement. It's a strong signal that we are part of a healthy group. Our limbic brain leads us to crave companionship for its own sake. To want to belong to and matter to those around us. To love, and to be loved in return.

Nature wastes nothing, and it never stops working, so let's give the limbic brain a hundred million years to grow up, and look what happens.

The Storyteller

Long, long ago, a wandering storyteller, powerfully built but dressed in ragged garments, joins your tribe in the small, close circle around the low, flickering fire. The night is clear and cool, and the stars are brilliant pinpricks of light in the darkness overhead. Beyond the light cast by the fire, the world is lost in shadow. Men and women sit together, their children leaning back against their knees, as the storyteller launches into his tale. Starting with a tone so low that you have to bend forward to hear him, he builds his tale of tragic love between a man and woman—a tale of passion, betrayal, war, and loneliness. As he speaks, he looks slowly and deliberately around the circle. His eyes meet yours across the fire, and you feel the physical shock of the connection. His eyes are deep-set, and as you look deeper into them his soft words become real and the story becomes yours. You fall in love. You feel the anguish and anger. You lose yourself in the direct, primal connection with the storyteller, and you are moved to tears by fictional characters in a tale told by a stranger.

So what happened around that fire? Why can we connect so deeply with others? Why can the person across the fire — or the table — affect your mood so powerfully, stir you to passion, anger, laughter, or tears? You've had this experience. You know that friends, family, storytellers, musicians, actors — and audiences — all have this effect on your own moods and emotions. How does this work?

The explanation is, in the end, simple and physical. Because of the limbic way we're made, we are not emotional islands. Simply put, *we complete each other*. In both good and bad ways, to be sure, but we do complete each other, and therefore we cannot make it alone. This is such a magical part of being alive that it seems almost sacrilegious to look behind the curtain. But the biology turns out to be just as magical as the experience, fairly simple, and critical to the rest of your life.

Your limbic brain reads the real world and makes emotions out of it. We read hundreds of subtle signals in each encounter: body language, tone of voice, the flickers of facial expression that give nuance to each sentence, the glances that speak their own volumes. Neurologically, we are profoundly visual creatures. The visual processing centers in our brains are enormous — far out of proportion to our eyesight, which is about average as animals go. So why build all that extra brainpower around fairly puny signals? And what are you looking at, anyway?

It turns out that you don't devote much of your brain to looking at trees, or rocks, or even prey. You look at people.

Specifically, you look at faces with a hungry intensity. Standard visual information about where the doorknob is, or how fast the tennis ball is moving, goes to a few, relatively small areas of your brain. When you look at another person, however, and specifically when you look at a person's face, functional MRI scanning shows massive sections of brain waking up to process the information. It's like someone throwing the switch for a night game at Yankee Stadium; a huge, brightly lit image shows up on the scan, totally separate from the area that processed the image of a rock, and it's all devoted to absorbing and interpreting every nuance of facial expression. You have millions of brain cells called "mirror neurons" whose job is to pick up the emotions of others and mirror them within your own limbic brain. That's the biological infrastructure for empathy. You literally read minds, or at least emotions.

Sadly, autistic children (and, to a lesser degree, severely abused or neglected children and severely depressed patients) don't do this. The faces of those who love them register in the standard vision areas—in the most severe cases with no more limbic content than a street sign. Yankee Stadium remains dark and empty.

We are primarily visual creatures, but further floods of information come from sounds, from touch, smell, temperature, from all our myriad sensors, internal and external; the limbic brain is constantly supplied with an astonishingly rich stream of information about every aspect of what's happening inside and outside our bodies. There are millions of signals to the limbic brain, every second, and each one gets a tiny chemical tag, a minute emotion, as it moves through the brain. Scientists have yet to find *any* brain signal that does not get a specific emotional tag from your limbic systems.

How can your brain make sense of this staggering, impossible ocean of information? The solution is brilliantly simple. Your brain makes maps. And not just a few maps, but maps of everything—thousands of them every second. Physical, social, and intellectual maps streaming in, emotional maps streaming out. To a large extent, you navigate your world and your life from emotional maps.

Sensory maps come up from the physical brain below: one map for temperature around the body, another map of light touch around the body (the feeling of a gentle breeze on your skin, or a light caress), another of visual information, a listening map, a map of salt concentration in your blood, of muscle position and tension, of bowel function, of bladder fullness, of saliva secretion, of scent—thousands more maps of individual, discrete physical patterns.

In addition, thousands of *social* maps come down from the thinking, social brain above—the brain that makes you human. Where do you stand in the pack, who owes you food or favors, whom can you trust, whom can you not, who likes you, whom do you like, what is every member of the group feeling, thinking and doing each second . . . hundreds of social calculations going on all the time.

And each map, each of the thousands of physical and social maps you create each second, also gets an emotional tag: a chemical feeling about your world. Each map contributes a slight chemical nuance to the limbic chemistry, a dash of serotonin, morphine, or adrenaline—each one a dash of relaxation, anger, anxiety, love, excitement, fear, or optimism. Part of your map right now relates to your experience reading this page, but there are hundreds more. Are you in a comfortable hammock or a commuter train? Did you exercise this morning or stay up late last night? Did you get a raise yesterday or did you get fired? Did your kid hug you this morning? Are your pants too tight? Bladder a little full? Gentle breeze blowing through your hair? If you take a moment to think of the flood of feelings that make up your emotions this instant, and then realize that there are massive, subconscious inputs that you're not even aware of (salt concentration in your bloodstream, for instance), you get a sense of what the limbic brain does for you all the time. The emotional mix of this instant, right now, reading this page, is the sum of all the individual maps you've generated around this particular experience, blended to create a single, complex, master emotional map of this moment in time. And it will be slightly different in a few seconds, or a few minutes, because your phenomenally complex inner and outer worlds will be slightly different, and you will have generated thousands of additional maps, and a different master chemistry of your mood.

Much of basic human behavior (not all, but an important part) turns out to be the result of massive automatic neurochemical chain reactions, and vice versa. There are also massive automatic neurochemical chain reactions in response to behavior—modulated to an extraordinarily high degree by learned and genetic influences, but powerful and inescapable.

The Dance of Life

There is one last step: modern life. Let's skip a hundred million years of mammals slowly building their brains, getting smarter bit by bit, and get right to you. Starting two million years ago, we began to climb out of nature. We started to leave evolution behind. Our brains exploded, tripling in size to create the subtle, thinking, calculating, problem-solving, tool-using, social-climbing, chatting, linguistic neocortical brain: the *thinking* brain. The *physical* brain speaks the language of sensation and movement. The *emotional* brain speaks the language of feelings and mood. The *thinking* brain, the conscious, thinking brain, our brain, *your brain,* speaks the language of . . . *language.*

Suddenly, in addition to our own brain maps of the environment, we had access to other people's brain maps as well. Group-dependent, collaborative activities like hunting, foraging, raising children, and sharing knowledge . . . teaching one another how to make things . . . took priority in early communication. Being part of a pack was good, but being part of a tribe, with real communication, was phenomenal: more food, better hunting, wearing clothes, using tools, taking a village to raise a child. In two million years, we expanded into every climate on Earth. Language and the opposable thumb drove this evolutionary explosion, but only because we already knew how to love and how to belong to one another. Of course, cheating, gossiping, stealing, lying, and plotting to kill each other weren't that far behind, but they were *not* the primary, driving force. Helping, caring, and loving each other were.

Now, with all three of our brains properly in place, we can step out of the evolutionary crucible and into our modern lives. Free to think our thoughts and act our actions. Free at last, you may be tempted to think, to lead a purely rational life. Well, not quite, because nature throws nothing away. Remember that the basic biological building blocks didn't change. You just figured out how to wire the whole thing up in a completely new way to make use of the torrents of information that started to come in. The conscious, thinking brain was superimposed on our primitive and limbic brains, but they were still left with responsibility for a tremendous amount of what we do, how we do it, and who we are.

We are primitives, we are mammals, and we are humans, all at once. And the three brains are intricately wired together. What that means for the limbic brain is that conscious thoughts and the actions they generate shoot back huge streams of information to the limbic system. Thoughts and emotions are partners in a never-ending tango: a dance of life, with no solos. Thoughts and emotions alternate the lead, but careful research has shown that, most of the time, our emotions take the lead. And our thoughts (in which we have such touching faith) follow. Maybe it "should" be the other way around, but it isn't.

Emotion literally precedes thought at the neural level. So a positive emotion will tend to generate a positive thought in response. And because it's an ongoing dance, having a positive thought will loop back through the limbic system to generate a positive feeling. The same loop works for negative thoughts and feelings, and research has shown that we have a remarkable ability to think and feel our way into happier or more depressed states, regardless of external reality, and you can train yourself to live in either an optimistic or a pessimistic frame of mind *regardless of your external circumstances*. Six months after winning the lottery, most people are back to their baseline mood, or a little below. And six months after spinal cord injuries, the majority of paraplegics rate their quality of life as better than average. Cognitive behavioral therapy, the science of teaching people how to train their thoughts into more positive patterns, is as effective as medication in treating depression, and with a lower relapse rate. It's not Dale Carnegie, but it's not that far off, either. How you view your life has a surprisingly large role in determining how your life goes, so there is a real premium on having *positive emotions*. The good news is that you can create positive emotions by *consciously* creating positive environments. You do this by deliberately driving away the modern versions of lions and tigers . . . stress, loneliness, and idle worry about status. By reaching out to good stimuli: exercise, decent sleep, rational diet, love, and *play*. Happiness comes primarily from building connections, from giving and getting love and friendship, and that just takes good old-fashioned work— hard, but deeply satisfying work. Connect and commit, in other words, to generate positive emotions and drive away despair.

Dancing with Strangers

Given the importance of the limbic brain, it's no wonder that you were touched when you looked into the stranger's eyes across the campfire, hearing his words . . . the sound of his voice. But the first intake of information to the limbic system, the visceral shock that you experienced looking into the storyteller's eyes, was just the beginning of a limbic dance. What happened next was even more remarkable.

Your response communicated itself instantly back into the storyteller's limbic system. Every nuance of your response registered deep in his brain through his visual connections and his mirror neurons. The slight dilation of your pupils as the adrenaline hit, your shift toward him, the slight straightening of your spine, the flickering of your facial muscles as you absorbed and mirrored the emotions of the story—all fed directly into his limbic system. He absorbed these signals from each person in the tribe, and each signal changed him a little bit. Remember, this was all chemical. He didn't control it; it just happened to him. The tribe tuned in to him emotionally, and his response in turn tuned you further in to him and to the collective rhythm of the group. A great circle of emotion and chemistry formed between you and the storyteller and with everyone else in that magic group around the fire. And that circle has a nice name: limbic resonance.

Remember that name: limbic resonance. And remember the concept, too, because this extraordinary process does not just happen on special occasions. It happens every second that you spend with other people. Experimental psychologists have known for decades that we share moods. There are people who bring us up just by walking into the room; now you know why. You are always tuning in to those around you: being changed by their moods and changing them in return, in a constant limbic dance. And the whole remarkable process feels good. Indeed, it feels so good (directly and unconsciously) that we cannot do without it. We wither, and we die. So do not underrate the emotional side of life. Connect and commit and be young.

It's accepted wisdom that women are naturally good at connecting to the emotional side of life. Beyond your experiences in daily life, think of all the books, TV shows, and cultural assumptions pointing to this. So it will come as no surprise that it's also scientifically accurate. Hundreds of research studies confirm that women are much better than men at creating and maintaining limbic resonance. Women are better at working to ensure that families stay connected as the years go on and at building lasting friendships and deep connections from the many different aspects of their lives. High school and college friends, friends from work, friends from raising children together, from neighborhood committees, from all the volunteer efforts at school functions, the shared vacations, the shared challenges. Some of these bonds and friendships fall away, of course, as part of the natural cycle of growing and changing. Because many connections remain, however, in the normal course of events new friendships grow.

But there is a cautionary note. Women are so used to having their lives filled to 110 percent capacity with connections and obligations that they often assume, on some level, that it will be that way forever. The mix of family, friends, and career provides such a huge level of commitment and engagement that the challenge for decades on end is how to fit it all in. During all those years of looking for bits and pieces of time for yourself, it's hard to plan for the day when having too little connection and engagement might become the danger.

The danger is real, however, because we can outlive so many of our connections. Women over eighty are the fastest-growing segment of our population, followed by men over eighty, and the *fact* of our new longevity has simply not settled in. We don't plan for it, so isolation can take hold. And if it does, the tide can set against you. Just as in our physical life there is a limbic choice to make every day: grow or decay. Be involved or die. The growth or decay in our social networks is cultural, but the effect on our bodies and brains is real, and often deadly.

It's hard to see the damage of isolation as it's happening, because it's so incremental. It's like watching paint fade on the side of a barn. Children grow up, careers wind down or change, friends move away, partners may sicken or die. All of that is the real and present danger—the steady tide eroding our limbic connections. If you don't steadily renew those connections and commitments, you can end up swept a long way out to sea before you realize what's happening. And don't think it can't happen to you. Surveys show that 60 percent of older American women live alone. Those who get out of the house and stay involved with their communities, activities, friends, and families do well; those who don't tend to decay. Telephone contact helps, but it's not enough. We are wired for *real* contact, for vision and touch and movement, and we are wired to be *working together*. To be doing things together and to be relevant to the tribe: foraging, hunting, taking care of our young, gossiping, playing, making clothes and tools. We need connections in real time. If you make this a job—by building new bridges, taking on new challenges, new involvements, making new friends and building new communities—you can stay connected virtually forever. You can do this at any age, but it's easier if you start early.

The Biology of Social Connection

Hundreds of studies confirm that isolation hurts us and connection heals us through the same basic, physical mechanisms as exercise and diet. Older people who have at least one close friend have cardiovascular systems that are younger by a series of objective measures than those of isolated people. Blood vessels are measurably more elastic, cardiac reserve is higher, cardiac inflammatory protein levels are lower, blood pressure response to exercise is better, and so on. More connected people also have stress hormone blood profiles that are measurably healthier than those of isolated people. Less cortisol, less inflammation, less insulin, lower blood sugar. Cardiac catheterization studies show that the less socially connected a woman is, the more plaque she has in her arteries. Women with fewer social connections have fewer circulating immune cells in their blood and weaker immune responses to vaccines. In one study, researchers swabbed viruses into volunteers' noses, and the most socially connected volunteers got markedly fewer colds than the least connected.

When you take a puppy away from its mother, there are immediate disturbances in heart rate, digestion, cortisol levels, blood pressure, energy, and sleep. The same is true for humans. The more a baby is touched and held in the neonatal ICU, the higher its survival rate; babies who are not touched at all are highly likely to die. That same limbic chemistry operates in adults, too. When nurses touch cardiac patients in the ICU, it brings an immediate reduction in the number of abnormal beats on the heart monitor. Your blood pressure falls when you hear the sound of another person's voice. Electrical resistance in the skin, a chemical marker for the fight-or-flight response, falls off dramatically with therapeutic touch or massage. The list goes on for pages and pages, and the point is that connecting is a biological imperative.

Connect to Live

Sadly, I see people in my practice who give up on connection, who stop living years before they die. These are women and men who feel so overwhelmed by the prospect of getting out there and building new connections that they stop trying. Our society doesn't help matters, with its emphasis on the nuclear family and the workplace as the centers of social togetherness. But the consequences of not making connections are so devastating that you cannot allow yourself to retreat into isolation. The stakes are too high. A study of 4,000 women and men in Alameda County, California, showed a direct link between the size of one's social circle and survival, with larger circles bringing ever greater longevity. Women with fewer than six regular contacts outside the house had significantly higher rates of blocked coronary arteries, were more likely to be obese and to have diabetes, high blood pressure, and depression and were two and a half times more likely to die over the course of the study.

Having either a good marriage or just one close friend cuts mortality by a third, and the benefit increases the more your circle broadens. It's reassuring to note that both quality and quantity count independently in this. Some people have a few close friends or family, while others have a broad network of involvement with their community. Either works well, though the best is to have both. There is a growing recognition that older Americans are turning friends into the new family as siblings and children scatter across the country and as people move to different communities with retirement. Marriage brings a major increase in longevity to men and a minor one to women, probably because men report that their main source of social connection is their wife while women report a much broader network of close connections. In one study, older patients, both women and men, were three times more likely to survive heart attacks if they were socially connected and supported. In another, women who had strong relationships with others were twice as likely to survive. Even the limbic connection to pets counts for quite a lot. Dog owners, for instance, have lower cardiac mortality.

Cultures can affect these connections, and in some ways coming to America can be dangerous. People who emigrated to America from Japan and lost the close connections of their homeland had a tripling of their rate of heart disease, even after factoring out the effect of diet, and this despite the fact that they smoke far more in Japan than we do here. Both Costa Ricans and Cubans have greater longevity than Americans do, despite poverty and higher levels of tobacco use. The leading theory is that both countries have strong, traditional family and community networks. In fact, *social connections are a more powerful factor in health and mortality than smoking, alcohol, exercise, nutrition, or age.* Researchers enrolled fifty isolated women in a program of involvement in community support groups and organizations. A year later, half of them had become active participants, with marked improvements in mood and health. The other half had stopped working at it, with predictable results.

Interestingly, staying physically active also increases your likelihood of staying socially connected. In a study of 6,500 older adults there was a linear relationship between levels of walking, biking, or gardening and the number of social contacts.

We all know this in our hearts, and we see it in the lives of those around us. Talk to any nurse about how much it matters to have visitors in the hospital—about the difference in outcome for those people who have a steady stream of visitors, the wall covered with get-well cards, the flowers obscuring the monitors and tubing. But the thing is, you can't wait until trouble strikes to build your community. You have to work at it day after day, year in and year out; make the calls, make the effort, be the hospital visitor years before you need one yourself.

Beyond mortality and illness, isolation can breed depression, which has reached epidemic proportions in our country, through a complex mix of predispositon and culture. Somewhere around 15 percent of our population suffers from clinical depression; many more have depressive symptoms that do not rise to the level of a diagnosis. And women are twice as susceptible to it as men. Age is *not* a risk factor for depression, but isolation is. Decades of research have shown over and over again that low levels of social connection can lead to depression—and depression in turn can lead to heart attacks and cancer.

Clinical depression is an illness beyond the scope of this book, and I am not suggesting that all depression is caused by limbic factors, or that limbic connections can protect all patients from illness. But they clearly play a deeply important role. While isolation and pessimism are the equivalent of opening the gates to the barbarians, connection and optimism are massive bulwarks against letting depression in. Remember that most isolation is decay, and most decay is *optional;* growth is the other choice.

Make Connecting a Job

t takes steady work to stay connected to friends and family. I am lucky that no one in my family has shied away from the effort, and so I couldn't imagine any other way until I became a doctor and saw the isolation and decay that define aging in our society. My mother and father each care deeply about building their passions and connections. They work hard at staying in touch with friends, and they're critically important people in their children's and grandchildren's lives. They have made living, caring, and connecting their job.

Beyond the gratitude I feel for being on the other end of this, I see it enriching their lives. Driving four hours each way to be at Grandparents Day is a chore, the hour-plus in the folding chairs at assembly is probably not the highlight of the day, and the ten minutes with the grandchild is wonderful but short. Ten minutes of limbic connection for ten hours of time may not seem like such a bargain. But they have almost always been there, and their grandchildren know it, and they feel it. So now, as they get older, the kids have real conversations with their grandparents. About friends, school choices, rap music, and all the myriad details of teenage life. They would love one another no matter what, but they have wonderful, deep, important relationships because my parents built them, brick by limbic brick, over the years.

Sex and the Limbic Life

f isolation is limbic death, sex is limbic life, bringing with it the benefits of touch, emotional connection, love. And, not surprisingly, it's a healthy thing to do. Interestingly, studies suggest that men live longer in direct proportion to the *frequency* of sex, while women live longer in direct proportion to the *quality* of sex. Sexuality, which is the limbic component of touch and emotional connection, is more important than physical sex, and if you can't have sex for some reason, snuggling works almost as well.

For couples where both partners remain physically active, the only predictor of an active sex life as you age is an active sex life in your forties and fifties. By that time, sex has already gone out of many relationships (not always to the detriment of the relationships, which can remain loving if not passionate). But if you make it to forty with a good sex life, you are statistically set for the long haul. Sexually active older couples have sex about six times a month, a frequency that continues into their nineties! Sexually active couples live longer and their marriages are more likely to last. Sex may become somewhat different with age, but people consistently report that there is just as much pleasure in it.

Of course, the loss of a partner is a major blow to anyone's sexuality. And 60 percent of women—many of whom will see a slightly older husband die at a slightly younger age (if they haven't divorced already)—will be alone at some point in their lives. But both research and anecdotal reports suggest that increasing numbers of women (and men) are finding new partners as time goes on. Lots of my female patients find old boyfriends coming back into their lives in their sixties, seventies, and eighties. Others enjoy sex or nonsexual companionship in more open relationships. Some women fall in love and remarry after years alone. Some find happiness in same-sex relationships; some remain open to that possibility but never meet the right person. There is no predicting it. You just never know.

Assuming you have a partner, and assuming that you never lost or can reclaim your sexuality, there is one final potential barrier, which is the physical ability to have sex. The fact is, if you can climb a flight of stairs, you can have sex. Maybe not athletic sex, but satisfying sex. Bad hips, weak knees, and sore backs pose challenges but not insurmountable obstacles, as long as there is tenderness, affection, and a good sense of humor. Vaginal dryness and pain during sex are obstacles, but ones your doctor can almost always help you with. Vaginal moisturizers like Replens and good lubricants like Astroglide work very well; if that's not enough, estrogen therapy, either in pill or cream form, is a good option for many women. And if the problem is his, Viagra is remarkably effective. Even though we use far more medications than we need to in this country, this is one area where they can make a real difference in the quality of your life.

Illness knocks everyone's sexuality for a loop, but lust has a few billion years of evolution going for it. Very few physical disabilities actually preclude sex in the long run, but broken bones, cancer, heart attacks, and obesity all deliver antisexual messages. No one feels particularly sexy during chemo, but millions of women reclaim their sexuality after strokes, mastectomies, hip replacements, and long stays in rehab hospitals. While physical aging poses challenges, it very rarely imposes barriers. A sense of humor and tenderness go an awfully long way toward keeping us sexual as we age, and so does a stubborn refusal to give up on it.

The mantra of this book—grow or decay—should have you fighting hard for the quality of your life. It is the only sensible way to approach aging, and certainly the only way to keep your sexual self awake. If not, you'll give in to our culture's relentless message that youth and sex are synonymous. This is particularly true if you let yourself go (a big blow to your self image and sexuality). Besides, the decay of sedentary living creates a subtle form of physical depression that affects your libido as much as your heart and immune system. Your sexual energy ebbs, an event all too easy to see as "normal" simply because it's a common occurrence. It's sad that it's common, but it's tragic that we have come to accept it as normal. Luckily, this particular blow against sexuality can be reversed at any age. All the signals you send for growth with exercise, nutrition, and connection have a sexual component; physical fitness in particular is strongly linked to libido and sexuality.

Attitude Counts

O ptimism is an extraordinary limbic resource and available to everyone, because it's a learned skill. You can *decide* to be optimistic with remarkable success. Not Pollyanna optimistic, but glass-half-full optimistic, and it's worth the effort. Women who are optimistic about motherhood before pregnancy have a much lower risk of postpartum depression. Optimistic women have lower mortality rates from cancer and heart disease. If you approach illness with a positive, optimistic attitude, you have lower blood pressure, better immune function. You recover from bypass surgery faster and better, you get out of bed sooner after back surgery, and you go back to work and regular exercise sooner. Anger doubles your risk of heart disease. But perceiving your work as satisfying cuts your risk of heart disease in half.

One of my favorite studies of optimism and social connection involved a group of older nuns. It turned out that those who used more optimistic language in autobiographical essays they wrote as young women remained highly functional as they aged, lived longer than those who carried a more pessimistic attitude through life, and were much less likely to develop Alzheimer's. The most optimistic nuns were two and a half times as likely to survive from age seventy-five to age ninety-five as the most pessimistic. And researchers could predict the risk of Alzheimers for each nun, with 90 percent accuracy, based on her lifetime level of pessimism or optimism. Consider Sister Mary, who was highly optimistic and involved in her community throughout her life. When she died at the age of a hundred and one, her autopsy showed fairly advanced Alzheimer's lesions in her brain, but her cognitive testing had been normal and she had shown no signs of dementia in her daily life. It appears that somehow her optimism and involvement protected her from the disease itself.

Another nun in this study provides one of my favorite quotes about aging. Sister Esther, at age one hundred and six, getting around fine on a walker and still going strong as an active member of her community, was quoted as saying, "Some days I feel like I'm a hundred and fifty, but I just make up my mind I'm not going to give up." Not surprisingly, the autobiographical essay she'd written eighty years earlier was optimistic and showed the same spirit. It's a great quote to tape to the bathroom mirror: *"Some days I feel like I'm a hundred and fifty, but I just make up my mind I'm not going to give up."*

Despite all the horrible stories about aging in our country, Sister Esther's attitude is more the norm than the exception. Most older people feel good about their lives; the majority of people in one survey felt that the best years of their lives came somewhere *after* age sixty. You just need to make up your mind to be part of the majority. To do that, you need to matter to others; it's our limbic imperative, and it's deadly serious. You need to connect to people who need your help, your nurturing, and your support—not as much as a newborn needs it, but enough to engage your limbic muscles. And you need to get at least a little dose of all of those back in return. Without this give-and-take, you decay.

Generations ago, we didn't have to go looking for this. Extended families and villages provided rich, lifelong limbic safety nets and connections to the group. In the days before TV, telephones, electric light, automobiles, and convenience stores, this wasn't a choice. There was nothing to do *but* be with the group! It wasn't always fun and games . . . villages and tribes can be cruel, harsh communities, and it's not so clear we would want to return to those days. But we should be able to save the best as we move forward. The great gift of traditional societies was that you were a *necessary* part of the community the whole way through your life. Okinawans have the greatest documented longevity of any population on earth, and in their culture older people are integral parts of the community until they draw their last breath. At ninety, or a hundred, they are respected for their life experience and they are relevant to the group. That's all changing with the younger generations, who have the blessings of daytime TV and fast-paced lives, and it seems as if that model is vanishing from the face of the earth, like an endangered species headed for extinction. There's a disturbing amount of truth to that if you look at our society as a whole, but that's just the view from afar. Close up, it's a different story for each individual. Our society still has all those limbic connections, but they are informal and hidden from view, so you will have to find them and put them together for yourself. Work, recreational activities, and volunteering are the major routes to limbic connection for most of us.

Work can be an important source of connection and gratification, and studies show that increasing numbers of Americans of both sexes are choosing to work past retirement. Part of this is financial, of course, but part of it is the increasing recognition that work has a value beyond the paycheck. Part of the value is simply in the structure—in having a reason to get out of bed and out of the house in the morning. Part of the value is in the social interactions that come automatically with most jobs, and part of it is the importance of still having a role in the tribe: a defined niche in the great social order.

A Fitness Community

You can build connections and communities through fitness. Think of it as making friends to play with, because playing is a wholly limbic activity. Watch children at recess or puppies tumbling over each other. That's pure limbic C-10, and recreation should be as much fun as you can possibly make it. The activities can be fitness-related or sedentary. Both work from a limbic perspective, but fitness-based activities have the major advantage that exercise itself wakes up your limbic connections. Bridge, fishing, and golf are wonderful examples of more sedentary pursuits that still work limbic magic. Bike groups, walking groups, and tennis are examples of physical limbic activities.

Chris and I recently met a woman named Pat who started a health club in New Jersey back in the early 1980s. She now has 8,000 members, and the average member stays for two and a half hours on their workout days. Far more than a gym, she has created a community where the first shared interest is fitness, and it builds from there. She has even started a grade school, fully accredited by the state, with yoga first period and ninety minutes of serious sports or PE at the end of the day. Her members have found a limbic community. One that you can pay for with a credit card and that works.

Whether it's skiing, hiking, biking, yoga, or a host of other possibilities, the chemistry of exercise is the chemistry of alertness, optimism, and increased willingness to connect. It's my informal observation that sedentary interests tend to segregate themselves along age lines, but the physical activities only sort themselves out by your willingness to show up and your stamina. Ski clubs, for example, generally sort out into two groups: young singles in one group and everyone else in the other, all the way up to your eighties. The only limbic requirement is that you chat on the chairlift and at the end of the day. Tennis clubs pair you up by ability. Apart from the truly gifted athletes, most of us are limited by our stamina more than our eye-hand coordination, so a fit seventy-five-year-old might well be playing with thirty-year-olds.

Volunteering: Replenishing Our Social Capital

Scientists have discovered a biology of altruism and extensively studied it in both mammals and birds—all in the interest of explaining the conundrum of why an individual does good for the community when it has no immediate Darwinian benefit. Why, for instance, do some species of birds raise orphan chicks in their own nests? The simple answer is that if everyone is wired to do at least some good, the community as a whole benefits, and average survival increases. You can spend your energy squabbling over whether you get 5 or 6 percent of the communal pie, or you can just accept the slightly smaller percentage and spend your time and energy working together to bake a much bigger pie. There are times when this gets you substantially more pie, and nature figured that out hundreds of millions of years ago. Investing some of your own time, energy, and resources in the health of your community is a natural imperative, controlled by the limbic system, and as much a part of your basic health requirements as going to the gym or brushing your teeth.

Economists have a term for the broad limbic net we weave as a society: *social capital.* It's the time and care we invest in a community, whether through faith-based programs, soup kitchens, literacy programs, environmental initiatives, or zoning boards; as poll watchers, museum docents, or registration workers at the League of Women Voters; supporting local efforts for the homeless, for the homebound, for the sick, and thousands of other efforts large and small. Each is just a group of ordinary people who have come together because they care about the same thing *and* because they want to work on it together. Working on it together is where the limbic magic happens. Writing a check to your favorite charity is a worthy act, but it does you little good. It's the hours working together with other people who share your interest that creates the limbic network ... you are back in the tribe. You are needed, and you are connected. You are back in the limbic sea, swimming against the tide.

Another major advantage is that charities tend to attract volunteers spanning a broad age range—an important counterbalance to the alarming amount of age-based segregation in our society. Maintaining friendships and connections across many different ages is *normal*. It's the way it always was, until recently. Your best friends might be your own age, but you spent your life in a community where you connected with people of all ages, all day long. *That's* normal.

So whether you've stepped out of the economic mainstream or are still working and bringing in a paycheck, look at ways to contribute some social capital. Do it for your limbic health. You need to matter to the group. As you get older, you're often told, in subtle and not so subtle ways, that you don't matter anymore. But that's ridiculous, and you know it, so do things that matter. If you have a faith, go back to church or temple or the pagan altar of your choice.

Get involved. Volunteer. Read to kids. You might not always like it; you might sometimes find it boring, tedious, or frustrating. Frankly, your limbic brain doesn't care. You need to matter, you need to give back, and you need to care—it's biological.

Spirituality: Being Part of the Greater Whole

The final component of a limbic life is that place where we somehow soar beyond evolution and nature into something more than the sum of our parts. Spirituality is too profound and too personal for us to give you any advice on which road to take, but we do know that for limbic reasons alone you should be on the journey. The growing number of reasonably well done studies on spirituality all point to its importance in our lives for both mental and physical health. People who search for meaning in their lives and their experiences survive loss better, cancer better, heart disease better, and have healthier immune chemistry, lower C-6 markers of inflammation, and lower risks of stroke and Alzheimer's disease. People who report that faith is an important part of their lives have mortality rates a third lower than average. They have lower blood pressures and lower blood sugar levels, spend fewer days in the hospital, and report substantially higher levels of life satisfaction and emotional well-being. You can decide for yourself how much of the positive effect stems from the increased social connections offered by organized religion and how much from something ineffable, but the simple message is that it is important to look for the meaning in your life's experience.

Limbic Pitfalls

There are two pitfalls that are so common they warrant a special discussion. The first is having health problems that drain your energy as you try to maintain the involvement and connection we're talking about. The second is having the emotional, physical, and logistical challenges of caregiving to contend with.

By age sixty-five, the majority of Americans have developed at least one chronic health problem. Somehow, we have developed the crazy idea that this lets you off the hook for exercising and living an active emotional life! The reality, of course, is that it puts you far more firmly on the hook than ever before. It is a simple fact of nature that the more difficult your life, the more important it is that you take care of yourself. It's when you face illness or loss that being fit and strong, both physically and emotionally, becomes critical. It is critical to get up every day and go take care of yourself, physically if you possibly can, and limbically no matter what, because the alternative is simply not acceptable. Nearly 50 percent of all women over sixty-five will end up in a nursing home at some point, which is a terrifying statistic. But here's an example of glass-half-full optimism: for most, it is a short-term rehabilitation stay. If you want to be one of those women who walk out the door, and back to their lives, you need to have two secret weapons in your repertoire: the physical strength to get up and walk out the door, and a limbic community waiting for you, pulling you home.

The other great stumbling block is the responsibility of caregiving, which is an increasing reality for a generation sandwiched between aging parents living longer and children spending more time dependent. There are some excellent books on caregiving, and we have listed some of them at the back of the book, but the bottom line is the same as for chronic health problems. The harder life is, the more important it is to take care of yourself. Without exception, the people I see doing the best job of caregiving somehow manage to carve out enough time for themselves. Often it's the bare minimum for exercise and for keeping close to a few friends, but it doesn't fall below that bare minimum. It should be clear by now why this matters so much and what the biology behind it is. If you feel guilty doing this for yourself, then do it for those who need you. The best metaphor is the briefing you get each time you get on an airplane: Put on your own oxygen mask first, so you don't pass out before you can help those who depend on you.

Courage

There's an old saying that aging is not for the faint of heart. Since we age no matter what, it might be more apt to say that aging *well* is not for the faint of heart. Courage is an old-fashioned virtue, but it plays a vital role in aging well. Not the momentary courage of rescuing people from burning buildings, but the bedrock courage to start over again, to reengage whenever necessary, no matter how late in life. It's my observation that women have this courage in abundance, and it can make all the difference. My paternal grandfather died in 1985, the year I graduated from medical school, after a long siege with Alzheimer's. My grandmother had cared for him at home the entire time, and for the last few years he did not recognize her, or anyone else. By the time he died, they had been married fifty-seven years, and my grandmother was eighty years old and worn down by nearly a decade of caregiving. She was living alone, in an empty house, coping with emphysema and loneliness. And she was visibly dwindling. Her trajectory was heading steadily downward, and I think we all half expected her to follow in Grandpa's footsteps. But that was not her temperament. She sold the big old house they had lived in ever since they were married; moved into a small, single-level house nearby and started her life over. A year and a half later, my sister walked in to find her doing sit-ups on the floor.

"Grandma, what on earth are you up to?" she asked.

"Oh," said Grandma with a twinkle, "there's a gentleman in my life, and I have to get rid of this tummy."

Six months later, at the age of eighty-two, she married a widower a few months her junior. My grandmother died five years later at eighty-seven from colon cancer, but she did not die at eighty-two from loneliness.

It's a fair caveat to say that she was lucky enough to meet someone, but it's also fair to give her a lot of credit for making her own luck. She rejected the limbic death that so often precedes the actual one. She had the courage to go back out there at age eighty. Not necessarily to find a mate, but to reengage with life.

Grab Hold

So that's your limbic biology in a nutshell: the mammalian imperatives of love and connection that run through our lives. Every single human being on the planet craves limbic connections. That means the opportunity to build them never goes away. There are limbic networks all around us. We just need to head out the door to build the connections every day, and we can continue to grow. Limbic decay is just as optional as physical decay. The tide of social atrophy—of limbic decay—is not that strong. It's just remorselessly steady. And the ultimate message is just the same as the physical message: Swim against the tide, every day. There are no universal road maps, but as with exercise, if you work at it steadily, it is almost impossible to fail.

CHAPTER NINETEEN

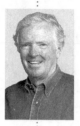

Connect and Commit

O ne of the nicest things that I have taken away from my years of working with Harry is the sense of the existence, power, and pervasiveness of our limbic brains and the importance of the emotional life. When I was a kid—and all through college, law school, and my years as a lawyer—there was a tacit assumption that reason, the thinking mind, should always prevail. The only life—for individuals, companies, and nations—was the rational life. There was an unspoken but fierce notion that if we could just get emotions out of the way, then, by God, life would be okay. Or at least a lot better.

Perhaps that was a sign of the times. After all, I grew up during an era when the thinking brain was not exactly in the saddle . . . the rise of Nazi Germany, lunatic racism in Europe and at home, and semi-tribal madness all over the place, culminating in World War II and the Cold War. Terrifying. I was around for the reigns of Hitler and Stalin, who were obviously crazy as bedbugs, yet wildly, inexplicably popular.

Want to see Harry's limbic resonance in a slightly different light? Take a look at a film of a Hitler speech in the 1930s . . . and don't miss the radiant faces in the crowd. Or watch Goebbels ask a hundred thousand folk, "Do you want the TOTAL WAR?" As he regularly did. His voice breaks on the last, rising scream . . . *"den TOTALEN KRIEG?"* And the crowd screams back, "Yes," in a desperate frenzy. And they got it, too; we all did. This is limbic resonance at the level of madness. And even after Hitler and Stalin were gone, there seemed an excellent chance that some successor lunatic would blow us all to smithereens with atomic bombs. People laugh, looking back, at the Eisenhower years . . . the Man in the Gray Flannel Suit, and the profound appetite for order and reason at any price. But it made a lot of sense in the 1950s. We'd had enough limbic fun to last a lifetime.

No, we hadn't. It doesn't work that way. The order we craved—and got for a while—was also suffocating, stultifying, and, yes, crazy-making in its own way, for the simple reason that, at the core, we are irreversibly emotional creatures. Rational, sure, but if we ignore our emotional sides, even for a short time, we will get sick. So, a conundrum: too much emotion and we go crazy; too little emotion and we get sick. *And* go crazy. Which sounds confusing but really isn't. As long as we know how we work and who we really are on these fronts, we can balance and cope. But the point of this chapter is not balance . . . it is alerting us all to the tremendous importance of the emotional life and of being connected and committed to others. It is that which we are more apt to forget or downplay in this age of reason (and as we age), and it is not a good idea.

As Harry eloquently points out, we are hardwired to be emotional creatures and yet we ignore our emotional side—especially the utter necessity for mammals of operating in packs and pairs and staying deeply in touch—at our peril. Personally, I find that a relief and a comfort—a coming together of my theoretical world view and reality. I can think pretty straight and even act rationally, if I must, but I am also profoundly emotional and it is relaxing in a way to know that that is a critical part of life, too. People talk censoriously about Bill Clinton and his divided character. Puh-lease . . . I am surprised that we all don't spend half our time rolling around on the floor together and licking each other's faces. It'd suit me. About half the time. The other half of the time, no. But it is a relief to know that we do not get "better," as I was taught, when we become less than emotional creatures . . . we shrink and we die.

You have had some of this from Harry, but I am so struck by some of the population studies that I want to give you a couple more, just to drive the point home. There are hundreds of these studies, by the way. If you're interested in reading more, a good place to look is a terrific book by Dean Ornish, the heart and diet doctor, called *Love and Survival*. His premise is that love saves lives. He's right.

Here's one example. There was a famously misguided effort early in the last century, when germ theory was new (and Sherlock Holmes was teaching that reason could solve all problems), to create a germ-free environment in nurseries for orphans. In the most advanced of these institutions, the foundlings were placed in aggressively sterile cubicles and never picked up or touched by anyone unless it was absolutely necessary. And they died in droves. In a 1915 study of ten such institutions, all the babies under two died. All of them. Being picked up, held, and cuddled turns out to be essential to life. Love saves lives.

It is our mammalian character at work here, as you now know, and it works just as well for lesser mammals as for us.

Rabbits, for instance. In one wonderful study, rabbits were stacked in cages up to the ceiling. They were being jammed full of cholesterol or something to study plaque buildup, but there were some anomalous results. The rabbits in the lower tiers did much better than the ones up high. Turns out the lab attendant loved animals. And she was short. She patted and fussed over the ones she could reach. *And they had 60 percent less plaque in their veins than the ones up high.* To check their suspicions, the scientists swapped the rabbits around, high for low. And the ones that were now reachable also prospered. It was the patting and touching, no question about it. Harry tells me that one has to be careful about drawing human inferences from animal studies, but my guess is, if you want less plaque, less Blacky Carbon and Gummy Sludge, get someone to pat you. If the person's short, sit down.

While we're talking mammals, you may want to remember that any mammalian contact helps. A study of recent heart attack victims also kept track of who did and who did not have a dog. As Harry mentioned in the previous chapter, the no-dog people were much more likely to die of a second heart attack than the dog owners. I sometimes used to get impatient with Aengus, our insanely demanding Weimaraner. But after I read these dog/health studies I went and got him a treat, which he took as his right, like everything else.

Here's the best one. There was a California study of women with metastatic breast cancer. They were divided into two groups, one of which met once a week for ninety minutes, for just six weeks, to talk about their cancer, how they were doing, and so on. The control group did not. The support group sessions weren't long, but there was intense bonding among the women. Not to put too fine a point on it, they came to love and care for one another. And guess what? The women in the support group lived twice as long as the women in the control group. Twice as long. Pretty big returns from a pretty modest investment in connection and commitment to one another.

It goes on and on. Studies showing that the lonely are twice as likely to have ulcers. Studies showing that unmarried men are two or even three times as likely to die of heart attacks as their married brethren. It is less true for women than for men, very possibly because women do so much better at creating networks of friends and other family, but it is true enough for women to act on it. Population studies are notoriously difficult to rely on. You can find one for almost any proposition. But there's no denying the logic of these studies, taken as a whole. Human contact, intimacy, is critical to good health. And the absence of it is devastating. Love saves lives.

This Society Makes It Hard

solation—which is one of the great perils in the Next Third—is hard. And in recent decades this society has done a lot to make it harder, not easier. Think of the big societal changes in my lifetime, starting with the family. When I was a kid in the 1930s and '40s, families were real, they were big, and they were very, very important. You knew who you were and where you stood because, most of the time, you were up to your armpits in family.

In my case, that meant three loving sisters and two parents who did not get divorced, plus a rich supporting cast of other relatives, many of whom lived with us at one time or another. My two grandmothers lived with us for a long time. And during the war Uncle Ben and his whole family moved in, because he was hard up. (Pa was the successful one and just assumed it was his job to take everyone in.) Later on, Uncle Esmond, whose life wasn't great, lived with us for his last five or six years. My sisters spent lots of time up in Castine with Aunt Kitty, the writer I mentioned at the beginning of the book. One of her conscious goals was to make her house in Maine "a haven for children and lovers," which she did. She also made the business of being an aunt into a conscious art form, and my sisters and cousins adored her and talk about her to this day.

At our house, as at hers, the notion of openness went beyond immediate family. In the mid-1940s, a friend of Ben's, a funny New Yorker named Max Schwebel, simply moved in, for reasons that are still unclear. I think he had done something for Ben, and Pa was devoted to Ben. Anyhow, there he was at the dining room table for almost a year: "the man who came to dinner," we joked. Awful good company, though. And there was distant cousin Edward, a six-foot-five Seabee, Cousin Emma's boy, who turned up at our door at age eighteen during the war and stayed after, when he was in college. Then there were all the relatives who lived nearby and were constantly in and out of the house. Aunt Kitty, of course. And Pa's sister Gladys, who was married to Mother's brother Fergus. Think we saw a little of them and their kid? I guess. Oh, and dogs, too. Six big, black Newfoundlands at one point. Plenty of cats. And a pig for a while. For the war effort, you know. The whole thing was a limbic feast, I tell you, and a joy for all of us.

If I could resurrect a household like that, I would do it in a heartbeat and never worry again about what to do in retirement. I'd just run the hotel. Cook the meals, call out the amusements, and make sure everyone got enough pats.

One of my long-term projects is to see if I can't do something like that before it's too late. A handmade retirement community for some of our close pals and relatives. We'll see. Hilary and I bought our big old house in the Berkshires with something vaguely like that in mind. Fill the sucker up with people and pets . . . sit in the limbic bathtub all day long.

Another societal change that makes retirement less cozy is the weakening of small city and town life. Towns like Salem, Massachusetts, where I grew up, have not ceased to exist, but the guts have been sucked out of them by the malls and the super-stores and the fast-food places. When I was a kid, a small city like Salem was the authentic center of its world. Locally owned and locally operated, for the good of those who lived there. We knew everyone, or at least Pa did. Cops, teachers, people in the stores, and a lot of the folks on the sidewalks.

People stayed put more than they do today. My relatives had lived in Salem and surrounding towns since the seventeenth century, most of them. All of them, in fact, except for one courageous Irish grandfather who showed up in Danvers, two hundred years later, to revitalize us all. Today, I'm in New York, two of my kids live on the west coast, my sisters are down south, and only two of my relatives live within a hundred miles of Salem. I'm grateful I left and lived the life I've lived so far. It's been fascinating and a world of fun. But I tell you, there are prices to be paid. Some of them are coming due now.

Maybe my family had it a bit thicker than some, but seventy years ago most people lived in towns and in families something like mine. And we all left. We just up and left. And changed the whole country. We left to start our nuclear families and move to impersonal cities like New

York or L.A. Where we could maybe make love to strangers or make more money. Get more stuff. And not know much of anyone outside of work and a small circle of pals. Funny thing to do, wasn't it?

Small wonder, then, that we gobble up books about traditional societies, like Peter Mayle's *A Year in Provence,* about a part of France where everyone knows everyone else and is in and out of one another's life all the time. Small wonder that we want to sit with Frances Mayes in her home *Under the Tuscan Sun,* in a part of rural Italy where the commitment to work is so much weaker and the commitment to family and community is so profound. Small wonder that we spend hundreds of hours watching reruns of *Friends* or *Seinfeld,* where the characters live rich, interconnected lives. We miss the connection of family and friends, so we watch surrogates, hour after hour, on television. Often alone.

Television is a little like those experiments where they put an orphaned baby chimp in a cage with a clock wrapped in a pillow . . . see how he does. And the poor little thing hugs it all day long, because it has a "heartbeat" and he hopes that maybe it's his mother. And because he's so damn lonely. We watch life on TV like that chimp with the clock in the pillow. Makes you weep, if you think about it.

All right, that's enough heartbreak. What do you do about it? Well, do what women have always done: Forge close bonds with lovers, friends, and family. Get more rather than less involved in community groups and projects. If your time isn't already eaten up with work, family, and friends—and an awful lot of women are going to be working for much of the Next Third—do volunteer stuff. Get involved. And, as Harry says, we're not talking about writing checks here. We're talking about you dishing out the food at the soup kitchen . . . you suggesting and starting the new organization to do something that urgently needs doing . . . you offering your own time and energy and caring to get important stuff done.

Limbic Giants: The Role of Grandmothers and Aunts

Talking about the possibility of limbic connections in the Next Third, there is almost nothing more obvious, important, and satisfying in that line than the business of being a grandparent. Or an aunt. If you have grandchildren, investing heavily in that relationship is one of the smartest and most satisfying things you can do. First of all, it could scarcely be more important to *them,* the kids. In a society where families are increasingly nuclear and distracted . . . where children see more of their iPads than their relatives . . . it is terribly important to remind them that they come from somewhere besides that nuclear core. It is *so* important to have that sense of roots. We all hunger for it.

Do you remember, back in the "kedging" chapter, how I mentioned going up to Stowe, Vermont, as a kid in 1941 with Mother and seeing "the Bigelow Girls," the old Quakers who had helped to raise her, long before my birth, in another century? That trip was *sixty-five years ago,* and I still think about it often. As I said then, the sense of that Vermont farm—and other family farms like it—purred away in memory, just below the surface, making me feel a little less scared. That's what that's all about, the sense of rootedness. The sense of coming from somewhere, of permanence . . . of coming from a tribe that goes back beyond your immediate life. And you can give that sense to your grandchildren, just by spending time with them and being kind. What a gift.

I don't know how good you are at "kind"; I could be better. But it's pretty easy to be kind to those grandchildren. They're not "yours" in the sense that you have to worry about disciplining them and all that. You don't have to *judge* them, ever, which their parents must do. But they *are* "yours" in the nice sense that they *came* from you, and they hunger for your company. Just be there, and you're doing a hell of a job. Oh, and be interested and kind.

My mother was a brilliant grandmother, one of the best I've seen. All her grandkids absolutely revered her. Her one great trick was that she never judged them. Ever. Up at that place on the island in New Hampshire I sometimes talk about, all the grandchildren would troop down to see her, on their own, every single day, all summer long. Usually, several times a day. Sometimes they'd just touch base . . . "Hi, Granny." In and out. Sometimes they'd hang for a while . . . watch her paint or whatever. They hungered for her company . . . loved to know she was there. They still do. Love to know she *was* there, even though she's been dead for twenty years. They have a better sense of who they are, and of their own *worth,* because they know they came from her and that she valued them so much. You can do that for someone.

Incidentally, if you are an aunt, rather than a grandmother, the potential and the importance of the relationship are the same. I mentioned my Aunt Kitty, the one who wrote *The Little Locksmith.* Well, she did not marry until later in life, and she never had children. However, she took the business of being an aunt with utter seriousness . . . thought it was one of the important roles in life and acted accordingly. I was too young, but my three sisters spent a lot of time with her and absolutely adored her. She had the great gift of treating them like equals (she was about their size, which helped) and never condescended. That's a trick. My sisters are in their eighties now, and when we're together they mention Aunt Kitty, oh, once a week. And don't think for a second that Aunt Kitty didn't get just as much out of it as she gave. Probably more.

Oh, and don't forget to touch them, those grandchildren and nieces and nephews. Remember the story about the girl who picked up the rabbits in the research place? Do that for your grandchildren. Pick 'em up. Hug 'em. Set 'em on your lap and fool with their hair. Hold their hands when you read to them. Limbic loops, man. Making limbic loops is a good use of our time. And kids love 'em.

Don't Retire at All

Here's another idea—maybe a necessity—which we hear about all the time. Keep on working until you drop at your regular job or as close to it as you can manage. It's particularly appealing for men: If the job is the flywheel of life, just don't let go. But it works for women, too. And often it has to, because there's not enough dough to live on. Or there will not be when you're too old to work unless you do something now. Whether amusing or not, whether part-time or full, work seems to give great satisfaction, even to the very old. Almost everyone who does it seems to like it. Not all, but an awful lot. And it doesn't seem to matter much what the work is. The other night, we went to a restaurant I've gone to forever. I said hello to Jimmy, the bartender, a nice guy in his early seventies whom

I've known for twenty years. I told him how this book was coming along and remarked on his good health and cheerfulness. Without waiting for the question, he said, "Work. No question about it. I don't have to be, but I'm here three nights a week and it keeps me going."

I forget where I saw a piece . . . *60 Minutes,* I think . . . about a factory that makes it a practice to hire old people, mostly women. Including some really old women. Works wonderfully for both employer and employed, apparently. The test of whether they're *too old* is whether they can walk up the steps. That's it. If they can walk up the steps, they can keep on working. And they do. I think the people who run that business are geniuses, and they should be imitated.

Same advice from a very different quarter. My law firm mentor, who has been one of the joys of my life for the last forty years, turned ninety-five last night (as I write this), and what a joy that was for the hundreds of friends and family. He gave a speech that any top lawyer in the country today would have been proud of. And warm? Wow! He's a legendary litigator, but he has more limbic force than a room full of golden retrievers. What a knack.

It was no surprise when a former associate and longtime friend gave a toast remembering her first year practicing with him. She had had a baby on the eve of a big trial, but trials are trials and eight days later she was in a hotel in Utica or some damn place with my mentor, the new baby, and some help. Trying the case. Remember, this man was born in 1910, and she assumed he might have a little trouble with this scenario, as much as he needed her. Not a bit of it. He went into limbic overdrive without giving it a thought. Tried the case, helped some with the baby, and made her feel absolutely terrific. She adored him all the rest of her life. Me, too.

Anyhow, when I first started on this project, I asked his advice generally. He didn't miss a beat. "Work!" he said with his usual intensity. "You have to have jobs or you'll die. I had to retire at seventy, but I've kicked around and dug up these projects: that environmental business [a pro bono suit to preserve the Hudson River], my little library [fund-raising and planning and politicking to build a public library], and so on. It keeps me alive. That and the boat. Thanks partly to you. I can't tell you how much that boat still means to me."

The boat is a nice story. He loves to sail, but in his mid-eighties he decided to sell it. It was getting to be too much for him.

"You know," he said, "I could be cranking a winch and slip and go over the side."

I paused for a few beats and said, "So what?"

He laughed for a long time. And kept the boat. He still sails it all the time. At ninety-five. So hobbies count, too.

Another irrelevant piece. He damn near died a few years ago, and when he recovered I asked him what it had been like and was he scared. He paused a moment, interested in the question. Then, "No, not really. I was concerned, of course, but oddly enough it wasn't particularly scary." He shrugged. "It seemed . . . all right. It wasn't a surprise. It was just . . . I don't know, I don't think about it much." Later, when we were about to break off, he said, "Listen, be sure to tell them about work. I know you're big on exercise. I am, too. But work, a project, that's the thing!"

One of the hard things about the "work" solution is that even mildly successful people are used to having a certain responsibility, whether in an office or at home, that's hard to get in a retirement-type job. The work is not as intense, and there can be a fair amount of envelope licking. Well, get over yourself. My mentor gave his last great "oral argument" to the board of a tiny library in his little town. Did a great job, too. Blew their socks off, I'm told. So think about regular volunteer work. It is one of the most satisfying things a lot of people do, and it does them a world of good. One study on the subject showed that those who did volunteer work once a week during the study period were *two and a half times* less likely to die. Dr. Ornish draws a nice conclusion: "Just as chronic stress can suppress your immune function, altruism, love, and compassion may enhance it." You have all read your Harry, so you are not surprised by this. But isn't it fascinating how closely our limbic lives are tied into our physical health as well as happiness? Limbic brain, hard at work.

There's a lot to be said for a paying job. You *know* you're appreciated when you're paid for it. And Lord knows, all of us are short of dough in retirement. Most part-time jobs are pretty modest, and for me it would be hard to get over my ego. But I think I'm wrong about that. A fancy pal of mine drives a school bus. My wonderful brother-in-law, a graduate of Harvard and a Navy Cross fighter pilot in World War II, is in his late eighties and is bagging groceries in Florida. He loves it. Loves the contact, loves having something to do. And is glad to have the few bucks. One of the nicest men in America, an authentic hero, and he's bagging groceries. They love him in the store. Why wouldn't they?

One promising area: the schools. They need aides, and they certainly need mentors. One of the traditional things for the elderly is the care and guidance of the young, and we could all do worse than to have a finger in that important work.

Have a Second Life, Using the Other Side of Your Brain

Personally, I think there is much to be said for making a job out of your hobby or your private passion. More specifically, do something entirely new and different. If, for example, you have even the trace of the artist in you, nurse it along and live in a different world for a while.

I particularly like the idea of using a different side of your brain, different gifts, in a different part of your life. A number of us had to suppress something in us to be successful at something else. Many of us gave up the book or the painting or the study to be lawyers or teachers or parents. Well, take a look and see if there's anything left of that abandoned side of you. I have a pal who has become a good watercolorist. Travels all over the place to paint, and loves it. Another has become a guide at the Metropolitan Museum of Art in New York. Others write, and several have become scholars.

Turning to the other side of your brain does not necessarily mean the arts. All it means is that it's *different.* And it will nourish you. New, different. Like rotating crops in your fields. Rotate your crops. You'll get a better yield.

Make a Job Out of Your Social Life

Women are good at this, too, but even women have to work at it. There is a terrible temptation for all of us, as we age, to close up shop and narrow our lives. Well, don't. It's killing us, for the reasons Harry explained. We have to "exercise" our social, pack-animal gifts as vigorously as we exercise our bodies, if we're going to lick that pesky tide. That means adding friends, doing more stuff, getting out there, and being involved. (If you need inspiration, go back and read about my friend Jessica in Chapter Two.) And nurturing and preserving the friends we have. Same, of course, with family members. They're not all perfect, and we tend to get a little more judgmental and petulant when we get older. We're tempted to say, the hell with so-and-so. Well, don't; we can't afford to lose a one. You remember how Old Fred used to howl at you for being on the phone all the time? Well, he was wrong. Get back on the phone. Call everyone. Use e-mail. Connect and commit.

Just Say "Yes"

There's a terrible temptation to say "no" to stuff as we get older. It's a hassle to do this or that. We don't really need to. Except of course, that we do. We need to do almost anything that gets us involved with other people. Because, as you now know, connection saves lives. So, default to "yes" when anyone suggests doing something or asks for help. Say "yes" to the dinner party, "yes" to the request for help organizing the potato race. Say "yes" to everything.

Simple example: A while ago I was asked to head up my fiftieth high school reunion. Well, there's a dull, thankless job. Besides, I didn't have the very best time of my life in high school and had not stayed in touch with many of my school friends. I said "yes" anyhow. And made a real meal of it. Wrote lots and lots of letters and hundreds of e-mails, made dozens of phone calls, and so on. Even organized six pre-reunion dinners around the country. Surprised myself. Met some new people and reconnected with some old ones. It was a lot of work, and it may not have made much difference in the grand scheme of things, but I loved it.

Shy Girl

f you're shy, you may think: It's all well and good for him, thumping about like a golden retriever, to talk about defaulting to yes, going out and doing things without a care . . . but I can't do that. It's painful for me to be in company. It's painful to say yes, to go to lunch or dinner or to this party or that. What am I supposed to do?

Well, I have no idea, since I am, as you say, a golden retriever, with a dog's limited vision. But I think the rule is the same. I think you default to yes. You "get over it," as people like me so cruelly, casually, say. You take a deep breath and make the connection, say yes to the offhand invitation . . . make the offer yourself, with whatever horror such an idea evokes. And try to bear in mind that, to the golden retriever, shy is infinitely interesting, infinitely surprising and strange. The dog wants to nuzzle you, to lick your face . . . see what this is all about. I spent an awful lot of time, over the years of my rottenness, with shy girls, endlessly fascinated, charmed by their distance, their remove.

I remember seeing an acquaintance standing in the hall outside a big cocktail party years ago. She was literally gathering her courage. As if anyone cared whether she went in or not. I was flabbergasted . . . asked her to dinner on the spot. We're still friends, all these years later. True, we're not close any more, but that, I submit, is okay. Get involved anyway. Have lunch with the woman. Go to the church supper, where the "barriers to entry" are probably lower. Go to the movie with the guy. Don't think of yourself as pathetic, think of yourself as brave. Which you are. Connection is as valuable for you as for anyone else . . . more so. So say yes to whatever comes up. Or *make* things come up, if you can bear it.

I once had an accountant, Smart Barbara, who was

"legally shy." That was the joke we made later on when we became close pals. We got past the shyness eventually and had about as much fun together as I've ever had. She was so smart . . . there was so much going on in there . . . so much to talk about and do. Try to bear in mind, shyness is an aphrodisiac to some. So, painful or not, you should default to yes, even more than your boisterous sisters. That's my brutish advice. Just do it. And if you are rejected or forgotten by this one or that, fine. Get over it and do it again. You are a mammal, and you have your needs.

Be the Organizer

Take it a step beyond the default-to-yes mode, and be the one who suggests stuff. Be the one who does the asking. You've got the time. So start making the calls and don't get irritable because your pals say "yes" and then forget about it. Keep after them, make it happen. You're building a life here. There's nothing wrong with the fact that it's hard. Of course it's hard. Look at the stakes . . . what did you expect?

All it takes is one person or one couple to make big stuff happen. You know the bike group I talk about all the time? We're in our twelfth year now, and it's one of the best things a lot of us do all year. It's all the result of an idea and a lot of work by a single couple, and much of the work has been done by one woman. The two of them thought it up, but he's working more or less full time so she does the heavy lifting. She makes all the phone calls. She organizes the food, the lodgings, the transport. And we go. Well, there's no magic to it. Sure, she's a forceful woman with more than the standard ration of charm, but it's just initiative, hard work, and, okay, charm. Do it. What else are you doing with your time that's so much more important? Let me take a guess: nothing.

Incidentally, money is not a big part of all this. Organizing a bike group—or a cross-country ski group or a swimming group—is not money-intensive. It can be done at any level you want. It's the work and the drive that are hard to come by, and they're free. In general, there's little correlation between having dough and having a rich social life. After all, kids right out of college are best at it, and they don't have a dime. What they do have is a huge incentive—to meet and make love to one another. Well, you do, too. Maybe not to make love to one another, but to put together the groups—to make the connections that are going to save you in the Next Third. So go to work. Start a bike group, a book group, a poker night, a yoga club, a political action group. Any damn thing. It all counts.

Another thing that counts is the spiritual side of life. Harry and I are perfectly aware of how important it is in your life and ours, but for once we did not have the confidence, the presumption, to take it on. And besides, that's a book all of its own, not a chapter in this one. Suffice it to say that a meaningful spiritual life may be almost all you need. And it may make everything else you have a lot better.

Well, that's kind of a cat's breakfast of ideas, but there may be some nourishment in there somewhere. The one thing I can promise you is that the basic notion—that you should make a steady and deadly serious effort to connect and commit *more* rather than less as you age—is rock solid. Love saves lives. You're a mammal. Cuddle up.

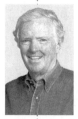

CHAPTER TWENTY

The New, New Thing: SMARTER NEXT YEAR!

W hen I was a little chap, everyone *knew* that we were given a certain number of marbles at birth and that was it. Worse, we were warned that it was critical to complete the basic work for our Nobel Prize or whatever by the time we were thirty-two, because starting at thirty-two, we inevitably start *losing our marbles.* Saddest thing in the world. There you are, you know, sitting at the kitchen table when you hear a rattling behind you. Sure enough, it is one of your marbles, rolling across the kitchen floor toward the rat hole. And when you get to be my age, you're sitting in that same chair and your poor spouse is wiping the goo off your face because you, sir, have lost your marbles. *Awful!* The deep knowledge of that fate cast a pall over all aging and much of life. Death is no walk on the beach, but for a lot of people (including me), dementia is worse. And the threat *seems* to have been getting more severe and more real. Partly it's because we are living so much longer and dementia—a disease of aging—has a much better shot at more of us. Partly, we are better at spotting it. But for whatever reason, Alzheimer's and other forms of dementia are reaching epidemic levels among growing numbers of older people in this country. And younger people, too, because it sets in earlier. Worst of all, we have been reliably told that we can do absolutely *nothing* about it. *Terrifying.* Talk about the dark pall over all aging. *Yowie!*

Well, here's some good news: A lot of that is horseshit. Not all, but a lot. And—contrary to the old view—you have a tremendous amount of control over how well your brain works as you age and whether you go completely to hell (i.e., Alzheimer's). There are indeed profound forces at work to sap your intelligence as you age—just as there are powerful forces that want your body to fall apart. But, as with your body, there are things you can do—behavioral changes you can make—to radically slow and, in some cases, reverse the loss, whether of psychomotor skills (aspects of coordination) or cognitive skills (rational thinking). Also, it is not true that you do not grow any new marbles. You grow a bunch of them. It's just a matter of maximizing the growth of new cells and taking steps to make sure they *work* hard once they pop up. In short, there is a lot you can do to fend off dementia and maximize cognitive effectiveness. *That* is extremely good news. It is the analog to what you learned about keeping your body young in the earlier chapters. Do nothing and your body goes to hell as you age. Make some serious behavioral changes and it does not. Or at least nowhere near as much. It is almost exactly the same with your mind.

On the matter of losing your marbles, the fact is that you grow new marbles all the time. How many you grow is significantly up to you because it is affected by that core

Younger Next Year consideration, how much aerobic exercise you get. The more aerobic exercise you get, the more new brain cells you generate and the smarter you become. By the way, it is as wrong to call them *brain cells* as it is to call them *marbles*; it is more complicated than that. *Everything* about the brain is more complicated than that, but brain cells will do for us. Then there is the question of how well those new brain cells work, and that, too, is significantly affected both by exercise and by that other *Younger Next Year* imperative: how much you *connect with and commit to others*. And how much time you spend *using your brain, at the high end*. The effect on out-and-out dementia is remarkable: This is a soft number, but the best thinking these days is that *you can reduce your own risk of Alzheimer's—regardless of your genes—by about 50 percent*. In a world where we were told we were helpless in the face of Alzheimer's, that's not bad. And it sure is worth going to a lot of trouble. At my age, you see ever so many friends with Alzheimer's, and it's grim. I don't want to go there. And all my doctors—from Harry on—have taken a look and said I won't. Good for me. And it ain't genes, kids: My father had devastating dementia for five dreadful years; I don't, and (I am told) I won't. Because of my lifestyle. It's all that dumb exercise I do and living a highly engaged life. Give it a shot. It works.

The advice in this chapter (and, more importantly, in Allan Hamilton's chapter right after it) is not just about aging and dementia; it is also about people of any age and how they can be significantly smarter and more effective *right now* through behavioral change. This is perhaps the biggest news in our new chapters, because it applies to everyone. Doing serious aerobic exercise (and connecting with and committing to others) can increase your cognitive effectiveness at any age—that is to say, *how smart you are*— by 10 percent. Ten percent smarter . . . Can that really be true? Yeah, it can, and it is.

Do you think getting 10 percent smarter is important? Of course you do. Executives, lawyers, doctors . . . all of us . . . would practically kill for that competitive edge. There's more to success and the good life than raw intelligence, but it sure doesn't hurt. If there were a pill we could take that would increase our functional intelligence by 10 percent, would we pay *any price* for it? And risk terrible side effects? You bet. Happily we don't have to face that little dilemma because there is no pill. But there is serious aerobic exercise, and it works like a charm. It has no side effects, except wonderful ones. The best of them you may already know about from the original *Younger Next Year* books (avoid 70 percent of aging until almost the end of life and cut the risk of major diseases and accidents permanently by an astonishing 50 percent). But there are some new ones, too. Which are the subjects of these new chapters. They may be of particular interest to those of you who are still in the thick of your careers.

Raise the Basic Executive Attributes

Here's the amazing deal: Exercise—especially intense aerobic exercise, but strength training, too—radically boosts what I think of as the basic executive attributes: energy, optimism, decisiveness, interest, resistance to stress, and resistance to depression. *And intelligence.* Read that little list again. There is nothing more important to your professional or business effectiveness and your joy in life than these attributes. Nothing. And you get a huge boost in all of them by making behavioral changes that (as you already know) make other astonishing differences at the same time.

Let's get prosaic for a minute. Think about the alternation of "good days" and "bad days" that we all know so well. Some mornings you wake up and feel great. You think, *Wow, what a nice day!* And that's true whether the sun is shining or there's a storm blowing through. You're full of energy, full of excitement about the new day, full of hunger for life. Energy may be the most important part of those days. When you wake up full of energy, you are just a different person. When you have the blahs, you should almost stay home. A serious exercise regimen creates cascades of energy and transforms most of your days. I sometimes think energy is *the* key executive or professional gift. But, I don't know; maybe it's cognitive intelligence, sheer thinking power. I have a sneaker for that because it mattered a lot in my kind of law. But you don't have to choose, because the same behavioral changes affect all these areas. It's a "hat trick," a combination of increased cognitive effectiveness, *and* increased energy, optimism, decisiveness, caring, and the absence of the blues. Put all that together and *pow*: You are your best self. And you can be that way most of the time. Almost all your days can be good days.

Think again about waking up on a "good day" and just reading the paper. Almost everything interests you. Several things trigger ideas that might be useful in your business or private life. It's not just a newspaper now—it's a menu for action. That's the energy edge.

Now think for a second about optimism, caring, and decisiveness in general. There are a million lousy ideas out there, as we all know. But there are a few beauties, too. And the person who is going to latch onto the good ones is the person who has the gift of *caring* and of *optimism (Hey, I can see how that might work for us!);* the gifts of *interest and decisiveness (I'm gonna cut this piece out of the paper, talk to Sarah and Billy)*. Openness to the new. Huge.

Now think about a "bad day." On those days, "there's nothing in the paper." You can barely bother to read it. At work, you soldier along, but it's a struggle and not amusing. New ideas do not bubble up. And if they do, who gives a shit. I mean, really, who cares? One could go on, but you know bad days; we all have 'em. Serious exercise helps get rid of a lot of them.

Harry Saw This Coming

Bringing out this "first revised edition" of *Younger Next Year for Women*—and spreading the amazing news about behavioral change and the brain—is a joyous business for all of us, except for one thing: Harry's not here. I talk about it a little in the introduction, but the short of it is that despite living the *Younger Next Year* life to the fullest, Harry had some appalling bad luck and died young. But he had already shown great interest in the subjects of the new chapters and written a fair amount about them in his usual, compelling way.

In the introduction to our 2016 book, *Younger Next Year: The Exercise Program* (with exercises by Bill Fabrocini), he talked about the new ideas quite a lot. At one point, after talking about the familiar notion of your body getting younger, he went on to say, *"Your brain will get younger, too*. Newer research shows that there are enormous cognitive benefits of exercise. The data and individual biology vary, but when you are fit, you are 10 percent more cognitively efficient [read 'smarter'] than when you are sedentary." I think that is a revolutionary insight, and Allan Hamilton—who truly knows this field—agrees.

Harry said that the brain, with its 100 billion neurons, is "the most complex, sophisticated object in the known universe" and that it dwarfs the Internet in information flow. The question, he said, is, What can you do to turn it on? The answer is, Give it challenges. And, he said, "There are only three great challenges that are hard enough to keep the brain healthy and growing. True emotional engagement with others, cognitive and social engagement with tasks that matter, and *exercise*. Motion. Moving your body through space is unbelievably complicated. . . . Movement is at the heart of evolution, it's key for improving our cognitive and emotional brains."

Then there was this lovely quote with a different emphasis:

"Exercise releases a powerful brain chemistry that in turn creates the energy, optimism, and mood elevation you need in order to engage with life at your best."

There was none of this in the original book, because no one really knew about it back then. Laura Yorke and I—Laura was the extraordinary agent for the original book, became Harry's true love, and is his literary executor— eventually concluded that it was important to have a new, expanded edition of the original book, just because this material *belonged* in the book. Laura got in touch with Allan Hamilton, a very busy man and a giant in the field of neural—or brain—science, and persuaded him to do a chapter. We—and you—are lucky. Harry was a serious *student* of brain science; Allan is a serious *teacher*, a leading figure in the field. Read his chapter closely. And rejoice.

And here's an interesting thing about this edition:

Nothing had to be changed. There's wonderful new material, but the old stands up astonishingly well. And the advice just gets more true and more important. Nice.

"UNTIL YOU'RE 80 AND BEYOND"

So, what else is new? Well, one question that the original *Younger* raised but did not address is, How long does this stuff work? The original hardback cover said, "A Guide to Living Like 50 *Until You're 80 and Beyond.*" Excellent! But my question these days is, Um . . . how *far* beyond? A lot of my older pals ask the same thing, and I have to say I don't really know. But I have some ideas.

I am afraid there is no new science, but I can tell you a little about my own experience, which I think may shed some light, because it is consonant with the basic message of the original book. With adjustments. I am now eighty-five (to my utter astonishment), and *Younger Next Year* has treated me pretty well. You would not take me for fifty, that's for sure. But you probably wouldn't take me for eighty-five either. And my life is awfully full and sweet. Which is one of the things I want to stress. We all have a picture in our heads of what it is like to be in our eighties, and that picture is pretty grim. The books on the subject are dark, the advice of most professionals is namby-pamby, and the sight of most of our elders is terrifying. Because most of them are a mess. So of course, we have a grisly picture of the eighties in our heads. Well, I know something about this subject, and I'd like to adjust that picture a bit. Because I think it is nonsense. Being in your eighties is not all beer and skittles, but it can be way, way better than most people assume. Change the damned picture; change your life.

Here's a quick Harry anecdote to set the scene. Harry and I and a heart-doctor pal of his were biking in the Berkshires when I was in my late seventies. We were climbing a hellish hill, and I was out front, pulling us up a 12 percent grade. That's *steep* . . . knock-you-off-your-bicycle steep. I have always been a wretched athlete, but—by following Harry's Rules—I was fit, and I was perfectly happy to take the lead for a while for two fit men who were twenty-five years younger. Here's the point: Harry later told me that his heart-doc pal expressed considerable surprise at what I was doing. Harry told him it was nothing . . . *it should be the new norm.* Harry said he wished *every gerontologist in the country could take this ride with us, with me.* Because they all radically underestimate just how good aging can be. They set the bar too low. Eventually things are going to go to hell in your eighties, maybe nineties. Duh. But that's no reason to live like a mutt in the meantime. Change the picture in your head. Go for it.

Okay, here's a little more in that same vein, if you can bear it. It looks shamefully like boasting—and of course it is—but that's not the point. The point is to change the picture in your head.

I am a wretched athlete, always have been. But I am still skiing the (single) black diamonds at speed and rowing joyful distances in my single scull on our sheltered mountain lakes. And riding my fancy bike thirty to fifty miles in comfort (not "centuries" in the Rockies anymore, but hey, what did you expect?). As I write these words, we are in a plane, flying back from a ski trip to Aspen. And I can tell you with deep pleasure that I was skiing with as much control and speed and *joy* as ever. Okay, I skied with a little less speed and spent a little less time on the blacks, but I was going for it. And if my knee weren't on the fritz, I'd be in the bumps in the trees. (I'm getting the knee replaced this Wednesday, just so I can ski.) It took me forever to learn this sport, fifty years ago, because I'm so uncoordinated, but I finally got it and then practiced like crazy. I became quite a good recreational skier, which for me was a miracle. *Me,* being that graceful, that athletic. How I loved it! But here's the real miracle: I can still ski about like that. I am swooping around with easy control, a lovely "feel" of the skis, my feet, and the snow. It's a wonderful sensation. Not like a kid but not like an eighty-five-year-old, either. I love it. It tells me I am alive, and I rejoice. Someday I'll have to go to all cross-country; fine. Harry told me that, the first day we met. But not this year. Or next.

If sports aren't your thing, that's fine. The good life extends to everything. A big piece of it for me is work. I'm still writing books, six since I turned seventy (do read *The Younger Next Year Back Book,* with Jeremy James, which came out in 2018; it's a beauty). I just finished my first novel, *The Practical Navigator,* a legal mystery, a retelling of the Minotaur myth and a serious contemplation of addictive sexuality (*what!*). It was a ton of *hard, mind-stretching work* and my favorite book. I loved doing it. On a very different front, Jeremy James and I recently started a business (almost all Jeremy) . . . a video-based protocol to teach people to heal their own backs: BackForever.com. Try it. We raised several million dollars, if you please, and it looks as if it is going to do well and change a bunch of lives. Did I mention that I am eighty-five? Good. Change the damn picture.

I am still giving keynote speeches, which lifts me up like nothing else. My wife, Hilly, and I still entertain all the time (I'm the cook, she's the charm), and we travel with pals and alone, mostly bike trips with Butterfield & Robinson, a bicycle travel company, and others. A sweet life and a fairly intense one. Is the end in sight? Of course it is; we're all heading for the waterfall, after all. Especially me. But not yet. And my goal—as always—is to go out like Wile E. Coyote going over the cliff. Never look down, never look back.

Here are a few details that may be worth knowing. You should know that the temptation to slack off as you get older gets much stronger. But the importance of *not* doing so gets way, way more important. How come? Because the tide of aging gets much stronger. And we feel less like fighting back. Odd but true. But here's the thing: If we're going to continue to live the good life, we have to work out with even greater resolve. I have tried (with limited success) to double down on exercise. That has not really worked, but I haven't really slacked off, either. And it helps tremendously. I see it every time I run into a pal who's gone the other route and every time I do *not* work out for a stretch. That is striking: Whenever I dope off, even for a short time, the effect is dramatic. My aerobic capacity trails off noticeably. But the most striking effect is in the "new area": My energy, optimism, mental sharpness, and ability to give a damn fall off sharply. Which scares the daylights out of me. It makes me think I am living on the edge of the abyss and I have to work *hard* not to turn into a dope. Which is absolutely true.

Hard mental work is key to maintaining your cognitive intelligence, as Allan and Harry stress at length. That may sound a little ominous, because it is hard for most of us to find serious, mental work in retirement. Two things: First, it's not impossible. You can find a new job or part-time job that pushes you to do serious cognitive work. Or you can do things for pleasure that do the same thing: Take courses, write books whether they will be published or not, learn *new* things you care about, and so on. *Use your mind.*

Second and a little surprisingly, serious, complex exercise itself is *extremely* hard work for your brain. Think about it: The brain has to do all kinds of exquisitely complex adjustments and tunings, at lightning speed, throughout exercise, especially *hard* and complex exercise. It is known that complex physical activity "grows" your brain. And not just the parts that are directly concerned with physical movement. It strengthens and grows the frontal cortex, too . . . the thinking part. So, if you don't feel like whiling away a quiet hour with Nietzsche or Schopenhauer, go to the gym and do some serious, whole-body exercise. That'll help, too. If you want some wonderful guidance, read Bill Fabrocini in *The Younger Next Year Exercise Book* or *Thinner This Year*. He's awfully good, and he'll show you exactly what to do. Sorry for these "plugs," but it's not commerce; it's the best advice I can give you.

The Margin for Error Narrows

et's have a candid moment. No matter how hard you work out, and no matter how vigorously you pursue mind-stretching activities, you are going to suffer some reversals, both physical and mental. Remember, in *Younger,* we said you could put off 70 percent of aging until almost the end, not 100 percent. That's still true. You can do a ton to maintain strength, balance, and coordination. But you don't keep it all. Be realistic and think *all the time* about these words of wisdom from Bill Fabrocini: "The margin for error narrows as you age." And you have to take steps to account for that. Your reaction time in the car is slower. No matter what a hell of a guy you've always been. So go a little slower. And be really, really careful in tight spots. That applies to skiing, too. And biking and everything else. Lots of things you used to be able to do automatically? You can't do them anymore. You have to stop and think. I hate to say this because it sounds so dopey, but you have to *think as you walk.* You do not always pick the right course anymore. Or lift your feet high enough. And you don't notice stuff you spotted before.

Here's a sad little story. Out in Aspen two weeks ago, I was walking along the sidewalk and took this dreadful header . . . landed flat on my *face—hard.* I never fall down; I mean *never.* I have never gotten hurt skiing or biking or driving. My instincts are good, and I'm careful (by the standards of reckless people). And here I was on the ground with a horrendous black eye and a broken rib. Had to go to the hospital to check for brain bleeding. I ask you! The ultimate explanation was weird: I was wearing a very old pair of heavy, "rocker" sneakers, the soles of which had almost worn through. The floppy sole caught on a bump in the sidewalk and down I went. Well, ten years ago, I would have noticed that my sneaks were dying. And if I had started to fall, I likely would have caught myself. Not now. I do the "fast foot" and other fine-muscle exercises Bill recommends for balance and coordination, and they help a ton. But there is still some decline. So . . . slow down, look over your gear from time to time, watch where you're going. Sorry to tell you, but that's the deal now. The margin for error shrinks.

Here's another nasty one. One of the most popular chapters in the original book was "The Drink," about the pleasures of temperate drinking. Still true, still a wonderful chapter. But less so now for you and me, babe, if you're really old. As you get into your eighties, you just can't drink as much with impunity. Maybe you can't drink at all. Alcohol kills brain cells, as you doubtless know. Well, you cannot afford that anymore. I find that I am okay if I hold it to one drink a night, but when I go over that, I feel it in the morning. Not hung over, but *stupid*. I am measurably more stupid. Good grief! I love to drink and mean to do it forever, but I hate stupid. So I don't drink very much. Harry was a bear about this, and he was right. Pity. By the way, cutting back or quitting helps enormously with sleep, which, as Allan says, matters tremendously.

Here is some general advice for the eighties (and maybe the seventies): Lighten up! I am the last one on earth to be making this sensible point, but it is my strong sense that you have to temper your ambitions some in your eighties. Still do stuff. . . . Do stuff like crazy. You're Wile E. Coyote, after all. But think a little about stress. I used to think I was immune to stress, and that was partly true. But I can see—to my horror—that that's less true now. After a simple flight across the country, I feel a little goofy the next day. I have to take it easy. I hate it, but there it is. In general, I try consciously these days to space out the stressful stuff—the speeches, the killer bike rides, and so on—and have more downtime. Not a ton, but some. Naps, my man, naps. I always was a napper; I'm even more of one now. Fine. The margin for error, kids. It's shrinking. If you're going to have fun and do stuff, you have to baby yourself just a little bit.

Okay, here's the wrap-up: You have a tremendous degree of control over your mind and mood throughout life and especially as you age. You have to be mindful of the darned old margin of error as you get really old. And you have to do the exercise and so on all the way through. But it makes you *smarter,* for heaven's sake. And stronger. And better looking (a little). And happier (a lot). So make serious exercise—and serious commitment—*your job*. It's as important as anything in your life. Be sane. But go for it, too; it's fun.

CHAPTER TWENTY-ONE

Protecting the Female Brain for Life

by Allan J. Hamilton, MD

am a Harvard-trained brain surgeon. So what am I doing here in the middle of a new fifteenth-anniversary edition of *Younger Next Year for Women*?

Early in my career, I became disheartened by how hospitalized patients were left so dismally unprepared for discharge and rehabilitation. In my case, I was dealing with brain tumor patients (who often had significant neurological deficits) as they were getting ready to go home or to a neurorehab facility. It bothered me that the whole notion of being discharged, of getting better, was made to sound like a litany of tedious chores rather than an upbeat send-off to getting better and healthier. I kept asking myself, *Where is the enthusiasm?*

I was searching for something to help motivate patients to recover fully. I felt like doctors were framing the process of rebuilding the body and mind back to wellness and strength as a fragmented, boring, and almost trivial part in the recovery process. I wanted my patients to approach their mental and physical conditioning with drive like athletes. I wanted them to train themselves to recover. I wanted them to have a coach with an inspirational whistle, not some geek staring at an iPad. I found that coach's voice in *Younger Next Year*. I loved the way Chris Crowley focused on how life had to be visualized as an endurance event for which one had to train, heart and soul. Meanwhile, in his own down-to-earth, simple, and wise way, Dr. Harry Lodge, as the medical coauthor, boiled the science down into an approachable program of rational encouragement. I had to warn patients that although the book talked about "older folks" in their fifties, sixties, and beyond, that was not the point. It talked about life—a long life, whether you were twenty or seventy years old—where you put yourself in the fittest body you could manufacture for yourself. That was the focus I cared about. Not one line in the book(s) even hinted at the possibility of giving up. I wanted Chris and Harry to be the ones who gave advice to my patients. I started handing out copies of the *Younger Next Year* books like after-dinner mints. Above all things, I wanted to leave my patients with the notion of inexhaustible optimism atop practical, measured, and effective resolution and discipline to encourage their recovery. So *Younger Next Year* became my bible. I even told patients they would get a copy only if I saw them in their sweatpants and sneakers as they made their way out of the hospital.

Both Chris and Harry were role models for me, one in life and one in the practice of medicine. Harry passed away. He was far too young and had much more to accomplish. But when approached to add a chapter on brain fitness for this fifteenth-anniversary edition (because the one area of *Younger Next Year* where we have new, pertinent information fifteen years later is the brain!), I jumped at the chance. First, because it fed into all of my own ideas about preserving and enhancing brain function even into the most senior years. But, more importantly, because I could get sandwiched in next to Chris and Harry's body of work and continue to cheer them on.

For centuries men maintained that women were the weaker sex. Nothing could be further from the truth when it comes to the science of aging and maintaining cognitive and psychomotor functions into our senior years. Cognitive capabilities refer to abstract thinking, and psychomotor skills relate to fine-motor movements, equilibrium, and eye-hand coordination. In this chapter, we are first going to look at the so-called "normal" aging of female brains and contrast it with that of their male counterparts. In the process, we will uncover some of the great strengths and resilient powers of the female brain with respect to aging. We will then discuss relevant scientific and clinical research that bears on what is now called "superaging." Superagers are people who maintain a physical and intellectual capacity well into their senior years of sixty to eighty and beyond that can match that of people decades younger—in their mid-twenties or thirties.

Differences Between Male and Female Brains

For centuries, anatomists noted that men's brains weighed more and had slightly larger volumes than those of women of the same age. Consequently, men took that as some indeterminate indication of male superiority. The notion that weight equated with superiority was as stupid as insisting that your heavy four-wheel-drive SUV is better than a Porsche 911 simply because it is bigger and weighs more. New brain-imaging data[1] from approximately 2,500 men compared with that from 2,500 age-matched women sheds light on this old anatomic question: What is it about male brains that explains these differences? Yes, male brains are bigger and weigh more, but there is far more to the story. Neuroimaging has demonstrated that female brains have thicker cortices than their male counterparts. The thicker the cerebral cortex or mantle, the greater the number of neurons (called "gray matter") in that cortex and the better those people tend to perform on cognitive and intelligence tests. Men, on the other hand, have thicker "white matter" fiber tracts connecting the different regions of the brain. Think of these gender differences like an art museum. The male brain is designed with specialization in mind. Distinct rooms make up the cortex, with each room holding, say, a magnificent period painting collection. Each room hangs in cerebral space as an isolated room. In the woman's brain, there are still all the rooms with the collections, but each room is massively interconnected with the others. So, you might gain access to a "historical passageway" that links the artwork by its place in history and its relationship to its predecessors and its successors. Or they might instead be geographically organized (say, artists who painted in the Côte d'Azur) or suddenly be connected by their ability to use colors in bold, unusual ways. Where the male brain has its rooms linked by a single corridor, the woman's brain offers a multitude of passages that can crisscross time and space with ease.

When it comes to interconnectivity, women's brains show some distinct advantages over men's. Men use their *left* hemisphere predominantly. It is dedicated to linear processing, focusing on language, calculation, and logical or deductive reasoning. Women, on the other hand, are much more adept at using *both* hemispheres. This means they can also access the right hemisphere, which dedicates itself to creative networking, combining processes such as shape and design with notions of color and form and seeing issues from the perspective of an integrated whole—as a gestalt— rather than as a series of linear challenges that must be confronted in succession.[2] That means men are more prone to approaching matters with linear processing, from a single perspective, in terms of allocation of resources. This would lend men a bit of a logistical advantage. Women, on the other hand, are more adept at parallel processing where they are pursuing several approaches in combination with each other, giving them a strategic advantage in problem-solving.

None of this affects intelligence; adult men and women usually score about the same on IQ testing. Because of the greater dependency on the left hemispheric functions, the male brain is slightly more geared toward math, whereas the female brain harnesses both the left and right hemispheres, giving women a distinct advantage in using language and artistic creativity. Women also show more activity and interconnectivity with the limbic lobe (LL), that area of the brain that lends emotional weight to our experiences and responses. This may explain why women are more adept at putting statements or conversation into emotional context than men. So, for example, I was recently at a meeting where a male speaker projected a large and somewhat complicated table summarizing peri-partum morbidity and mortality data among different racial groups of women. It was a long series of numbers and footnotes. As participants were scanning all the lines of data for meaning, the woman who led the break-out session jumped in to highlight three or four key differences, pointing out that black women were, in some cases, five or six times more likely to die from pregnancy-related complications. Suddenly, everyone was scrambling to jot down the key stats because they suddenly had a powerful context to frame their meaning. Of course, these are gross, overarching generalizations, and within each sex, exceptions abound at the individual level but as a rule the male brain is quick to grasp content while the female's brain interconnectivity permits access to contextual impact as well.

Rather than looking at these variances in terms of one sex's brain doing something *better,* we should look at them as demonstrating ways of doing something *differently.* Male brains are inclined to use more clusters of neurons in the cerebral cortex, whereas women are more likely to use association-fiber networks. The areas of brain cortex are dedicated to processing information—to extracting its content—and the association fibers are used for creating linkages and associations between the different kinds of information. This enhanced networking capability may explain why women are more successful at linking tasks than their male counterparts. Again, these are always gross generalizations about the gender differences in brain function but the male brain has a tendency to work on problems in serial fashion while the larger and enhanced volume of association fibers in the female brain can facilitate approaching problem-solving in a more parallel fashion. Naturally, no one approach is the exclusive domain or gift of a single gender.

In the past, much of the observed sex-related differences in thinking, proficiency, and intelligence were assumed to be "nurture"-related, meaning caused by educational, external socioeconomic, and educational factors. Now there is a distinct swing in the pendulum of scientific thinking, and many of the anatomical differences between the male and female brain have been determined to be the result of genetic programming[3] (i.e., to be "nature"-related) and are reflected in significant architectural and functional divergence between the sexes.

The Genetics of Brain Aging

When scientists examined the so-called *transcriptome* of men and women, there were some telling insights. The transcriptome is essentially a record of the messenger RNA (mRNA) being produced by genes that are either activated or deactivated by the genes encoded in an individual's DNA. It is sort of the equivalent of looking at the incoming and outgoing emails (mRNA) of a corporation as a way of determining what corporate decisions and initiatives are being pursued within corporate headquarters. In short, the transcriptome is a record of the genetic "initiatives" taken by our DNA. What scientists have found is that aging-related genetic changes directed by our DNA seem to be more accelerated in women than in men, especially in the prefrontal cortex (PFC). The PFC is where critical, executive thinking and planning occur, and it is especially hard-hit by aging and dementia. In fact, after reviewing the activity of more than 13,000 genes in various regions of the brains of men and women, scientists were shocked at the size of the differences. For example, in one area of the PFC, nearly 700 genes demonstrated different activity by sex, and 98 percent of them would suggest that faster aging occurs in the brains of women.[4] But there were significant differences among women within this analysis: Only half the women showed the accelerated genetic changes associated with faster brain aging. Here, the difference appears to be more environmental: Women exposed to increased levels of stress showed increased activation of genes coding for inflammation markers. The effect of stress upon the activation and expression of damaging brain inflammation markers has also been extensively demonstrated in animal experiments and speeds up the aging of neurons. So it would appear that stress plays an important permissive role in accelerating mental decline in women.

Genetics play a central role in cognitive decline, dementia, and developing Alzheimer's disease. It is estimated that 40–80 percent of our individual risk of developing Alzheimer's disease lies within our genetic makeup. The possibility of developing Alzheimer's disease, irrespective of our own sex, appears to be tied more strongly to genetics derived from our mother's side of the family than our father's. Early research has shown that if our mothers suffer or have suffered with dementia related to Alzheimer's disease, we are more likely to show atrophic changes in brain size and cortical thickness much earlier on brain-imaging studies than scans taken from people whose mothers were without symptoms. However, as we shall see in later sections of this chapter, we need not be resigned to letting the simple laws of genetic proclivity set the agenda. Instead, we can set our own agenda to prevent mental decline.

Potential modifications in our personal lives directly or indirectly influence the expression and effect of such genetic factors. Certainly, environmental factors such as higher socioeconomic status, attaining a longer and higher level of academic education, lower numbers of siblings, and growing up in a suburban (rather than urban) setting are all elements that *lower* the likelihood of developing cognitive decline. One possibility is that such factors establish a greater cognitive "reserve" that is better able to buffer and adjust to assaults on memory and intellectual functions later in life. Senior women who displayed sustained cognitive function well above that of their counterparts showed substantial correlations with the following health factors: a lack of diabetes, nonsmoking status (although many had been smokers earlier in life), lower levels of depression, good visual function, a lack of physical disabilities, low incidence of hypertension, better social networks, and moderate alcohol intake.[5] Another interesting difference between men and women is that women who reach their mid-eighties are more resistant to declining cognitive function than men.[6] Similarly, the U.S. National Institute on Aging reported that women appear to be more resilient and able to call on cerebral reserves to maintain cognitive function in the face of age-related decrements in intellectual function later in life.[7]

Molecular and Cellular Aspects of Brain Aging

The brain is filled with genetic switches that get turned on or off during development and throughout our adult lives, but they are affected by environmental factors as well. Our brain cells do not operate in a vacuum, and age-related changes can help induce or prevent brain dysfunction or dementia as we age. One of the more interesting genetic factors being evaluated in cognitive dysfunction is called repressor element I-silencing transcription (REST).

REST protects aging neurons throughout our entire lives by mitigating oxidative and toxic damage, and inhibiting excessive accumulation of amyloid proteins associated with Alzheimer's disease. REST is very active in infants and childhood and is dramatically reduced or even shut off as people age.

REST plays a big role in dementia. Studies have shown that people who suffered from Alzheimer's disease had virtually zero REST protein in their brain tissue. On the other hand, seniors who maintained high levels of cognitive function during their life spans showed high concentrations of REST. Higher levels of REST activity help our brain cells resist stress and, thus, actively sustain neuronal longevity, preserve cognitive function, and protect us against Alzheimer's disease.

Another factor that plays an important role in preventing or mitigating cognitive decline is brain-derived neurotrophic factor (BDNF). BDNF is one of a family of nerve growth factors that help neurons grow and thrive. It has proved to be a major player in modulating brain plasticity. What's plasticity? Well, for starters, it has nothing to do with plastic. It has to do with the brain's ability to adapt and reorganize itself by rewiring or establishing new connections. It is a natural part of how the brain circumvents deficits or deficiencies (like those produced by a stroke, for example). So, we know that someone who is blind develops heightened senses of touch and sound. In fact, some blind people's sense of hearing is so highly developed that it functions as a kind of acoustic radar. BDNF is an important element in inducing compensatory connections like this. Low levels of BDNF predispose people to develop degenerative neurological disorders such as Huntington's and Parkinson's diseases and Alzheimer's dementia. One reason exercise may help preserve mental function is that it is a powerful stimulus for increasing BDNF.

Differences in Aging in the Brains of Women Versus Men

A number of subcortical (i.e., structures lying beneath the cortical surface) areas of the brain are the targets of neurodegenerative disorders. So, for example, the *hippocampus* is the area responsible for the storage and retrieval of memories. It is one of the unique targets of Alzheimer's disease. Similarly, Parkinson's disease attacks a subcortical structure called the *substantia nigra*. These subcortical areas seem more susceptible at an earlier age in men than in women.[8] This could be because male brains shrink faster than female brains as they age.

In terms of degenerative disorders that can lead to dementia, the female brain appears to be more susceptible to Alzheimer's disease, whereas male brains are more prone to degenerating to Parkinson's disease. Studies indicate that women may experience age-related declines in cognitive functioning in their fifties (post-menopause), which is earlier than their male counterparts. Mental function appears to decline in the normal population at a rate of about 5 percent per decade. This means that a woman in her early fifties could expect as much as a 20 percent drop in cognitive capabilities by the time she is in her eighties.[9] This decline is separate from comorbidities such as cardiovascular disease, hypertension, or diabetes and any neurodegenerative process such as Alzheimer's disease. But there's far more to the story than just waiting for our brains to fail us. Although many of these statistics are daunting, there's no reason why we should stand by idly and let ourselves fall victim to them. If anything, it makes the adoption of lifestyle changes that thwart mental decline all the more compelling.

Brain Function: The Fruits of Aging

The good news is this: Not all vectors relating to aging brain function are pointed south. There are some things that older brains do better and for which they deserve to be celebrated. For example, although some people think a teenager's brain is in "peak" condition, it has a paucity of fibers between the prefrontal cortex (PFC), where executive thinking, risk taking, and restraint originate, and the LL, where emotional responses are generated. The significance of this is that teenagers have less ability to use PFC function to restrain themselves from risky and impulsive decisions. Sounds like adolescence, right? Well, as we age, our brains lay down more and more fiber bundles between the PFC and the LL and amygdala, the latter being the region where especially powerful emotional responses are generated within the LL. This explains why, although it once seemed to be a good idea for you and your teenage friends to get drunk and then see if you could outrun an oncoming train in your car, it now seems far more dangerous and unappealing. Those fibers from the PFC are the anatomical equivalent of wisdom; with white (or slightly graying) hair comes white-matter fiber tracts. So, with all that wisdom, seniors tend to be much better at assessing risks and pitfalls than younger people. Along with those white-matter changes between the PFC and LL, there are more fiber tracts in a structure called the corpus callosum that integrate left and right hemispheres. This enhanced interaction between hemispheres also brings greater cognitive assets to seniors[10] when it comes to problem-solving.

Seniors can also remain more focused on a project. As we age, multitasking proves harder to pull off. First, the brain really never multitasks. It can handle only one task at a time. What the brain does is try to dart back and forth from one task to another. There is a pause between each task as the brain recalibrates itself. As we age, that recalibration takes longer and longer. So older brains learn to stay focused on one task, finish it, then move on to the next. Another finding is that older brains excel at inductive reasoning, which ensures that there is less of a tendency toward reactive and impulsive actions. Verbal abilities improve as we age. Our vocabulary grows, and our ability to use language to better express ourselves improves. It is also far easier for older brains to compartmentalize, so seniors can more easily park an issue off to the side while they move on to something more enjoyable. Seniors are also able to extract greater contentment and well-being from their activities than younger subjects.

Mental Decline Is Not Inevitable

As happens in the field of medicine with embarrassing regularity, sometimes we're just plain dead wrong. And we were wrong in our understanding about mental decline in the brain as we age. We assumed that decay in the brain was inevitable and could not be prevented, forestalled, or treated. In fact, once upon a time we claimed that the brain stopped growing after age eighteen and that it was all downhill from there. Boy, did we get it wrong! Why? Because there was an implicit bias in the neurosciences. It began to take shape almost as soon as history began to be written. In the Bronze Age, the average life expectancy was twenty-nine. By 1950, it had climbed to forty-eight years—an additional nineteen years over the course of almost 5,000 years! So you can begin to understand the bias: On average, people simply did not live long enough to undergo the effects of degeneration of the central nervous system (CNS).

It is not an accident that the neurodegenerative picture of Parkinson's disease was not even described until the nineteenth century and the dementia of Alzheimer's disease not until the twentieth. These diseases became manifest only as the population became old enough that their brains could begin to suffer cognitive and functional decline. It was assumed that brains were likely to show signs of wear and tear and degenerative processes once they reached a certain age and ran out of reserves. It is only in the last half century that the aging population has provided powerful new insights into the degenerative process. Even so, Dr. John Trojanowski, the director of the National Institute on Aging, initially summed up the general consensus among medical practitioners: "It's a very difficult thing to say to a patient that there is nothing we have for you, but that is the honest response. There are no disease-modifying therapies for Alzheimer's."[11] What Dr. Trojanowski also realized was that this meant steps had to be taken within the profession to ensure that the focus shifted from a traditional disease-based model of seeking "cures" to endorsing an aggressive attitude toward preventing or reversing premature brain aging.

Superaging: Strain, Train, and Sustain

t is easy for us as seniors to feel discouraged by daunting statistics that hint at a sort of inevitability about cognitive and psychomotor decline with advancing age. It is critical to remind ourselves that these are just averages extracted from large population-based studies. Aging, as I'll explain, represents precisely the kind of scenario where people can use their attitudes and wills to trump biology.

Superagers, a term that was coined by neurologist Marsel Mesulam,[12] make up the group of outliers in which we want to earn membership privileges for ourselves, right? We want to create the highest likelihood of placing ourselves in this group by making the right lifestyle choices. So we can begin to examine the question, What do superagers do that we don't? Examples of superagers include the likes of Mary Ann McGowan, an ultramarathoner, who started running at age forty-nine to help herself recover from the loss of her husband and, a year later, a mastectomy for breast cancer. She entered her first senior track-and-field competition that year and as of the age of ninety-two, had continued to qualify to compete in every single National Senior Games competition since its inception![13]

Ora Brooks is in her eighties and on a mission. She participates in Northwestern University's Superaging Project, which accepts only subjects who are eighty or older for its research study. Ms. Brooks is a retired schoolteacher who scored very high on physical fitness (she works out five times a week) as well as in psychomotor and cognitive pre-enrollment testing. Only 10 percent of all applicants qualify to be enrolled as superagers. Ms. Brooks is also a penguin aficionado who has taken dozens of trips to regions in the Southern Hemisphere and

Antarctica to help track and carry out ecological research on all seventeen species of penguins on Earth. Her recent non-penguin-related travel itinerary called for her to journey abroad to some of the most remote regions in Asia, such as Kazakhstan, Kyrgyzstan, Tajikistan, and Uzbekistan, for several weeks.[14]

Dame Judi Dench is a proclaimed Academy Award–winning actress who has starred in innumerable movies and plays and maintains a schedule that would exhaust an eighteen-year-old Olympian. In her mid-eighties, she was scheduled to star in three movies and a play this year. It is hard to imagine the feats of memorization she must carry out to maintain such a demanding acting schedule, but she certainly qualifies as one of the entries in our pantheon of female superagers!

Superagers are not common. Their numbers are believed to represent less than 5 percent of the senior population.[15] What makes them stand out is that their brain functions often are closer in performance to that of people decades their junior. One study,[16] for example, compared seniors in the fifty- to eighty-year-old age group with a control group made up of young adults between the ages of eighteen and thirty-two. We can determine the adequacy of brain functions by employing computer games or standardized assessment tools. What made this study stand out was that the researchers evaluated the neuroanatomy of the senior subjects and found that (1) they had thicker brain cortices than a cohort of normal seniors and their cortices most closely resembled the cortical thickness seen in the group of eighteen- to thirty-two-year-olds, and (2) hippocampal volumes were similar in young subjects and superagers. This also was seen in other areas such as the temporal lobes, the PFC, and the anterior cingulate area, all of which are involved in memory and retrieval. The conclusions of the study were that superagers stood out precisely because their brain functions and brain anatomy closely resembled what was seen in youngsters in their prime. Their brains defied aging rather than being ravaged by it.

Other traits also set superagers apart. They consistently exhibit three traits that I sum up as *strain, train, and sustain.* By *strain*, I mean that superagers use their cognitive abilities to stretch their intellects to their maximum. In essence, first and foremost, the trait that sets superagers apart from the rest of the aging senior population is that they *think*. In fact, they *think very hard*. Secondly, they *train* physically to stay extremely fit in comparison with their contemporaries. The third factor is that they eat to *sustain* their brains in the best shape they can. Consistently, these are the factors that place individuals in this select group of cognitive and psychomotor overachievers. A handful of additional factors need to be tweaked, including sleep regimen, social connectivity, and what I term a downright "ornery" resistance to growing old.

As neurologist Lisa Feldman Barrett, who has studied superaging extensively, puts it, "You may hear that you can exercise your brain by playing sudoku and visiting 'brain game' websites. These relatively mild activities are not likely to increase your odds of becoming a superager, because the level of difficulty is too low. You have to work hard enough to feel the strain of effort." In fact, the medical literature and television commercials are replete with brain-training games, puzzles, and exercises, but the scientific literature demonstrates that although playing those games improves your ability to play those games (so you naturally see the subjects' scores rise), it does nothing to improve your overall cognition.[17] No, we are talking about pursuing new lines of intellectual interest, learning new languages, undertaking a new career where you must study loads of new information, resupplying your intellectual toolbox, or undertaking a whole new line of research. In short, to become a superager you must be willing to take on the challenge of learning new material and information that takes you way out of your usual comfort zone.

How to Maintain Brain Function in Aging Women

ynn Posluns, the founder and chief executive of the Women's Brain Health Initiative, explains, "You're never too young to start looking after your brain health. . . . There are lots of things you can do to help delay the onset, rather than just figuring, 'if I'm going to get it, I'm going to get it.'"[18] Despite the structural evidence cited above, women still score better than age-matched men on verbal memory tests. There is, however, a downside to this advantage: Because verbal memory tests are some of the most widely used to assess for dementia, women may be able to compensate longer and therefore progress further in their cognitive decline before it is detected.[19] Again, it's possible that women's demonstrated better abilities to communicate between both hemispheres might allow them to more efficiently harness both hippocampi when encountering memory tasks. Also men's brains show pronounced shrinkage in the frontal and temporal lobes—where personality restraint, executive planning, and impulse control occur—whereas women show preferential shrinkage in the hippocampus (involved with memory) and the parietal lobes dedicated to visuospatial memory and language.[20] This selective atrophy may explain why women suffer from Alzheimer's disease. Many women report feeling mentally "slower" after menopause, when estrogen levels plummet, but estrogen replacement therapy appears to offer little or no protection against the development of Alzheimer's disease itself.

Exercise and Brain Fitness

Throughout this book, we have been singing the praises of exercise. The first three of Harry Lodge's Seven Rules in the original edition of *Younger Next Year* were dedicated to exercise, and he made it very clear that you were to make a solemn commitment to exercise six days a week (four sessions of aerobic activity and two of strength training) *for the rest of your life.* Well, here's another hallelujah to shout out on Harry's behalf: *Exercise for life is the single most important factor in maintaining your brain fitness.* Period. If I can leave you with only one single pearl of medical wisdom, it is that. A lifelong healthful regimen ensures the mental and physical conditioning to safeguard a high-quality, independent lifestyle. One of the biggest issues is that normal cerebral function does not degrade very much before the age of sixty. In part, this is because people under sixty are more likely to remain active; it is only with advancing age and inactivity that the effects of chronic conditions such as cardiovascular disease, hypertension, and diabetes on the brain are more likely to manifest themselves and affect brain function. *Recent studies show that a good exercise routine can lower your risk of dementia by more than half!*

Aerobic Exercise

S trenuous physical exercise is a powerful tool in preventing or slowing cognitive decline. People who have maintained active physical training regimens or continued to do strenuous outdoor activities exhibit a lower incidence of cognitive dysfunction and dementia later in life compared with a cohort of sedentary subjects of the same age. As Dr. Lodge said, aerobic training (running, cycling, hiking, swimming) has the most demonstrable effect in this regard. Recent studies have shown that aerobic training also appears to exert a potent preventive effect on cognitive decline, and especially with respect to higher level executive functions. It produces a pronounced effect on the ability to maintain attention and focus. More convincing, however, was the fact that if *previously sedentary* subjects between the ages of sixty and seventy-nine were introduced to a six-month program of moderate aerobic exercise, their brain scans showed significant increases in brain volumes, especially in the areas dedicated to executive functions in the PFC and, in the temporal lobe, associated with emotional processing and memory storage. The increases in volume were seen both in the number of neurons in the gray matter and in the fiber bundles (i.e., white matter) connecting different areas of the brain. This brain-volume-enhancement effect was not seen in a similar age-matched controlled group that allotted the same amount of time to tonal exercises such as yoga and stretching. This makes it clear that aerobic fitness plays a special role in enhancing central nervous system (CNS) health and function[21] as we age and that it has a direct, sustained effect on our very neuroanatomy.

Adopting a new aerobic training regimen was accompanied by improvement in overall cognitive function, informational processing, and psychomotor skills on validated tests. Magnetic resonance imaging (MRI) scans showed increases in cerebral blood flow and oxygen delivery to the brains of subjects who had undergone six months of aerobic training. Another exercise study demonstrated that elderly subjects in a retirement community who progressively increased their tolerance for aerobic conditioning showed all the same changes with increases in volume but also showed higher levels of BDNF, which maintains neuronal health and encourages the growth of new neurons, especially in the hippocampus and PFC.[22] In addition, aerobic exercise regimens encourage more afferent sensory nerve signals from exercising muscle groups to reach the spinal cord. This can help produce profound improvements in peripheral neuropathy,[23] which is one of the primary contributors to poor muscle coordination, increased risk of falling, and worsening equilibrium issues in the aging population.

Mechanisms of Exercise

For more than fifteen years, the *Younger Next Year* series has been trying to inspire people to exercise in a serious and sustained fashion. And we have been advocating for exercise in this chapter to prevent mental decline. But why does it work? In a nutshell, you could sum it up thus: Exercise prevents cognitive decline because it boosts growth factors that sustain existing nerve cells and encourage new ones, and it curbs the toxic effects of inflammation on the brain. Exercise boosts not only BDNF, as we discussed earlier, but a whole host of other growth factors such as neurotrophin 3, synapsin, and growth-associated protein 43. All of these have been shown to accelerate the growth and maintenance of not only nerve cells but also the long fibers (called axons) that link nerve cells together.

Exercise regimens that include both aerobic conditioning and strength training turn down the chemical signals within the brain (like tumor necrosis factor-α and local cytokines) that trigger inflammation and ultimately underlie many of the mechanisms of pain sensitization leading to chronic pain. These training programs also dramatically increase the level of anti-inflammatory cytokines (such as interleukin 10 or IL-10) and reduce inflammatory markers such as IL-6 and TNF-α, thus reducing the neurotoxic inflammatory effects that increase incrementally with advancing age. Exercise also has a dramatic effect on C-reactive protein (CRP). CRP can be measured with a simple blood test and is a good, generalized marker for the body's overall systemic inflammatory health. Elevated CRP levels are associated with increased rates of cerebral atrophy[24] (brain tissue loss), and a consistent exercise regimen lowers CRP levels, leading to less inflammatory damage to the brain and cardiovascular system.[25]

So exercise turns out to be the "old folks' friend." It is like an elixir from the gods, because it addresses the very areas where we see brain and nerve deficiencies with both age-related cognitive and sensorimotor decline. It goes to the heart of preventing brain deterioration with advancing age! It also makes you feel subjectively younger (which is the only age group that counts). Researchers evaluating the notion of subjective age determined that younger subjective age and cognitive function were closely linked with a person's body mass index (BMI), which is an indirect measure of body fat and fitness, and the frequency of physical activity. BMI correlated not only with subjective age but also with how people performed on standardized tests of cognitive and psychomotor performance.[26]

Strength Training

Does strength training play any role in preventing cognitive decline? You weren't hoping to get out of lifting weights, were you? The scientific literature[27] on strength training (ST), also called resistance training, has been slower to emerge but is beginning to accumulate. After only a two-month regimen of ST, subjects in one study were able to demonstrate improvements in memory. These improvements were seen in both immediate and delayed recall. Even though the training intervention lasted only two months, the memory improvements persisted for more than a year after the end of the experiment. Furthermore, the more subjects incrementally increased their resistance levels, the more memory improved. So get back on those weights. Resistance training may have some gender-specific effects: It appears to improve memory and verbal conceptualization in men and enhance executive functions more in women.[28]

Cognitive Training

As I have said, a person's level of formal education correlates with cognitive function later in life. There may be some protective effect from having the brain undergo sustained cognitive challenges as part of higher education activities. In any event, as noted, participating in intellectually challenging activities also maintains or improves cognitive function. Similarly, sustained playing of a musical instrument for ten years or longer is predictive of preserved cognitive and psychomotor skills later in life.

Numerous studies now support cognitive and intellectual challenges as part of the superaging program. A large study conducted at the Center for Brain Aging at the University of Texas evaluated the effect of a challenging cognitive training program (known as SMART, which stands for Strategic Memory Advanced Reasoning Training) on a group of subjects between the ages of fifty-six and seventy-one. The SMART program introduced the participants to intense and demanding problems that required logical and deductive reasoning, extensive problem solving, and the creation of imaginative and novel solutions. It was carried out over a period of twelve weeks while its effect was compared with a similarly age- and gender-matched group that underwent more than 150 minutes of aerobic conditioning. Whereas the aerobically conditioned group demonstrated improvements in cognitive functioning, the SMART group showed a greater effect on cognitive efficacy and processing speed than the exercise group, as measured on MRI scans.

One almost universal finding in dementia studies is this: Leading an intellectually challenging lifestyle seems to sustain neuronal health even well into advanced old age. As one dementia researcher implored, "This is not the time to retire. It is the time to rewire!" A randomized-controlled double-blinded trial of cognitive training of more than 5,000 volunteers from around the United States was known as the Advanced Cognitive Training for Independent and Vital Elderly (ACTIVE) trial. Subjects enrolled in the trial were randomized to (1) a no-contact control group, (2) a group focusing on tasks to improve memory, (3) a group focused on advanced reasoning, or (4) a group concentrating on enhancing brain processing speed. Training in any of the three cognitive groups showed enhanced cognitive function compared with the control group.[29] One concern raised in both the SMART and the ACTIVE trials is that although cognitive training (and especially memory training) produces improved results on testing performed in the laboratory, it is less clear that such improvements extend to the subject's functions involved in active, daily living.

Iatrogenesis Imperfecta

atrogenesis imperfecta is the pseudo-medical term we use to refer to a situation where a patient's problems or illnesses have been caused by doctors practicing medicine imperfectly. In other words, "your doctor hurt you." Believe me, that's a very real problem today throughout the field of medicine: Medical adverse events (MAE), which is medicalese for *mistakes*, are the third leading cause of death in the United States. You will rarely see it listed that way, but actually twice as many people will die from MAEs as from Alzheimer's disease this year.

The reason one must be so vigilant about iatrogenic injury is that the leading cause — by far — of confusion, mental slowness, and forgetfulness is the inappropriate use and side effects of medications prescribed by one's doctor. Let me give you a real story to illustrate. A seventy-six-year-old woman had difficulty sleeping (we will talk about this subject later in the chapter), and her doctor prescribed zolpidem (trade name Ambien) to help her sleep. Zolpidem is a commonly prescribed sleep-inducing medication; in 2016 about twenty million prescriptions for it were written.[30] This particular patient was placed on a prescription of five milligrams every night before bed. She began to fall asleep more predictably and stay asleep for a longer period throughout the night. She was also on blood thinners because of a prior stroke. One very common side effect of zolpidem usage is that it can make the person forgetful, even to the point of becoming amnesiac about events during the night. It can also make you feel a little wobbly with light-headedness. So, you can imagine how important it is to screen for drugs (see table, next page) that commonly cause memory problems before evaluating someone for cognitive decline! One of this lady's problems was that she would often wake up in the middle of the night and have trouble falling back to sleep, so she would occasionally take the dog out for a walk in an attempt to make herself feel sleepy again. In the morning, she would often have no recollection of having gone out with the dog, although she could see that the leash was on the breakfast table and her sweatshirt had been hung on the back of one of the chairs.

On one particular night, she took the dog out and was coming home when she stumbled on the steps to the house and fell. Her coordination and balance were off because of the zolpidem. She hit her head and lay there unconscious until morning. Her husband finally found her, with her hand still through the dog's leash, when it was time to go out and get the morning paper. Ultimately the patient went on to die. Her death certificate listed an intracerebral hemorrhage as the cause of death. What it did *not* say was that her death was the result of a sleeping medicine recommended and prescribed by her physician that made her forgetful and confused, and affected her balance. In other words, the prescription for zolpidem that was written by the decedent's physician was never listed as the primary cause of the woman's death. The death certificate never made that critical connection that set events into fatal motion.

Classes of Medications That Can Cause Mental Status Changes, Confusion, or Cognitive Dysfunction in the Aging Population[31, 32]

Delirium or Psychosis	Tricyclic antidepressants (e.g., Elavil)
	Sedatives (e.g., Valium)
	Anti-cholinergics (e.g., Benadryl)
	Antacid medications that use H2 receptor antagonist (e.g., Zantac)
Confusion or Cognitive Impairment	Sedatives (e.g., Valium)
	Anti-cholinergics (e.g., Benadryl)
	Antacid medications that use H2 receptor antagonist (e.g., Zantac)
	Sleep medications (e.g., Ambien)
↑ **Risk of Falling**	Pain medications (e.g., opiates)
	Anti-hypertensives
	Cardiac anti-arrhythmia medications
	Diuretics

It is vital for each of us to scrutinize our list of medications to ensure that they aren't inadvertently contributing to some cognitive or psychomotor impairment. A good person with whom to screen your medication list is your local pharmacist. First, pharmacists are usually more knowledgeable about prescribed drugs than most doctors. Second, they have very elaborate machine-learning-based algorithms that screen prescribed drugs for side effects and potential interactions.

Sleep Habits

As we get older, a good night's sleep can be a hard commodity to find. In fact, research has shown that just about every aspect of sleeping can become problematic as we age. That includes falling asleep, staying asleep, and getting enough sleep. Nonetheless, *adequate sleep is essential for brain health.* The amount of sleep we need declines with advancing age: For example, babies need up to sixteen hours of sleep per day, whereas most adults need only about half that on a daily basis. But from these adult levels of sleep requirements, our need falls by ten to twenty minutes per decade until we reach our sixties.

There are several reasons why sleep is so important for protecting the brain against impairment. First, many of our brain functions—especially memory—rely on sleep to permit consolidation of learning and recall. Second, inadequate sleep is a significant source of stress, which sets off inflammatory markers that damage cells and neurons in particular. Recent research[33] has demonstrated the function of the so-called *glymphatic system.* This is a fascinating new discovery. During sleep, there is an increase of flow in cerebrospinal fluid (CSF), the fluid that bathes the brain. It appears that this increase in CSF flow is directed to flushing out toxins and metabolic by-products that can interfere with neuronal function. This may explain a phenomenon that has puzzled doctors: Why do we need so many hours of sleep? The detoxifying process would naturally require enough time to flush the brain clear of an entire day's worth of by-products from high-level, high-speed functioning. The second question the glymphatic system may help answer is, Why is a lack of sleep so impairing? We know that losing sleep can become associated with marked cognitive impairment. For example, losing one night's sleep produces the same amount of psychomotor and cognitive impairment as two shots of hard liquor. No one would let you drive in such a condition, and yet it is commonplace for night-shift workers, doctors, truck drivers, and people having to work more than one job to carry out their job functions in just such a state. It is for this reason that pilots must comply with very strict regulations over how long they can fly in terms of consecutive hours, how many days they can fly per month, and how much rest they must get between flights. A last finding about the glymphatic system is that it plays an important role in specifically removing β-amyloid, one of the agents that causes neuronal death in Alzheimer's disease!

There are several things you can do to help yourself achieve a good night's sleep[34] for your brain's health:

1. **Short naps.** Keep your naps to thirty minutes or less. A short nap is restorative, but a longer nap may actually make you groggy and cause your body to feel like it has slept so much that falling asleep at nighttime is difficult.
2. **Burn it.** Keeping your body and mind active means you are expending a lot of calories during the day. That means your energy levels during the day are good, which cues your body to get into a more pronounced circadian rhythm.
3. **Schedule sleep.** Tailor your sleep schedule in such a way that you develop a bedtime ritual. Say you always hit the sack around 10 p.m. You brush your teeth, change into your pajamas, read for ten to twenty minutes, and then turn off the light and tuck your pillow under your head.

It might take you about a half hour to do all that. You want to create a ritual around the time and sequence, because each of those events will serve as a cue to your brain that it is time to shut down for the night. Even if you are having trouble sleeping in, stick with the same bedtime routine.

4. Fast a little. Get in the habit of eating your dessert at the end of your dinner so that afterward, you are fasting for the whole night. That way you are not giving your body a jolt of energy as you are getting ready to sleep. (It will also minimize the potential for aspiration during sleep.)

5. Reserve your bed. You want to reserve your bed for, as one sleep expert put it, "sleep and sex only!" Period. The bed is not a machine shop or an office or an artist's studio. In this day and age of laptop computers, many people are working on their beds while watching TV or talking on their phones. That's all fine (although, I will caution you, the brain actually does not multitask efficiently), but now the bed is serving as a cue to get to work rather than to get to sleep.

6. Don't! Don't drink alcohol or caffeine in the evening. They disrupt your body's intrinsic mechanisms to prepare for sleep.

7. Be cool. The human body sleeps better in a room that is slightly colder than the environment in which we work. Again, the body needs to shut down and conserve energy, and snuggling under a comfortable blanket is another cue to add to your routine. Just remember to turn the thermostat down first.

8. No time. Do not have clocks prominently displayed in your bedroom to remind you how long it has been since you started trying to fall asleep. Obviously, if you need to, you can check the time on your cell phone, but

clocks and focusing on the passage of time (or the lack thereof) can be frustrating and get you fuming rather than relaxing.

9. No TV. If you want to help your mind go to sleep, don't get involved in the plot of your favorite sci-fi flick or murder mystery. You can turn on the white noise generator, or listen to a story or some soothing New Age music to help you sleep instead. There are a number of apps, such as Calm, that are wonderful sleep aids.

The overarching principle is that you have to help your brain find sleep so your brain (and the rest of you, too) can remain healthy. If you are having trouble staying asleep long enough to feel refreshed when you awaken, then you need to discuss matters with your doctor to ensure that you don't have any health-related issues that might be contributing to your sleeplessness.

Brain Nutrition

We know that food is a form of medicine for the body, and eating for brain fitness is one of the hottest trends in brain health. Max Lugavere is a young filmmaker and journalist who also happened to be taking care of a loved one with Alzheimer's disease. He went to many doctors while looking for treatment of the disease but ran into what he called the "diagnose and adios"—i.e., "we've told you what you have and there's nothing that can be done for it"—school of medicine. Understandably, he became frustrated and began investigating nutrition from the standpoint of sustaining, or improving, brain health. He researched the connection between nutrition and neurodegenerative disease for the next seven years, which led him to write a book, *Genius Foods: Become Smarter, Happier, and More Productive While Protecting Your Brain for Life*. Lugavere admits to a lifelong obsession with nutrition, but this search was motivated by helping his own family and launched him into developing a coherent and extensive document that helps us decide how to supercharge our brains with what he calls "genius foods."

Some of his findings[35] recommend the inclusion of phospholipid docosahexaenoic acid (phospholipid DHA) to ensure adequate membrane structure and repair. Oils can be a rich source of phospholipids (including phospholipid DHA) and come from foods that are rich in lecithins such as eggs, olive oil, wheat germ, soy milk, and almond milk. Lugavere also highlighted the carotenoid astaxanthin, a marine carotenoid found in wild salmon and lobster, so these are excellent for inclusion in a superaging dietary regimen because it helps activate pathways that promote longevity and enhance brain cell survival and neuroplasticity. Another genius food is the avocado, which has the highest concentration of antioxidants of any food. Antioxidants are vital compounds that inactivate agents that cause cell membrane damage and early cell death. Lugavere likens eating the grenade-shaped fruit to dropping an antioxidative "bomb" to protect your brain. Some other genius foods are organic, grass-fed meat (an important source of creatinine), eggs, leafy vegetables, dark chocolate (*not* milk chocolate, sorry), and mushrooms. Mushrooms contain high levels of powerful antioxidants, and high mushroom intake is associated with increased life span and lower risk of developing Alzheimer's disease. Another food with which we need to augment our diets is extra-virgin olive oil. Lugavere recommends up to one liter of the oil a week, because studies have shown that consuming high levels of extra-virgin olive oil improves cognition and processing speed.

Another aspect of brain health is modulating fasting periods. Ketones, which increase rapidly as we fast (even for a few hours) are excellent fuel for the brain, whereas we know high blood sugar from excessive carbohydrates actually inhibits maximal brain function. Folks who consume excessive amounts of carbohydrates are known as "bread heads." Lugavere recommends postponing the first food of the day by several hours and avoiding food consumption after eight p.m. to give your brain the longest period of fasting each day. There is also literature that recommends occasional twenty-four-hour fasts, again to promote brain health.

Finally, brain nutrition matters. Richard Isaacson, director of the Alzheimer's Prevention Clinic at Weill Cornell's Alzheimer's Disease and Memory Disorders Program, is involved in custom designing nutritional "prescriptions" for people whose genetic testing indicates they are at increased risk for developing Alzheimer's disease. Isaacson puts great emphasis on nutrition; he says, "One of the most important things is that anyone can take control of brain health by changing the food they eat. There isn't a one size fits all."[36] The Mediterranean diet provides olive oil as well as flavonoid-rich fruits and berries, and the Paleo diet provides omega-3-rich fish and carnitine-rich meats.

Mindfulness and Brain Function

From a narrow neuroscientific perspective, I could describe mindfulness, as it was derived from Eastern meditative tradition, as a repetitive training regimen aimed at amplifying and expanding a person's ability to intentionally direct and apply attentional control. There. That doesn't sound very "om"-like, but practicing mindfulness is really an exercise in heightening one's ability to selectively attend to discrete amounts of data while resisting attempts to let other perceptions interfere with that focus. This means that the person is attempting to exert control over connectivity and informational inflow. So, for example, if I am practicing the *zazen* meditative technique (typically conducted in an erect, cross-legged position), I must work at developing my attentional habits and skills to ignore initial issues with minor discomfort or intrusions as I maintain that position (I know from experience!).

It should come as no surprise that interest is increasing in the clinical applications of mindfulness practices and their effects on aspects of aging and cognitive decline.[37] As we discussed earlier, stress and inflammatory markers play a powerful role in the modulation of growth factors that govern neuronal health and longevity. Psychosocial stress has been shown to contribute to structural changes in the brain along with later cognitive impairment.[38] Because meditation focuses specifically on changing attentional habits, it allows us to accept aversive or noxious experiences without necessarily generating excessive anxiety and improves coping mechanisms.[39,40] It may be precisely for this reason that meditative practice has been demonstrated to reduce a number of circulating inflammatory markers such as cytokines and cortisol and may explain why mindfulness practices seem to improve both cognitive and memory functions.[41]

In a randomized, controlled study, meditative relaxation techniques were shown to improve the quality of sleep and cognitive and memory function in older subjects.[42] Studies evaluating brain activity in accomplished meditators demonstrated heightened connectivity in areas of the brain that were cued to self-monitoring and reducing distractibility. A similar study showed that practiced meditators demonstrated enhanced gray- and white-matter volumes in the brain as measured by MRI, suggesting that sustained meditative practice appears capable of inducing significant structural modifications over time. In general, although the actual mindful practices in these clinical studies varied widely from transcendental to yogic meditation, improvements were demonstrated in attention, executive function, memory, processing speed, and overall measures of cognition.

Finally, in the digital age, it is important to practice mindfulness because our central nervous systems are being incessantly bombarded with distracting data. Text messages. Beeps signaling incoming email. News alerts. The constant scroll of the global conversation. This barrage of information rains down on us irrespective of what we are doing and where we are, so I suggest that each of us practice "recentering" ourselves daily. This means turning everything off for fifteen to thirty minutes at least twice a day. Let yourself off the hook for a while: Take a stroll. Listen to the wind. Go sit by a body of water (a stream, a lake, or even just a fountain). Or take in an open vista for a few minutes.

Connect and Socialize

One of Harry Lodge's important rules about health, well-being, and aging was that a healthy lifestyle includes a vibrant, connective social network. Social bonds of kinship and friendship belong in our superaging formula for several reasons. First, maintaining complex social relationships keeps our minds fine-tuned to be good listeners; we need to catch nuances of intonation and the secrets of body language and to practice empathetic listening, which requires full cognitive engagement. Second, people who have strong social networks have fewer cardiovascular events and experience less stress, both of which impede brain processing. Finally, the brain's internal milieu works best when there is a rich and satisfying emotional life. It amplifies the secretion of neurotransmitters (such as oxytocin, endorphins, and dopamine) that lead to enhanced sharpness of focus but also streamline regional interactions within the brain. Again, Harry Lodge's seventh and last rule is "Connect and commit." This turns out to be not just social wisdom but true physiological guidance, because the brain needs happiness. The neurochemicals that lead to happiness and stability of mood not only help protect you from stress and inflammatory damage, but actually make the brain work better. Studies confirm across cultures that significant loneliness is associated with greater cognitive impairment later in life and is predictive of more advanced mental decline as a separate risk factor apart from its health effects.[43] Long-term studies evaluated senior populations and discovered that the greater the measure of an individual's social isolation, the greater the likelihood of that person suffering cognitive decline and dementia later in life.[44] Socialization and connectivity have effects that go far beyond just feeling good; they directly affect our ability to sustain enhanced cognitive brain function!

An Ornery Disposition

There is another quality that one sees in superagers. I would just boil it down to being ornery. Superagers do not see obstacles or setbacks as indications that they should slow down or give up. Rather, they see them as an inspiration to redouble their efforts in pursuit of their goals. As the saying goes, "Growing old is not for the faint of heart." It is for the strong in mind, spirit, and body. A close friend of mine, Jimmy Salk, used to say, "The trick to growing old with grace and dignity is to get up in the morning, stare Death straight in the face, and then spit in his eye and tell him to f--- off!"

When Could It Be Early Dementia?

How can we tell what's just normal aging and what's worse? A normal amount of vexing forgetfulness can go along with the aging process. Why? Because some gliosis, or scarring, takes place in the hippocampus. There is a gentle decrease in cerebral blood flow. And finally, the ability of neurons to repair themselves diminishes with age. A lot of these processes, as we have seen, can be prevented or reversed, but let's put to rest what is normal, nonpathological forgetfulness and what isn't.

You are allowed to forget a name now and then. You are allowed to substitute your daughter's name for your sister's. You are allowed to experience the "tip of the tongue phenomenon," where you can't remember the name of that actress or the word for the thingamajig you use to figure how much to turn that bolt. For such matters, my rule is simple: I get ten minutes to try to remember, and then I google it. The ten minutes are a requirement, because usually the recollection will come to me if I am patient. Plus, it is good to make your brain work to remember! Then, of course, there is the "You don't remember where I left my glasses, do you?" phenomenon for which no good GPS application exists to date, although it would be a wonderful Bluetooth app if any of you app developers are listening. All these kinds of things are normal.

So, when is it dementia? My first question is this: Is it just annoying or is it interfering with your ability to function? Second: Is it more than one thing? Are you having problems remembering names *and* balancing the checkbook? Or do you notice you are having a hard time following the plot in TV programs? These are more worrisome. Third: Do your family members and/or close friends notice? Family members and close friends know you very well and can often pick up subtle differences that might go unnoticed by more casual observers. The more intrusive the memory lapses, the less likely they are to simply be the result of the more benign age-related loss of memory. The best way to be vigilant about memory loss is to bring the matter to your doctor's attention so that formal neuropsychological testing and brain scanning can be carried out.

Time for Hope and Action

t is true that Alzheimer's disease, Parkinson's disease, and other neurodegenerative diseases are being diagnosed more often than at any other time in history. That is because of the shifting demographics, with the huge mass of baby boomers moving into their older years. However, times have changed and attitudes have changed. First, after a half century of research and development, no cure for Alzheimer's disease or other dementias has been found. Some drugs can help slow the progression of dementia for some patients, but there is no cure. Nor has one been found for Parkinson's disease, so the emphasis has shifted from intervention to prevention. That change in focus has begun to open whole new perspectives on aging, superaging, and the ability to keep the mind fed both physiologically and psychologically to help preserve it and keep it running at maximal capacity. This is a time for hope and for action if we wish to grab the title of superager for ourselves. It is a time to rally to the cry of "strain, train, and sustain." We have to strain our minds by plunging into demanding intellectual pursuits, we have to train our bodies to permit our brains to work at peak efficiency, and finally, we have to eat to sustain our brains, to keep them working at supernormal capacity and be able to use them to create, reinforce, and expand our personal web of connectivity to family, friends, and community. It is from the web of life that the brain draws its power.

Let's Join Ulysses

My favorite poem is "Ulysses," which was written by Alfred, Lord Tennyson. The subject of the poem is the old, spent, and weary warrior Ulysses as he sails toward his home in Ithaca after twenty long years away during the Trojan War. Ulysses ponders what life may hold for him as he returns home, where the old warrior finds new inspiration.

> I am a part of all that I have met;
> Yet all experience is an arch wherethro'
> Gleams that untravell'd world whose margin fades
> Forever and forever when I move.
> How dull it is to pause, to make an end,
> To rust unburnish'd, not to shine in use!

As tho' to breathe were life! Life piled on life
Were all too little, and of one to me
Little remains: but every hour is saved
From that eternal silence, something more.[45]

So we reach out and link our arms with those of Ulysses, knowing we too sail ahead, traveling bravely through that same arch, and navigating the high seas as resolute super-agers, never content to rest.

Footnotes on page 425

CHAPTER TWENTY-TWO

Relentless Optimism

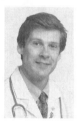

Harry

This has been a deeply optimistic look at aging—and for good reason. First, you are likely to live for a long, long time. And second, you make a daily choice in how the rest of your life goes, and it can be great. The rules are straightforward: Exercise hard and you will grow younger. Care about other people and you will grow happier. Build a life that you think means something and you will grow richer.

Chris has tremendous optimism about getting older, and he's right. The new science outlined here is radically different from what we thought a decade ago. And the lessons are pretty simple when you get right down to it: Exercise, care, and connect. We've tried to show why this is so profoundly important . . . and why it's a biological choice you make every day. Our bodies are still part of nature, even if we're not, and they still run like railroad trains, on tracks of steel laid down over eons. The train keeps moving forward, but we control the switch. We can choose left or right, growth or decay. The choice we make by being sedentary or isolated is as powerful as the choice we make by exercising or connecting. Remember tonight, before you go to sleep, that you chose just a little bit of growth or decay today, and you get to choose all over again tomorrow.

Personally, I find the evolutionary biology of this comforting. I like knowing that I have a place in nature and that my body operates according to predictable rules. And I certainly like the idea that I have so much control over just how I age. But mostly I like looking around the natural world and seeing echoes of my own biology everywhere I turn. Chris had to edit out large chunks of the book where I went off on tangents about the biology of squid, moose, worms, snails, fruit flies, and bacteria. Still, the point is that we are all part of something much larger than ourselves. You are not alone as you swim against the tide. You have all your ancestors on your side, rooting for you—three and a half billion years of family portraits hanging on the walls, urging you forward. It's a huge genetic retirement account that you can start drawing from right now.

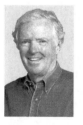

Chris

Harry is quite right about my optimism. We're finishing the book as I'm getting into my seventies, and my dominant mood is optimism about the next decade and, if I have a touch of luck, the ones after that. In a way, that's the most important thing we hope you will take from the book: optimism about just how different—and how good—the Next Third of your life can be. My view of aging had been the traditional one ... that grim arc of disconnection and decay I mentioned in the first chapter. With the experience of the last few years behind me, and an understanding of Harry's science under me, my view today is entirely different. I am enormously optimistic for myself and even more optimistic for you. Not just because you're going to live longer. That's nice, but that's not it. I am more optimistic for you because most women have a deep flair for the connection and commitment that men find so difficult. Hell, that I find difficult. Put your gift together with the physical regimen that has revolutionized my life and, by heaven, you're going to be a rocket ship. Then if you can also hang on to that sense of empowerment and purpose that so many women start to feel in their fifties and sixties, you can have a hell of a life.

But for heaven's sake, don't assume you've got it made and don't have to do the physical stuff, just because you have that flair. The physical side has been so important to me, and it will be to you, and you simply have to get it right. It is, as I say, the engine that drives the train. With that engine in place, everything else has been possible. For me as for you.

Today, I am more physically fit than I was twenty years ago. I am stronger, more flexible ... *doing* more. My personal life is fuller and much more intense, it really is. I have far more things to do and people to do them with. I have frankly worked hard at creating projects like this book and networks of new pals. As a result, I have more things to do—things that I urgently want to do—than I can finish in my lifetime. And because it wasn't always that way, I know what a luxury that is.

So here I sit, in my seventies, full of projects, curiosity and optimism. I believe I am going to have an interesting life, maybe even a useful life, in my very last years. I am not going to pass them in idleness, petulance, and anxiety, which is the way it looked for a while. Not bad.

I know . . . I may wake up some morning with a tangerine in my brainpan. Or ski into a tree. Fine. But I don't assume for a minute that I will be in radically worse shape ten years from now than I am this evening. Some decay, sure, but not significant. And certainly not debilitating. All the core dread about that is gone. And optimism and curiosity stand in its place. Not so many folks, I'll betcha, have gone into their seventies and eighties with those as their dominant emotions. And the bedrock of all of that is this lunatic exercise program, which turns out to be the only sane way to approach the rest of your life.

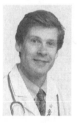

Harry

Exercise is absolutely the most important message of the book, because movement *is* life, and because it's easy to structure. Just make it your job. Chris, who is not a lifelong athlete, has chosen to grow a bit, just about every day, for the past few years. He has been steadily swimming against the tide, getting a little younger every year. At seventy-one, he says he has been sixty for longer than anyone he knows. That's a nice line, but based on his last stress test and physical exam, he's actually a healthy forty-nine-year-old today. The biology and the message would be just the same if Chris were Christine. The world is full of fit, vigorous older women who are on the same journey. It has nothing to do with gender; it has to do with growth or decay.

Always remember this: Most of our aging is just decay, and decay is optional; it's under your control. Some of life's changes are not under your control, but this one is. Taking charge of your life, physically and emotionally, is the best possible antidote to standard aging.

And it all starts with exercise. Exercise reverses the bizarre message our society sends older women and men that they should retire not just from work, but from life. The message that there is something unnatural about living a young life as you get older—something unnatural about being strong, fit, mentally and sexually active, and emotionally involved. That message is just plain wrong. Growth and life are the most natural things in the world. Decay is what's unnatural. Chris is optimistic because getting into good shape has freed him from this social construct. It has given him the enthusiasm and drive to build a full life, physically and emotionally, heading into those renaissance years.

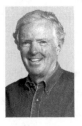

Chris

I passionately agree about exercise, but it's hard to overestimate the importance of connection and commitment. When I was turning sixty, my greatest fear was not that I would fall apart—although I worried plenty about that. It was that I would be useless and idle and bored. And ashamed because I was not doing anything. When I first retired and found myself walking along the streets of New York at midday with nothing to do, I felt as if I'd just walked out of a porno movie. I didn't want my friends to see me, because they'd know I had no job, that I wasn't *doing* anything. I felt that weird guilt for a ridiculously long time. It was silly, but it was a near-crippling, isolating phenomenon. Women don't seem to have that, thank God. They seem to be able to turn more easily and smoothly from a job—or an empty nest—to the critical business of broadening and deepening their circle of friends, finding stuff to do, and getting on with their new life. Lucky. That's lucky. But even for women, finding something new and worthwhile to do, after life's regular tasks are behind us, seems difficult.

In fact, it's not all that hard, it's just unfamiliar, which *reads* as hard. Harry uses this wonderful metaphor about how the paths for the young are actually superhighways, carefully marked with huge, legible signs: GO TO COLLEGE. TAKE THIS EXIT TO PROCTER & GAMBLE. STOP OFF TO HAVE A CHILD. STAY HOME OR BECOME A COG IN THE AMERICAN ECONOMY. Your pick. But, he says, the paths after sixty are back roads or country lanes, with no signs to tell you where to go. Or who to be. No role models. No norms of behavior and no support organizations. In time, if you do it somewhere near right, you'll come to appreciate the beauty of the back roads, their comparative calm—and the fact that you have so many, many options to do whatever you want. But it takes a while. And it takes some work.

You have to get used to the idea that, as with any meandering road, it is less a matter of getting someplace and more a matter of enjoying the trip. It means rethinking our ideas of success. Getting over them, as a matter of fact. Most of us gave up far too much when we decided to live vicariously through our kids or our work and got back far too little in quality of life. Eventually, you'll wonder why you spent so much of your life on that noisy, unrestful highway. Take the scenic route. And worry less about getting somewhere.

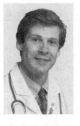

Harry

That's a great way of putting it, because building the complete package of a healthy body, mind, and spirit is the real end goal of this regimen. We see a new generation of very fit older people unlike any that has gone before, a generation living complete lives almost all the way through, with all the challenges, successes, sorrows, and joys that implies. Good to the last drop, to borrow a phrase. Actually, lots and lots of people are already living those lives, but they're hard to see because they're doing it on their own. They've gotten off the interstate, choosing to find their way on quiet, two-lane roads with light traffic. There are no traffic jams and no rush hours. If you join them, you may feel strange at first, as if you should be back on the interstate, rushing along. You will miss some things about the old life, but this is your new adventure. And you will be just fine on whatever back roads you take.

There are only a few basic things you need for this new, back-road life. You need some sort of transportation, which is your body. Take good care of it, because it's the only ride you've got. You also need some company on the road. If you're lucky enough to have one, wander the countryside with your spouse or partner; if not, work hard to get your friends to share the ride. Don't worry so much about where you actually go; if your partner or friends have different ideas, let them drive for a while and see how it works out.

Finally, you need some good old-fashioned courage. It can be scary on the back roads without a map. You might get lost—you *will* get lost, over and over again. The renaissance is going to be unpredictable. You won't have the familiar structure and support of the old life, but neither will you have a lot of the constraints and limitations. The possibilities are endless.

Our advice is simple. Stay young until you die. Work hard at the rest of your life, but do it your own way. Get into good shape. Then go out and take some chances. Get to know new people. Work hard at relationships and get involved in your community or some projects. This may not all be fun or rewarding at first. You will take wrong turns and hit some potholes. But you will also have great adventures.

So take matters into your own hands, no matter what. Become the organizer. Take some risks. Build bridges. Some of them will fall down, some will be bridges to people you find you don't like that much, but that's fine. Some of them will eventually lead to real friendships. Besides, even if you don't actually like everyone in your pack, you still need a pack.

Build your passions. We talk about finding passions, but I think building passions is more accurate. If you have passions already, that's great. If you don't, then fake it for a while. That's serious advice. Pretend you're enjoying things, no matter what, until your attitude catches up. It's clear from research over the past thirty years that being happy is largely a choice. It's a decision *you* make in your limbic brain, with very little regard to external circumstances and with virtually no regard to money. Deciding to be happy may be the most serious commitment you can make for the renaissance years.

One of the roads you should try in the next part of your life, if you haven't already, is the road to altruism. A lot of people have taken it, and they *all* recommend it. They simply do things that help other people—most often in small ways, in little shared moments that added up over time. So give something back. It is a natural impulse and feels good.

Chris and I hesitate to talk about spiritual matters. Not because they don't matter, but because they're so intensely personal. Still, we both feel that there's a strong spiritual component to our journey through life, and it becomes more pronounced with age. As Chris often says, a life fully lived is also a life fully examined. That's all we're going to say, but we would encourage you to pursue the deeper thoughts when they come to you.

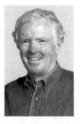

Chris

I agree completely, but good grief, Harry, we can't end on a note of sanctity. Let's make our last pitch a pitch for having fun as we close the covers. Let's leave 'em playing, like big children. They should be doing a lot of that now.

One of your nice points is that play is a great mammalian invention and that it's good for us. Good for its own sake, without thought or justification. Because we were built for it, and it makes us feel nice. The reptiles and the fishes and the birds of the air, for all their beauty and skill . . . they do not play, Harry, as you wisely point out. We mammals are the only ones. And we should revel in it. We should tumble like otters in our terminal days. Snuggle like puppies and tumble like otters. Isn't that the stuff?

One of the great sights of the past year was of some of the women on our Idaho bike trip, at the end of the day, playing on the lawn. Some preteen girls had been doing handstands and cartwheels in the long twilight, and sure enough, three or four of our pals—all in their fifties and sixties—thought that looked pretty good and they could do it, too. And they did. Rolling around, taking turns holding each other's feet . . . laughing, getting grass stains all over. Rolling around like puppies. That's what we need more of in the long, sweet twilight of our lives—more rolling around on the grass.

A lot of our advice is about "aligning ourselves" with our essential, Darwinian traits in useful ways. "Useful" is such a north-of-Boston, Puritan word. Remember the dreary sermons about "useful virtue," Harry, when we were kids? Well, play is "useful" in that high sense. It exercises our bodies and our minds in the most profound and useful ways. Play is virtuous now. It is its own reward. So, go do a cartwheel. Or a headstand. Throw a Frisbee. Play in the surf. Throw parties for yourself, every single birthday.

Just plain do stuff. Default to doing stuff. Learn to cook "fusion" food or some damn thing. Jump into some new sport, now that you're fit for it. Just do it. Darkness will descend, you darlings. We are going over the falls alone. But not this week. And probably not this decade. In the meantime, let us, by all means, play.

Okay, that's it. We're out of here. Last one over the waterfall is a rotten egg.

Appendix

HARRY'S RULES

1

Exercise six days a week for the rest of your life.

2

Do serious aerobic exercise four days a week for the rest of your life.

3

Do serious strength training, with weights, two days a week for the rest of your life.

4

Spend less than you make.

5

Quit eating crap!

6

Care.

7

Connect and commit.

Author Notes

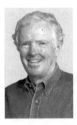

From Chris

Chapter One

"Instead of getting old and fat and ridiculous in the thirty- or even forty-some years after menopause, you can remain essentially the same person you are today."

When we sent an early version of our first book to friends for their thoughts, I was baffled when a similar line—and a similar promise—drew near-angry comments from two of the people I respect most in the world: S. Hazard Gillespie, ninety-five, my mentor and close friend for some forty years, and my sister Ranie Austin, eighty-three. Turns out they thought the book was too conservative. "Chris," Hazard said, "you make it sound as if the whole thing comes to an end at eighty, and that is simply not correct. Harry's Rules . . ." and now his voice gained some of the force, rhythm, and intensity that thrilled courtrooms for fifty years, "Harry's Rules apply as clearly at eighty . . . and at ninety . . . and, I dare to presume, at a hundred . . . as they do at sixty." Pause for effect. "You simply must explain that to people." My sister was every bit as insistent. I hereby passionately endorse what Hazard and Ranie said. The fact is that Harry's Rules apply with greater force and importance the older you get. Hazard and my sister are elegant proof.

We have not gone through this book and added new thoughts at every turn. But I do feel obliged to add this quick note here. As this new edition comes out, I will be eighty-five and I understand my sister's and my mentor's reactions a bit better. And I endorse Hazard's view with great passion. At eighty-five, I am no longer fifty, but I still do an awful lot of the stuff we boast about in this book. The one new insight from me: As you get into your eighties, Harry's Rules and all the rest matter *much more*, not less. Following them is hugely important, because the tide of aging is picking up speed. Do more, if anything. And, look, there will be some decline; what did you think? But the difference in quality of life and plain fun between those who follow these rules and those who don't is vast. Don't let up!

"Meeting Harry and Getting a New Start"

I talk about one skin surgeon, Desiree. In fact, there were two in the room that day, and the younger one, Dr. Robin Gymrek, is my dermatologist to this day. She also knew and recommended Harry, from whom she had taken some course in medical school. Most importantly, she has been the source of a lot of great advice about aging and skin care. Some of it is included in later chapters. She is a terrific doctor and inexplicably cute for someone who spends a lot of time cutting divots in your face.

Chapter Two

"Jessica Alone"

I didn't know how to reach "Jessica's" heirs, so she appears with a pseudonym. But believe me, she was every bit as wonderful as I say, and lots and lots of people adored her. Not, let me assure you, because she was anyone's idea of a nice little old lady. She was not. Once, when she was well into her seventies, she was clipped from behind by some idiot while skiing and knocked unconscious. When the ski patrol guy came up and found this old person in the snow, he was a little flustered. "Now, don't you move, miss. Just . . . just you lay there." She opened a baleful eye and said, "Surely you mean *lie* there!" Then she calmly got up and skied off. I miss her all the time.

Chapter Four

"Jump-Start Your Life"

These vacations (and the "kedging" vacations referred to in Chapter Nine) are easier to arrange than they sound. My pal George Butterfield started Butterfield & Robinson, the premier bicycle travel company in the world. Write them (70 Bond Street, Toronto, Ontario, Canada M5B 1X3), or email (*info@butterfield.com*), or pick up the phone (1-800-678-1147), and they'll send you a brochure that will blow your socks off. They command a premium, but they're simply terrific. Great exercise, super accommodations and meals, great fun. Take a peek at their website, *www.butterfield.com.* Hilary and I did two serious B&R bike trips—El Camino de Santiago in Spain and the Tuscan hills in Italy—back to back a couple of days after we put this book to bed. A huge reward to ourselves and the kedge of a lifetime.

For other ideas about biking, skiing, and other exercise vacations, look at the back of general magazines like

Outside or magazines specific to each sport. For less intense vacations, try mainstream magazines like *Travel & Leisure.* The woods are full of great places to go for a jump start or a kedge. Finding them is easy and fun. So is going.

"Do not delay because you do not happen to have a bath . . ."

Some time after our first book was done, I was sitting in the bathtub at the New Hampshire lake house, reading the autobiography of the incomparable Vladimir Nabokov, *Speak, Memory.* He mentioned that his father, a wealthy Russian aristocrat with democratic leanings, had been imprisoned by the czar in 1905. Put in solitary confinement, in fact. He said that his father had not minded it much because he had "his books, his collapsible bath, and his copy of J.J. Muller's manual of home gymnastics." The collapsible bath rang a very faint bell. I walked dripping to the bookshelf in my bedroom, and sure enough, my grandfather and Nabokov's father were both working out with the same mustachioed Dane a hundred years ago. How nice to have that link with Nabokov, whom I admire so much. I am sorry to say that the regimen did not make either of our forebears bulletproof. My grandfather died of cancer in Salem in 1904, and Nabokov's father was shot to death by an assassin in Berlin in 1922.

Chapter Eight
"Building your aerobic base is the most important aspect of this regimen."

The fact is that "building your aerobic base" works near-miracles. Here's another bit of proof. Last summer, I did that Ride the Rockies bike trip over the Colorado peaks. Think about this: I was seventy years old, I was ten pounds overweight and my only training was the daily regimen that we're pushing here. One of the more demanding days in that demanding, five-day bike trip is a hundred-mile pop over two peaks, which my pal and I did at a blazing fifteen miles an hour. That's some eight or nine hours, including rest stops and lunch. In prior years, I have been drained to a frazzle by doing a century at much lower speeds. When we finish this one, I am not tired or sore. I want to go out and have supper, wander around the town . . . boast to unlucky strangers. I could do another fifty miles, honest. And the only reason is this: I have a solid aerobic base and sound joints, which were created one day at a time with this program.

It really, really works. And it's easy, because you only have to do one day at a time. Then you get to go flying into old age on that amazing aerobic base, which is the envy of kids half your age.

A candid moment: At eighty-five, I am not doing Ride the Rockies anymore. But I do bike twenty to fifty miles all the time and love it. I still ski hard (both downhill and XC) and row. And those activities—which most people have given up decades ago—are central pleasures in my life and will be for a while.

Chapter Twelve

It has been widely pointed out by my friends that it is amusing to the point of appalling to have someone as irresponsible as I am about finances lecture *anyone* on personal economy. I have run through a lot of money. And I am very, very ashamed. Well, sort of ashamed; it *was* fun. And I *am* more or less over it. But look, if you have any serious tips about living within one's means, send them to the website. We could all use the help. Not Harry; he is a saint in this area. But I could go off the rails any moment.

Chapter Nineteen
"Make a Job Out of Your Social Life"

It turns out that one of the strongest motivators for men in our first book was the section where we urged them to treat exercise as their new "job" in retirement. Quite a few men said the book changed their lives and the tipping point was the realization that working out was a job now, not just fun or recreation. Very liberating for some guys.

I hope women have the same experience with exercise as a job and with the notion that your social life is also your job. Many women have a real flair for people, but I suspect that a lot of them tend to think of it as recreational and maybe a bit self-indulgent. It is not. In the next third of your life, it is deadly serious business . . . a real job. And should be seen in that light.

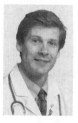

From Harry

The science of growth or decay ranges across many disciplines, and there are no standard textbooks on the subject, so the details in this book are drawn from hundreds of articles, papers, and reference books. To make the science accessible, we distilled all that material into a single, coherent story. It's accurate, though drastically condensed and simplified, with all the inevitable compromises that entails, but any errors in the science are mine alone.

That doesn't let Chris off the hook, though, because he's responsible for our writing these two books. He talks as if "Harry's Rules" were fully developed when we first met and he merely signed up as the demo model, but that's not the way it happened. I had been talking about the life-style issues with my patients and exploring the science for a long time, but Chris had been working on these ideas in his own life for a number of years before we met; he actually talked about doing this book together that very first day in the office. It took a few more years for the notion to sink in, but that's how *Younger Next Year* got its start. The science in the book comes from me, and the practical advice from both of us, but the experience of living it comes from Chris.

There are hundreds of good books out there on different aspects of healthy living and thousands more that are not so good. Some books, however, stand out as core resources for living the rest of your life, and we have listed them on the following pages. If you enjoy reading, my recommendation would be to buy them all at once as a cheap investment in the rest of your life. In general, we are huge fans of books. They are dirt-cheap for the amount of information you get, and they are fun. If you find books you think are good, email us at our website, www.youngernextyear.com.

By the way, the same goes for great ideas or specific suggestions you might have for jump-start vacations, gear, and exercise programs. Just drop us a line, and we'll put the best ones on the website.

Exercise

The books listed below are applicable to all sports and will give you a good foundation. There are good books on almost every sport you can imagine, so once you become passionate about a specific sport, read books about it—for fun, motivation, and advice.

The Younger Next Year Exercise Program, by Chris Crowley and Henry S. Lodge, MD (Workman Publishing)

This is simply the best exercise guide or how-to book out there for almost all of you. In a very short book, it sets out the critical rationale for doing both aerobic and strength training (they are very different, and you need both for different reasons). And it goes on to give specific guidance as to just what to do. (And, almost as important, what NOT to do.) I still take it with me to the gym *all the time*. The key ingredients are the superb instruction (and illustrations) from Bill Fabrocini, who—in my serious view—is one of the very best and smartest physical therapists and strength trainers in the country, and the guidance from Riggs Klika, PhD, who knows everything about aerobics.

—Chris

Precision Heart Rate Training, by Edmund R. Burke, PhD (Human Kinetics Publishers)

An excellent guide to the details of using your heart rate monitor. You really should buy it at the same time you buy your monitor.

Serious Training for Endurance Athletes, by Rob Sleamaker and Ray Browning (Human Kinetics Publishers)

This is the bible for people who want to take fitness to high levels, like marathon runners and Olympic athletes. Surprisingly, it's very accessible, and you will probably find it both fun and inspirational. If nothing else, it will give you a sense of how far you might want to take this, so read it even if you don't plan to set the athletic world on fire.

Long Distance, by Bill McKibben (Plume Books)

This one is just for fun. It's an engaging look at the ultimate jump start. The author, a middling athlete, had Rob Sleamaker take him through a year of intensive training on the same program used by the U.S. Olympic cross-country ski team. It's like a yearlong version of Chris's ski camp in Vermont.

Why We Run, by Bernd Heinrich (Ecco)

This is a wonderful look at the evolutionary biology behind running, by a biologist who is also an ultra-marathon runner. To my mind, he is one of the best nature writers around, and this is a great blend of science and story. If you like this book, Heinrich has written several others, and they are all worth reading.

Nutrition

Thinner This Year, by Chris Crowley and Jen Sacheck,
    PhD (Workman Publishing)

George Washington University professor of nutrition Jen Sacheck is a rock star nutritionist, an All American rower, and a lovely person to learn from. In the swampy (and sometimes corrupt) world of nutrition advice, she is crystal clear and rock solid. Follow her advice and you will do well. The second half of the book consists of detailed exercise advice, written with the invaluable help of Bill Fabrocini, PT, CSCS, on strength training and Riggs Klika, PhD, on aerobics.

—Chris

The Okinawa Program, by Bradley J. Willcox, MD,
   D. Craig Willcox, PhD, and Makoto Suzuki, MD
   (Three Rivers Press)

This is my favorite book on nutrition and one of the defining books on how to age well. It is a look at *one* ideal lifestyle. It is not the *only* ideal lifestyle, and you are not likely to adopt it, but the lessons are important for all of us. The dietary recommendations make a lot of sense, and the authors do a great job of explaining basic nutritional principles. Read this as an educational book more than an actual program to live by, but make sure it's on your shelf.

The Zone, by Barry Sears, MD (ReganBooks)

Skip the diet part of this one and read it just for the nutritional education. It's a pretty well-balanced diet, and the science is fairly good, though not perfect. The real advantage is that it's well written, and Sears does a good job of explaining how to get good nutrition in the modern world. Don't bother with all the variants of The Zone—just get the basic book.

Eat, Drink, and Be Healthy, by Walter C. Willett, MD
   (Free Press)

This is the Harvard nutrition guide that got Chris thinking about food labels, so he's a huge fan. It's a great look at the best current recommendations about what you ought to be putting into your mouth.

The G.I. Diet, by Rick Gallop (Workman Publishing)

Based on the Glycemic Index (a measure of the free sugar in food), this book divides the food you eat into three columns—red means "avoid," yellow means "use caution," green signifies "eat away." Makes it all very simple. If you want more, read Gallop's second book, *Living the G.I. Diet.*

Women's Health

Though we have not found a book that deals specifically with women's *health* (which is why we wrote this book), there are a number of truly excellent books on the health problems and illnesses women face as they get older. This is by no means an exhaustive list; rather, it represents some of my personal favorites.

Our Bodies, Ourselves: A New Edition for a New Era,
 by the Boston Women's Health Book Collective
 (Touchstone)

The classic against which all other women's health books are measured. Whether or not you're comfortable with its feminist perspective, the book is great on recognizing that the stages of a woman's life—including menopause—are not diseases. A wonderful resource.

A Woman's Guide to Menopause and Perimenopause, by
 Mary Jane Minkin, MD, and Carol V. Wright, MD
 (Yale University Press)

A straightforward and readable look at what is known about menopause. What I like best about it is the clear distinction the authors make between fact and myth, whether they're dealing with physical or emotional issues.

The New Harvard Guide to Women's Health, by Karen J. Carlson, MD, Stephanie A. Eisenstat, MD, and Terra Ziporyn, PhD (Harvard University Press)

This is a good, comprehensive reference manual—smartly cross-referenced, easy to use, illustrated. Keep it around for when you have any sort of question about your health.

The Silent Passage, by Gail Sheehy (Pocket)

Another classic, revised and updated. Based on extensive interviews with more than 100 women, Sheehy's book captures the wide range of experiences women have with menopause.

Finance

Getting up to speed on financial information is critical to spending less than you make. We suggest starting with this book, which is very detailed and helpful. It supports Chris's point that it's not hard to stop chasing iron bunnies—it's just hard to stop wanting to chase iron bunnies.

Your Money or Your Life: Transforming Your Relationship with Money and Achieving Financial Independence, by Joe Dominguez and Vicki Robin (Penguin)

Cognition Concerns

The Spectrum of Hope: An Optimistic and New Approach to Alzheimer's Disease and Other Dementias, by Gayatri Devi, MD (Workman Publishing)

Eminent neurologist Dr. Gayatri Devi rewrites the story of Alzheimer's by defining it as a spectrum disorder—a disease that affects different people differently. She encourages people who are worried about memory impairment to seek a diagnosis, because early treatment will enable doctors and caregivers to manage the disease more effectively through drugs and other therapies.

The Rest of Life

We hope we've convinced you that aging well can be the norm rather than the exception. Here are some books you might want to read along the way.

Successful Aging, by John W. Rowe, MD, and Robert L. Kahn, PhD (Dell Publishing)

I think this is the most important book on the science of aging ever written. *The Okinawa Program* (see page 414) comes in a close second. I'm going to leave it at that, as a mild tease to get you to buy them both.

Aging Well, by George E. Vaillant, MD (Little, Brown)

This is a good look at several of the most important long-term studies of health and happiness ever done. These studies enrolled large samples of young people from different backgrounds in the late 1930s and followed them through their lives for over fifty years. The studies are not perfect, but they're by far the best of their kind and directly relevant to the principles in our book.

Never Cry Wolf, by Farley Mowat (Back Bay Books)

This is also a classic, by a master nature writer, and a limbic feast throughout. It's a little dated, but absolutely worth reading and laughing over.

How the Mind Works, by Steven Pinker (W.W. Norton)

If you don't enjoy reading science, this is definitely not the book for you, but if you do, you have a real treat in store. This is a masterful look at the biology of the mind, especially the cortex, the "rational" human brain that we pretty much skipped over in the book. It can be a challenging book to read, but I think it's one of the best out there. And, in the end, it's a lot of fun.

What Your Mother Never Told You About Sex, by Hilda
    Hutcherson, MD (Perigee Books)

This is a great book about sexuality. It's written for women, but the men in your life should read it to learn more about your sexuality. The section on sex as you get older is especially worthwhile.

Pleasure: A Woman's Guide to Getting the Sex You
    Want, Need, and Deserve, by Hilda Hutcherson, MD
    (Putnam)

Finally, a book that takes the mystery, but not the romance, out of great sex. It's a little racy, but truly significant in its message.

Sex and the Seasoned Woman, by Gail Sheehy (Random
    House)

As Gail describes in her foreword to this book, she talked to women in their forties, fifties, and beyond and discovered that the Next Third can be the best third. It's very inspiring reading.

A Round-Heeled Woman: My Late Adventures in Sex and
     Romance, by Jane Juske (Villard)

This is a delightful and funny book about one woman's
sexual coming of age . . . at a certain age. I can do no bet-
ter than to quote the ad she placed in the personals of
The New York Review of Books: "Before I turn 67—next
March—I would like to have a lot of sex with a man I like.
If you want to talk first, Trollope works for me."

A General Theory of Love, by Thomas Lewis et al.
     (Vintage Books)

An intriguing look at some of the biology behind our emotions, with a good explanation of the emerging science that
is changing our perceptions of what it means to feel and to
care. If you like the science of emotion, you'll like this one.

Love and Survival, by Dean Ornish, MD (Perennial
     Currents)

Dr. Ornish, a pioneer in the influence of lifestyle on health,
summarizes a lot of the research on the importance of connections and emotional support. This book is well worth
reading.

Authentic Happiness: Using the New Positive Psychology
     to Realize Your Potential for Lasting Fulfillment, by
     Martin Seligman, PhD (Free Press)

When going into the Next Third, it's always good to focus on
your strengths rather than your weaknesses, and Seligman
convincingly argues that this kind of optimism can be learned,

no matter your age. Identify your strength—whether it's your kindness, your sense of humor, perhaps your generosity—and nurture it. The benefits to your health are enormous.

Triumphs of Experience: The Men of the Harvard Grant Study, by George E. Vaillant (Belknap Press)

This is a deeply valuable book that summarizes the findings of the seventy-five-year Harvard Grant Study, concluding that "love is it. Full stop"—not in keeping you alive, but in creating what one considers a "successful life."

Spirituality

Of course, no one can really recommend books on spirituality that don't reflect their own taste, and I don't recommend specific books to patients, but these are some of my favorites. If you don't like my taste, explore on your own, but explore!

Faith: Trusting Your Own Deepest Experience, by Sharon Salzberg (Riverhead)

Salzberg, a best-selling author and Buddhist teacher, does such a good job of writing about her own journey to faith that many people find this book something of a road map to finding their own.

Field Notes on the Compassionate Life: A Search for the Soul of Kindness, by Marc Ian Barasch (Rodale)

If compassion is hardwired into our nervous system, tapping into it can transform us—to say nothing of the world we live in. Barasch is particularly convincing when he argues that compassion is a "prescription for joy." Chris and I think it's also a prescription for health. This book is a particularly powerful read.

Why God Won't Go Away: Brain Science and the Biology of Belief, by Andrew Newberg, MD, Eugene G. D'Aquili, MD, PhD, and Vince Rause (Ballantine)

By studying brain images of meditating Buddhists and Franciscan nuns, the authors come to the conclusion that brain function and religious experience are linked. Their attempt to answer the Big Question—"Is religion merely a product of biology or has the human brain been mysteriously endowed with the unique capacity to reach and know God?"—makes for interesting reading.

Wherever You Go, There You Are: Mindfulness Meditation in Everyday Life, by Jon Kabat-Zinn (Hyperion)

This is a classic, mainstream exploration of meditation and a great place to start. And it's perfect for someone trying out our program: Kabat-Zinn likes to think of meditation as a workout for your mind. Just don't forget to go to the gym, too.

Caregiving

Mercifully, there are excellent resources for caregivers. If you are in this situation, make it a real job to read all these books and to work hard to find resources in your community. The books give very practical information on this, so take advantage of them.

How to Care for Aging Parents, by Virginia Morris
   (Workman Publishing)

AARP called this book "indispensable" when it was first published in 1995. Now it's out in a new edition that is truly comprehensive, covering the complete range of emotional, legal, financial, medical, and logistical issues involved in caring for the elderly. There's also a "Yellow Pages" guide at the back that will help you navigate the enormous elder-care industry.

Caring for Your Parents: The Complete AARP Guide, by
   Hugh Delehanty and Elinor Ginzler (Sterling)

Speaking of AARP, their website (*www.aarp.org*) is a great resource, as is this comprehensive guide, which goes to the heart of AARP's expertise.

*The 36-Hour Day: A Family Guide to Caring for Persons
   with Alzheimer's Disease, Related Dementing Illnesses,
   and Memory Loss in Later Life,* by Nancy L. Mace,
   MA, and Peter V. Rabins, MD, MPH (Warner)

This is the standard resource for families and is an outstanding book, with great information about outreach programs and other options.

What Your Doctor May Not Tell You About™ *Alzheimer's Disease: The Complete Guide to Preventing, Treating, and Coping with Memory Loss,* by Gayatri Devi, MD, and Deborah Mitchell (Warner)

An excellent look at the experience of Alzheimer's, this book is also strong in describing the difference between the disease and the normal memory issues of aging.

Footnotes

[1] James, G. (2017, April 8). Yes, women's brains are different from men's brains. *Inc.com*. Retrieved from https://www.inc.com/geoffrey-james/yes-womens-brains-are-different-from-mens-brains.html.

[2] Barclay, R. (2013, December 7). Men's and women's brains are wired differently, but what does it mean? *Healthline.com*. Retrieved from https://www.healthline.com/health-news/mental-mens-and-womens-brains-wired-differently-120713#4.

[3] I am including in genetic factors the more recent evaluation of epigenetic factors that can turn certain genes or gene products on and off but offer a bridge through which environment can affect the expression of our DNA.

[4] Slezak, M. (2012, July 26). Stress may cause women's brains to age prematurely. *New Scientist*. Retrieved from https://www.newscientist.com/article/dn22107-stress-may-cause-womens-brains-to-age-prematurely/.

[5] Barnes, D. E., Cauley, J. A., Lui, L-Y, Fink, H., & McCulloch, C. E. (2007, January 8). Women who maintain cognitive function into old age. *Journal of the American Geriatrics Society*, 55(2), 259–264.

[6] Van Exel, E., de Craen, A. J., M., Bootsma-van der Wiel, A., Houx, P., Knook, D. L., & Westendorp, R. G. J. (2001). Cognitive function in the oldest old: Women perform better than men. *Journal of Neurology, Neurosurgery & Psychiatry*, 71, 29–32.

[7] National Institute on Aging (2016, April 28). Age-related cognitive decline: Women are more resilient than men. Retrieved from https://www.nia.nih.gov/news/age-related-cognitive-decline-women-are-more-resilient-men.

[8] Nield, D. (2015, December 28). Male and female brains age differently, a new study finds. Sciencealert.com. Retrieved from https://www.sciencealert.com/male-and-female-brains-age-differently-new-study-finds.

[9] Gregoire, C. (2017, January 23). For women, cognitive decline may start much earlier than we thought. *Huffington Post.* Retrieved from https://www.huffpost.com/entry/women-age-cognitive-decline_n_588256bee4b070d8cad2387c.

[10] Harvard Health Publishing, Harvard Medical School, Harvard Women's Health Watch. (2015, March). Why you should thank your aging brain.

[11] Alzheimer's.net. (2014, July 7). Retrieved from https://www.alzheimers.net/quote-alzheimers-epidemic.

[12] Barrett, L. F. (2017, April 20). How "superagers" stay sharp in their later years. *The Guardian Observer—Neuroscience.* Retrieved from https://www.theguardian.com/science/2017/apr/30/work-on-your-ageing-brain-superagers-mental-excercise-lisa-feldman-barrett.

[13] Harvard Health Publishing, Harvard Medical School, Harvard Women's Health Watch. (2017, May). What does it take to be a superager? Retrieved https://www.health.harvard.edu/healthy-aging/what-does-it-take-to-be-a-super-ager.

[14] *Chicago Daily Herald.* (2014, September 11). Oak Brook woman travels world, finds ways to make a difference. Retrieved from https://www.dailyherald.com/article/20140911/news/140919959.

[15] Hillman, J. (2018, October 30). Investigators work to crack the code on superaging. *Will I Be Next.* Retrieved from http://willibnext.com/investigators-work-crack-code-superaging/.

[16] Sun, F. W., Stepanovic, M. R., Andreano, J., Feldman Barrett, L., Touroutoglou, A., & Dickerson, B. C. (2016, September 14). Youthful brains in older adults: Preserved neuroanatomy in the default mode and salience networks contributes to youthful memory in superaging. *Journal of Neuroscience, 36*(37), 9659–9668.

[17] Simons, D. J., Boot, W. R., Charness, N., Gathercole, S. E., Chabris, C. F., Hambrick, D. Z., & Stine-Morrow, E. A. L. (2016, October 2). Do "brain-training" programs work? *Psychological Science in the Public Interest.* Retrieved from https://journals.sagepub.com/doi/abs/10.1177/1529100616661983.

[18] Cited in Pearson, C. (2017, December 6). Six things you need to know about women, aging, and brain health. *Huffpost.* Retrieved from: https://www.huffpost.com/entry/women-brain-health_n_3899555; accessed April 10, 2019. Ibid., p. 4 of 7.

[19] Klein, S. (2017, November 28). Five ways women's brains age differently than men's and what it means for your health. *Prevention.com.* Retrieved from https://www.prevention.com/health/g20490580/5-ways-womens-brains-age-differently.

[20] Klein, S. (2017, November 28). Ibid.

[21] Colcombe, S. J., Erickson, K. I., Scalf, P. E., Kim, J. S., Prakash, R., McAuley, E. . . . Kramer, A. F. (2006). Aerobic exercise training increases brain volume in aging humans. *Journals of Gerontology. Series A, Biological Sciences and Medical Sciences, 1*(11), 1166–1170.

[22] Acheson, A., Conover, J. C., Fandl, J. P., DeChiara, T. M., Russell, M., Thadani, A. . . . Lindsay, R. M. (1995, March). A BDNF autocrine loop in adult sensory neurons prevents cell death. *Nature, 374*(6521), 450–453.

[23] Cooper, M. A., Kluding, P. M., & Wright, D. E. (2016, August). Emerging relationships between exercise, sensory nerves, and neuropathic pain. *Frontiers in Neuroscience 10*, Article 372.

[24] O'Bryant, S. E., Waring, S. C., Hobson, V., Hall, J. R., Moore, C. B., Bottiglieri, T. . . . Diaz-Arrastia, R. (2009, November 20). Decreased C-reactive protein levels in Alzheimer disease. *Journal of Geriatric Psychiatry and Neurology, 23*(1), 49–53.

[25] Ford, E. S. (2002, September). Does exercise reduce inflammation? Physical activity and C-reactive protein among U.S. adults. *Epidemiology, 13*(5), 561–568.

[26] Stephan, Y., Caudroit, J., Jaconelli, A., & Terracciano, A. (2014, November). Subjective age and cognitive functioning: A 10-year prospective study. *American Journal of Geriatric Psychiatry, 22*(11), 1180–1187.

[27] Gregory, M. A., Gill, D. P., & Petrella, R. J. (2013). Brain health and exercise in older adults. *Brain Health and Exercise, 12*(4), 256–271.

[28] Gregory, M. A., Gill, D. P., & Petrella, R. J. (2013). Ibid.

[29] Andel, R., Hughes, T. T. F., & Crowe, M. (2005). Strategies to reduce the risk of cognitive decline and dementia. *Aging Health*, 1 (1): 107-116.

[30] ClinCalc.com. (2016). Zolpidem tartrate: Drug usage statistics, United States, 2006–2016. Retrieved from https://clincalc.com/DrugStats/Drugs/ZolpidemTartrate.

[31] National Academy of Sciences. (2018). Cognitive aging: Progress in understanding opportunities for action. Chapter 4B: Risk and protective factors and interventions: Health and medical factors. Washington, DC. Retrieved from https://www.nap.edu/read/21693/chapter/7#186.

[32] Coggins, M. D. (2018). Medication monitor: Medications that increase fall risk. *Today's Geriatric Medicine, 11*(4), 30.

[33] Xie, L, Kang, H., & Xu, Q. (2013, October 18). Sleep drives metabolite clearance from the adult brain. *Science, 342*(6156), 373–377.

[34] Vann, M. R. (2013, July 23). The senior's guide to sleeping well. *Everyday Health*. Retrieved from https://www.everydayhealth.com/senior-health/seniors-guide-to-sleeping-well.aspx.

[35] Kwik, J. (2018, July 19). Kwik Brain 066: When to eat for optimal brain function with Max Lugavere. Retrieved from http://jimkwik.com/kwik-brain-066-when-to-eat-for-optimal-brain-function-with-max-lugavere.

[36] Crane, K. (2015, January 12). The brain preservation diet: Eating to save brain cells. *US News & World Report*. Retrieved from https://health.usnews.com/health-news/patient-advice/articles/2015/01/12/the-brain-preservation-diet-eating-to-save-brain-cells.

[37] Baer, R. A. (2003). Mindfulness training as a clinical intervention: A conceptual and empirical review. *Clinical Psychology: Science and Practice, 10*, 125–143.

[38] Brunson, K. L., Kramar, E., Lin, B., Chen, Y., Colgin, L. L., Yanagihara, T. K. . . . Baram, T. Z. (2005, October). Mechanisms of late-onset cognitive decline after early-life stress. *Journal of Neuroscience, 25*(41), 9328–9338.

[39] Linehan, M. M. (1994). Acceptance and change: The central dialectic in psychotherapy. In S. C. Hayes, N. S. Jacobson, V. M. Follette, & M. J. Dougher (Eds.), *Acceptance and change: Content and context in psychotherapy* (pp. 73–86). Reno, NV: Context Press.

[40] Kabat-Zinn, J., Massion, A. O., Kristeller, J., Peterson, L. G., Fletcher, K. E., Pbert, L. . . . Santorelli, S. F. (1992). Effectiveness of a meditation-based stress reduction program in the treatment of anxiety disorders. *American Journal of Psychiatry, 149*, 936–943.

[41] Gard, T., Hözel, B. K., & Lazar, S. W. (2014, January). The potential effects of meditation on age-related cognitive decline: A systematic review. *Annals of the New York Academy of Sciences, 1307*, 89–103.

[42] Sun, J., Kang, J., Wang, P., & Zeng, H. (2013, May). Self-relaxation training can improve sleep quality and cognitive function in the older: A one-year randomized controlled trial. *Journal of Clinical Nursing, 22*(9–10), 1270–1280.

[43] Zhong, B-L., Chen, S-L., Tu, X., & Conwell, Y. (2016, March 9). Loneliness and cognitive function in older adults: Findings from the Chinese longitudinal healthy longevity survey. *Journal of Gerontology: Social Sciences, 72*(1), 120–128.

[44] Cacioppo, J. T., & Hawkley, L. C. (2013, October). Perceived social isolation and cognition. *Trends in Cognitive Sciences, 13*(10), 447–454.

[45] Tennyson, Alfred, Lord. Ulysses. The Poetry Foundation. Retrieved from https://www.poetryfoundation.org/poems/45392/ulysses; accessed Dec. 11, 2018

About the Authors

Chris Crowley and Henry S. Lodge, MD, coauthored *Younger Next Year for Women: Live Strong, Fit, and Sexy—Until You're 80 and Beyond* and the *Younger Next Year Exercise Program*. They were also patient and doctor, and the enthusiastic creators of the Younger Next Year™ program. A graduate of Harvard and the University of Virginia Law School, Mr. Crowley was, until his retirement in 1990, a litigator and partner at Davis Polk & Wardwell in Manhattan. He is married to the portraitist Hilary Cooper. To hire Chris as a keynote speaker, go to Chriscrowleyspeaker.com. Dr. Lodge, who graduated from the University of Pennsylvania and Columbia University Medical School, was a board-certified internist in New York City. The head of a twenty-two-doctor practice, he was a member of the clinical faculty at Columbia University's College of Physicians and Surgeons and was the Robert Burch Family Professor of Medicine at Columbia University Medical Center. Laura Yorke was his partner in love and in life.

Allan J. Hamilton, MD, a Harvard-trained brain surgeon, is the Regents' Professor of Neurosurgery at the University of Arizona Health Sciences Center. He is also the author of *The Scalpel and the Soul*; *Zen Mind, Zen Horse*; and *Lead with Your Heart*. He lives near Tucson, Arizona.

THE YOUNGER NEXT YEAR® SERIES:
MORE THAN 2 MILLION COPIES IN PRINT

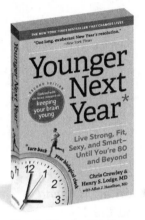

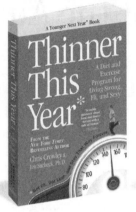

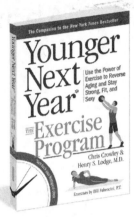

Share the *YOUNGER NEXT YEAR* program with the men in your life! The 2nd edition is updated with research on how to keep the brain young too. This *New York Times* bestseller shows how to put off 70% of the normal problems of aging—weakness, sore joints, bad balance; eliminate 50% of serious illness and injury; and now, become 10% smarter.

Here's the how-to book for the new revolution in aging. It's about how you move, with exercises that will be the greatest driver of positive change in your body. About how you eat, from avoiding foods with solid fats and added sugars to skipping the supplements. And the payoff is amazing.

A training program for the rest of your life, this guide not only shows you how to start an exercise regimen, but also provides the motivation and know-how to keep it going for life.

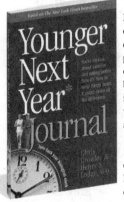

Is it a cardio day or a strength day? A 52-week, prompted fill-in organizer and date book that makes it easy to record what you're doing, and when, the *YOUNGER NEXT YEAR JOURNAL* is an essential tool for living the program day to day.

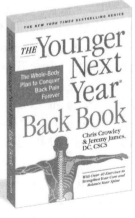

Eighty percent of Americans seek expert help for back pain. Coincidentally, 80% is Dr. Jeremy James's success rate, and now he brings his revolutionary behavioral/whole body approach to the book that will heal, and often eliminate, back pain forever with "Jeremy's Rules" and a regimen of simple exercises.

Available Wherever Books Are Sold

(workman)

workman.com